Gestational Diabetes Die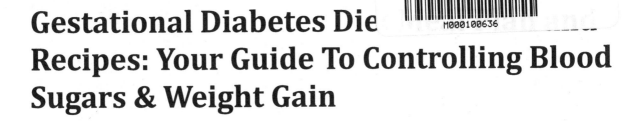 Recipes: Your Guide To Controlling Blood Sugars & Weight Gain

By Mathea Ford, RD/LD

Introduction and Disclaimer

I wrote this book with you in mind: the mom to be who has found out that she has gestational diabetes and does not know where to start or can't seem to get the answers that she needs from other sources. I am writing this book to help you manage your gestational diabetes and make it easier to live with by giving you answers [in general] to questions that you have and giving you a meal pattern and recipes that you can use.

Who am I? First and foremost, I am a mom who was in your shoes. I had gestational diabetes with both of my pregnancies and I found that solving the issues of high and low blood sugars didn't come easy to me, even with all my knowledge. I am also a registered dietitian in the USA who has been working with moms and other patients for my entire 15 + years of experience. I have a website that provides gestational diabetes information – check it out at http://www.gestationaldiabeticdiethq.com/gdm-mealplan-book/

I felt that I needed to help you travel down the road with a more helpful information than you had before. My goals are simple – to give some answers and to create an understanding of what is typical. It will not necessarily be what happens in your case, as everyone is an individual. I may simplify things in an effort to write them so that I feel you can learn the most from the information. This may mean that I don't say the exact things that your doctor would say. If you don't understand, please ask your doctor.

I want you to understand, I am not a medical doctor, and I do not know your particular condition. Information in this book is current as of publication, but may or may not have changed. This book is not meant to substitute for medical treatment for you, your friends, or your family members. You should not base treatment decisions solely on what is contained in this book. Develop your treatment plan with your doctors, nurses and the other medical professionals on your team. I recommend that you double-check any information with your medical team to verify if it applies to you.

In other words, I am not responsible for your medical care. I am providing this book for informational and entertainment purposes, not medical treatment. Please consult with your doctor about any questions that you have about your particular case.

Table Of Contents

What Do I Do Now That I Have Gestational Diabetes?

"I have gestational diabetes" can be a tremendously terrifying thought. You want to cry, scream, and yell, yet you don't know what else to do. You tremble when you just think about it. You were tested and diagnosed, and your doctor has given you some vague directions. You now know that you have a condition called gestational diabetes. And you are wondering what you should do about it?

First, it is not the end of the world. You can survive this and have a healthy baby with just a little planning and work. I had gestational diabetes just like you. I had to work really hard to control my gestational diabetes and keep my blood sugars under control. But I have two healthy children, and they are worth every moment of frustration and pain that I endured. I'm sure as a mom-to-be, you feel the exact same way.

My Story

I want to tell you for a moment about my experience. I have a family history of diabetes, so it didn't really surprise me that I developed gestational diabetes. Gestational diabetes testing was enough to make a person feel really nauseated – I have been through it, I know.

Either way, I was still mad about it. Perhaps you are past that stage, but it took me a few days after I found out to get past that. I wanted to be different and not have a problem. Then, I realized, it was something I could handle. I was already working hard at exercising and not gaining too much weight. I knew, based on my education, that I understood what to do – or so I thought. Sometimes gestational diabetes made me feel like I had no control over my body. It was like my pancreas had a mind of it's own.

After the anger wore off, the guilt started. How could I have this, I tried so hard to eat perfectly but maybe that one time… Get over the guilt. You are where you are, and you are going to be fine with a little help. One incident of bad behavior is not going to cause gestational diabetes – you got it and now you can move on from anger and guilt to acceptance. Accept that you are not perfect but you can do what is necessary to manage your gestational diabetes. You can do it!

I had the good fortune of feeling hungry every 3 hours with my first child, and only nauseated if I didn't eat a small bit of something when I got hungry. I tested my blood sugars as I was supposed to. The doctor instructed me to test 4-5 times per day and record the numbers. Even though I have counseled lots of patients, I have never had to take a blood sugar reading, so I went to a nurse who taught me how to do that. The pricking the finger was the hardest part! But the rest was manageable. And it got easier every time, and I felt good. I walked after meals to keep the blood sugars down, which really helped.

I took metformin instead of insulin to manage my blood sugars along with diet. I kept them in a normal range through diligent effort and close management of the food I ate. But, then again, I knew how to eat better because I am a registered dietitian, right? No, I don't think that it's something you know from reading a book. It's something I learned from the experience of how the food made me feel and how the numbers on my machine registered.

Sometimes I would be perplexed at how the food I ate reacted in my blood stream. I thought I had control, but the diabetes at times had a mind of it's own. I did have control over what I put into my mouth and how much and when I ate, so I focused on that.

And that is what I want you to see, that you can be mad, angry, guilty or accept what has transpired. However, you have gestational diabetes. And you can control what you eat and help your body deal with the food that you eat and have a healthy baby. You have a short time to learn and then manage your gestational diabetes, so that is what I am writing about to you today – shorten the learning curve and follow a meal plan.

Making Simple Changes

Some of the changes you need to make are simple, and some are complicated. But most of them start with a meal plan and number of calories for the day. Every single food you eat must be scrutinized for carbohydrate content and reviewed to see if it fits in your daily limits.

What are carbohydrates? Carbohydrates are parts of foods that break down in your digestive system into glucose for absorption into your bloodstream. Glucose (also called blood sugar) is then used by your body's cells for energy. But, the doors to your cells are locked, and insulin is the key to open them and allow the glucose inside. Sometimes your hormones from being pregnant affect your body's ability to produce insulin and you don't have enough. You don't have enough keys to let your glucose from your blood go into your body's cells and make energy for you.

Carbohydrates come in a couple of forms, simple sugars – like the sugar in the packet on the table you might put into your tea, and complex carbohydrates – like wheat bread and whole grain cereals (oatmeal, for example). Each carbohydrate serves a purpose in foods. Your goal should be to eat a certain amount of carbohydrate each day, and eat it throughout the day – not all at once. Another goal should be to eat more whole grain foods – replacing many of the simple sugar foods with foods that take longer to digest, make you feel fuller and allow your body to absorb the carbohydrate more slowly. The slower digestion gives the body more time to react with insulin to use for carbohydrate in your blood stream.

Better carbohydrate choices are going to be multi-grain foods and items that have a lot of fiber and are less processed, fruits instead of fruit juice. The fiber slows the absorption of the food and allows your body to respond a little slower, which is good. Eating whole grain pasta or wild rice instead of white pasta or plain white rice is a good choice. Whole grain wheat breads (make sure it has 2-3 gm of fiber per slice) make a much better choice than a slice of white bread. Your body can usually break down white bread almost as quickly as simple sugar, and white bread should be exchanged for whole grains in a gestational diabetes meal.

Carbohydrates are also found in juices, fruits, and vegetables. Much the same as whole grains, eating whole fruits and vegetables is a better choice than the juice. Juice contains fructose, which is a type of simple sugar that breaks down in your digestive system quickly. Sometimes women drink a small amount of juice or soda when they experience a low blood sugar so that they can recover more quickly. Whole fruits and vegetables are higher in fiber, make you feel fuller, and contain more nutrients than juices alone.

Portions And Patterns

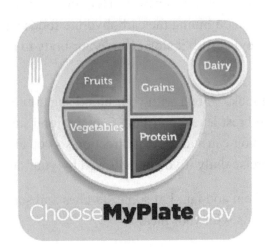

For women who are not over weight before pregnancy, it is recommended to eat 30 calories per each kg per day. 1 kilogram = 2.2 pounds, so divide your weight in pounds by 2.2, then take that number and multiply by 30. For example, if you weighed 150 pounds that is 68.18 kilograms. So you would estimate your calorie needs at about 2045 per day. Women who are overweight should multiply by 25 calories per each kg per day. As long as your baby is growing and your blood sugars are under control, you should be okay with the amount of food you are eating during your gestational diabetes treatment.

Distribute your carbohydrate intake throughout the day to make it easier on your body. Many women find that their body reacts very quickly to sugar in the morning. Some dietitians think it's prudent to not eat fruit or juice in the morning so you don't have a higher reading than normal. You can eat fruit after 10 am, but the recommendation is to avoid it in the early hours of the day. Your meal plan at the back of the book reflects that recommendation based on my experience with women who are gestational diabetic.

Eating 3 small meals and 3 small snacks is the best way to distribute your carbohydrate throughout the day. It will help with managing hunger and your body's reaction to glucose will be more proportional. Many women typically follow the breakdown of 40-50 % carbohydrate, 30% fat and the rest as protein. At snack time, it is wise to eat a meat or fat with a carbohydrate to slow the absorption of the food product.

Portion sizes of carbohydrate foods tend to be very small, much smaller than you think. Use a scale and measuring cup until you are absolutely sure you have the right amount. Eat off a smaller plate so you don't feel like you have to fill it up to get a good meal. Weigh out your cereal to get the right portion, and use a measuring cup for your milk that you put on it as well. It all counts as carbohydrates.

Your Doctor's Orders

Some women find that their diet is limited based on their bodies and their hormones. Your unborn child is your first priority, and getting your body's ecosystem into balance is a priority. Your body is unique, and how it reacts to certain foods is going to be slightly different. Take your medication as prescribed, exercise as you are allowed, and eat a balanced diet. Keeping a meal plan for your diet can keep you sane in the frustrated world you live in.

You need some carbohydrates, no matter what, so that your body can raise that child you are carrying. Complete avoidance of carbohydrate foods is not the answer. Helping your body to process the carbohydrate by eating more slowly and combining the carbohydrate foods with protein or fat foods will help you digest it slower and absorb it slower and your body to respond better to an influx of carbohydrate.

Make note of your blood sugar levels in your logbook. Along with your blood sugar numbers, make note of your stress, and rest level. Stress and rest level contribute to high blood sugar, and although you won't solve this problem in a day – you can start in that direction so you are not stressed out all the time. And don't forget to exercise daily if you are allowed by your doctor.

Each meal should contain some carbohydrate, protein and fat. Eat some starches and some simple sugars, and eat plenty of vegetables and fruits with your meal.

Checking Your Blood Sugars

One of the hardest things you will have to do is check your blood sugar level on a regular basis. It's something you can get used to, though, and you will find it easier to do as time goes on. But the hard part is not only checking your blood sugar levels, it's reacting to them as well.

To begin with, you <u>have</u> to check your blood sugars. Ignoring your blood sugar levels does not make it go away. It doesn't give you control over them if you don't monitor them. And you need to know what they are – if only for your baby's sake! It might feel like you are being judged when you measure them, but all they are is a number, a result of a test. And you can change the next test – but you have to face up to the fact that you need to change something. Sticking your head in the sand and ignoring it doesn't make it any better.

Make sure you know what your doctor, nurse educator or dietitian wants you to do. If they want you to take your blood sugar 4 times a day – do it! You will take it more often when you are on insulin.

The best practices for the doctor's that I have been in tune with are:

Take your blood sugar levels at least 4 times a day as listed below –

1. When you wake up in the morning (fasting)
2. One hour after you start eating breakfast
3. One hour after you start eating lunch
4. One hour after you start eating supper
5. **Any time you feel "funny" or different**

You can check less often as you get your diet into balance and figure out what your daily pattern would be. But – ALWAYS – check it if you feel "not quite right". (Side note: as a mom, you can start tuning into that feeling because it will work for evaluating your children as well) Our bodies do handle the sugar in our food differently and react with different levels of insulin, so go with what you know about your body after discussing with your doctor. I am only giving you some "rules of thumb". If you end up checking once a day, do it at different times so you can see how you are doing throughout the day – as your pregnancy progresses the hormones change and your body's reaction might change.

One thing women experience sometimes is the "dawn phenomenon". That means your blood sugar in the morning is higher than you expect it to be after fasting. This happens because your body gets low on blood sugar over night, then your liver makes blood sugar to compensate, and you may not have as much insulin – so it takes longer to go down. Many women find that eating a little larger bedtime snack can help with this – especially additional fat or protein in the snack – to even out the overnight reaction. It takes longer to digest fat and protein, so it's released into your blood stream at a slower rate and your body doesn't get as low in blood sugar over night. The reaction that you might have – to stop eating a bed time snack – is not the best choice! You can see that will only lead to your body making more blood sugar overnight because it gets even lower.

When you are documenting your blood sugar levels, make sure you are clear about what time you started eating and when you did the blood sugar check. Usually 1 hour post prandial (after eating) is the peak of your blood sugar, and you are aiming for a level of 140 gm/dl or lower. If your number is higher than that – look at your meal and see what hidden carbohydrate you might be eating. Ask your doctor how they want you to react to your blood sugar numbers – more insulin, taking a walk, or changing medications are all options. My recommendation is that if your blood sugar is a little high – take a 10 minute walk to decrease the number. A stroll around will help your muscles use the sugar in your blood more effectively and make your levels come down. And – change your meals a little for the next time and replace some of the carbohydrate with fat or protein.

Eating Out On A Gestational Diabetes Diet

You are not expected to eat at home all of your pregnancy. You do need to exercise caution during your excursions to ensure your meal goals can be met, whether it is at a friend's house or at a restaurant. Many foods have added oils, butters and other toppings that can affect your blood sugar and calorie levels.

Many restaurants and fast food chains offer "healthy" meals or "light" meals. Look at those first! You are not bound to those entirely, and you can choose off the ala carte menu as well – just picking a few items that you want to put together for a meal. Or eat an appetizer for your meal. Servers are very flexible and understanding of your special dietary needs. Some restaurants have "healthy nut" meals, which give you the meal that is grilled chicken and grilled vegetables and no starches (or carbohydrate choices). You could ask your server if the restaurant has those, or low carbohydrate meals, and just add a carbohydrate choice to the meal, like a bread or potato side dish.

Ask for these "special requests" to make sure your meal is a healthy as possible.

1. How is this dish made? Fried, Grilled, Broiled? What is put on it on the grill? (Many restaurants brush meats with butter while cooking)
2. How big is this meal? Ounces on the main entrée, cups on the side dishes if possible
3. If it seems large, ask for them to bring out a "to go" box with your meal and immediately put half in the box for eating later.
4. Ask for dressing and toppings (gravy, salad dressings, potato toppings) to be placed on the side so you can add the amount that you want.
5. At a fast food restaurant, the children's meals can be a good choice as far as portion sizes are concerned.
6. Many fast food restaurants now post calories on menus, but ask if they have a nutrient facts brochure so you can see the carbohydrate counts for meals and portion sizes.
7. Choose the grilled or broiled option over the fried option.
8. Stick to eating at your regular time, arrive early enough to be seated and start eating at a normal meal time.
9. Remove the chips or breads from the table so you are not tempted to eat them.

What If I Get Sick?

Becoming sick during your pregnancy is difficult whether or not you have gestational diabetes. You can't take most over the counter medications and just have to suffer through the virus. Aside from the first 12 weeks and morning sickness, getting a cold or the flu with gestational diabetes is important to be prepared for, especially if you are on insulin.

No matter how you are feeling, you should take your insulin. Make sure you take your blood sugar level and know whether you are low or high. (Sometimes having a high blood sugar can make you feel sick as well). Your body needs the extra insulin you inject to run normally. But if you have the flu and are vomiting, make sure you know your blood glucose level using your monitor and drink a non-diet clear beverage (7-up or Sprite) or juice and eat some crackers. Call your doctor about any other concerns and especially if you are vomiting and cannot keep food down. They may instruct you differently or even ask you to come in and get checked.

Testing more often and making sure you keep your insulin and blood sugar levels in check is the important part of being sick with gestational diabetes. Talk to your doctor or nurse educator about illness guidelines <u>before</u> you get sick if you can.

Common Mistakes in a Gestational Diabetes Menu Plan

You will need to plan a menu for yourself, and make some meals that are appealing to what you feel like eating that day. Easy enough, right? However, if you have never had to create a menu tailored for diabetes eating, you may have problems with knowing where to start.

1. A common mistake that many women make is "eyeballing" the portions. You know what I mean, you just look at something and say, "well, that's about ½ cup". Until you have measured that food several (and most likely many) times, you will not get it right. It's a mistake to think you know how much is 3 cups of popcorn, or how many carbohydrate servings are in the bagel in the package.

Start with soda, which is pure sugar just as juice can be for you. And many moms don't want to drink diet soda because of the sweeteners, which is fine. But my point right now is that a 20 ounce bottle of soda is 2.5 servings of soda. Over 300 calories, and over 70 gm of carbohydrate. If you drink the whole soda, you just had an entire meal and then some worth of carbs. I know, I know, you are not going to do that. Juice serving sizes are just 4 ounces, which is even smaller amounts.

Portion sizes of common foods are easy to compare to some common objects that you have readily available to compare to.

  a. 3 ounces of meat is the size of a deck of cards
  b. 1 teaspoon oil is the size of a quarter in diameter
  c. 1 cup of raw vegetables is the size of a light bulb
  d. 1 medium fresh fruit is the size of a tennis ball
  e. 1 bagel or roll portion is the size of a 6 ounce can of tuna

When everything around you is supersized, you have to be the one to do the right thing. You have to read the label and know how much a cup of popcorn is instead of guessing. And the huge chocolate chip cookie at the register in the cafeteria – more like 3 or more servings. Packaging can contain several servings, so read the label, and if you have to – split the item into the serving size portions so you know. For example, if a bag of popcorn says it has 3 servings, split it into 3 serving bowls equally and see how much you should have. Or weigh the food with an inexpensive food scale. To this day, I still weigh the amount of granola I put in my Greek yogurt I eat every morning so I don't overdo it. Cereal is a big thing that is easy to overdo as well. {Sounds like everything is easy to overdo – that's why you need a scale!}

2. Another mistake some women make is to not eat balanced meals throughout the day and maybe even skip some meals. Please don't skip meals, as it can cause you to overeat

later in the day. Many women think that eating automatically raises their blood sugars, and for some foods that is true, but your body works best when you feed it throughout the day so it can release smaller amounts of insulin and react to a smaller doses of food. Eat 6 times a day, 3 meals and 3 snacks.

Don't avoid foods just because they are made of carbohydrate. If you eat the right portion (see #1), you can manage to eat a little bit of the things that you want in the correct amounts. Instead of skipping meals and starving all day, you need to develop a plan for how much carbohydrate you will eat for the day and when – and stick to it for a couple of days while monitoring your blood sugars. Then you can see how your body reacts during the day as well. Many women find that at different times of the day they have higher blood sugars and sometimes their bodies seem to use the carbohydrate just fine.

Once you know how your body handles the glucose, you can adjust how much carbohydrate you eat at that time. So, follow the meal plan and adjust – because everyone is different.

3. Finally, another mistake is to not have your plan with you and follow it. Set yourself up for success by making a plan, and sticking to it. You should make a plan for what you are going to eat for the week so when you go to the grocery store you can buy the right foods and have them in the house. That way, when you start to make your meals everyday you don't have even MORE STRESS because you don't have the right foods to make your meals and snacks.

You will find the meal patterns in the back of the book that show you an entire day's meal plan and also a meal-by-meal plan. You can take that and the recipes you want to make for the week and create your grocery list. Then you go to the store and save yourself time with a list and not be too frustrated by not knowing what to eat. Once you have the plan, you are well on your way to controlling your gestational diabetes using the best tools possible.

Work on fixing these mistakes, and as you work with your doctor or dietitian, be sure to understand how you should eat throughout the day to make your pregnancy as problem free as possible.

Ways To Use Recipes In Your Meal Planning

When you are diagnosed with gestational diabetes, gone are the carefree days of eating all the chocolate and bon bons that you want. You have to watch what you eat and measure your food, or your blood sugars may stay high and that is hard on the baby. One of the reasons why women with gestational diabetes have larger babies is that the sugar passes through the placenta from the mother to the baby and the baby's body turns the sugar into fat because it's too many calories. So, just like what happens with you and I, too many calories make for a large baby.

But I am not here to scare you. I want to talk about ways to improve your meal plan. You bought this book and it has a ton of recipes in it. You will see that very soon. But you also need to use those recipes wisely. You have to portion out the food and eat the right amounts. Previously, I talked about measuring your blood sugars throughout the day to know what types of highs and lows your body naturally has. You can use that to your advantage. If your body does really well at lunchtime and after, or you are able to take a walk right after lunch to lower your blood sugar, then you can eat a little more at lunch. (I said, "a little more")

So, one of the best things that you can do is to start planning your meals to have a green, yellow or orange vegetable with it. The carbohydrate load of a regular vegetable is around 5 gm per ½ cup, so you can eat 1.5 cups of vegetables to 1/3 cup rice. Pretty filling, right? So make your plate with ½ of it filled with green, orange or yellow vegetables, and ¼ meat and ¼ starch. Your body will love you and you will feel fuller and stay full longer. In the meal plans you get we always balance out the carbohydrate to have some vegetables to make it healthier and allow you to eat more.

The second thing I will recommend is to stop using so much salt. You are pregnant and subject to random swelling at any time, and salt can contribute to water retention, so don't use it. Don't add it to your recipes unless it's called for. And in your recipes, use less. Sometimes you have to have salt for the chemical reaction to take place when you cook, but most of the time it's just for flavor. Learn to love the taste of spices and herbs so that you can add them to your meals and recipes instead of salt. Try the ethnic seasoning blends you see in the store as well to increase the variety, but check the sodium (salt) content on the label to make sure that it does not have hidden salt. And put a Mrs. Dash type shaker on your table and remove the salt shaker. (p.s. – don't go back to lots of salt after the baby is born – stick with the low sodium lifestyle)

The final way to improve the health of your recipes is to reduce fat and add fiber. How do I do that, you ask? You take your favorite casseroles and add beans! Beans are low fat and high in fiber plus they give you protein. Yeah! You can use black beans for pork or beef dishes, and white kidney beans for chicken products. Just add a can of beans and cut the meat in half. You will have a healthier meal with more fiber and no one will notice a few extra beans in the recipe.

You need to stick to your gestational diabetes meal plan so that you are able to have a healthy pregnancy, and I think the tips I just told you should help you get on the right track. You have a short time, depending on when you are identified as having gestational diabetes, to live with this and you can do it for your baby. Controlling that blood sugar is what it's all about. But the best tool you have in your kit is your meal plan. It will keep you on track and making good choices.

A Week At A Time

Meal planning can seem overwhelming, but it is something that will be a great help to you and your stress level. Starting your week with a plan will make the process much easier. Don't try to change a lot of things – like making food ahead or completely eating different foods – just get your plan on track and find out what you can eat. Make it your goal daily to eat to your plan and measure your blood sugar levels. You will see how the amount of carbohydrate you eat and your blood sugar levels are tied together.

Begin with reading labels. Look at the foods that you normally eat and read the label on the back. Look at the Nutrition Facts labels. Your nutritional facts labels tell you information about the amount of food in a serving, how many servings are in the container, and how much carbohydrate is in each serving. You want to start out with eating 30-45 grams of carbohydrates per meal, and see how your body reacts to the food. If you can't keep your blood sugars under control, keep it to 30, if you are doing fine, and you are still hungry, you can add a little more.

First thing in the morning, though, you need to keep it to 30 gm or less of carbohydrate and no juice or fruit.

What else can you eat besides carbohydrates? You can eat proteins and fats, in moderation. So, choose a sandwich and add lettuce, tomato, mayonnaise, and pickles. Eating more vegetables is always a good choice. Keep carrot sticks and ranch with you for between meal snacks. Eat a cheese stick or a salad with your meal to round it out without adding more carbohydrate.

Adding lots of green, orange and yellow vegetables will fill you up without increasing your carbohydrate load. Eat some peanut butter on celery for a snack if you need more food but not more carbohydrate. And keep in mind you have a certain calorie level that you should be eating, so while you can eat more of the proteins and fats, you still need to watch the portion sizes.

Try to eat 3 meals and 3 snacks for your day. Your meals can have 30-45 gm of carbohydrate plus other foods and your snacks should have about 15 gm of carbohydrate. All meals and snacks should have some carbohydrate, protein, and fat. Bedtime snacks might be peanut butter and crackers or a small serving of ice cream.

Overall, you should look at this as a short term problem for which you have a solution. It's not forever! You will go back to normal after your pregnancy. But you will be at higher risk for type 2 diabetes later in life, so you will need to have your doctor continue to monitor your blood sugar and hemoglobin A1c levels over time. In this book, you will find two sets of meal patterns that you can use right now to get started on a meal plan that will help you control your gestational diabetes.

Gestational Diabetes Complications And What To Do

You have gestational diabetes, and I am not going to get into the definition here because your doctor should have told you why you were diagnosed. But once your concerns are answered, you leave and you think, "what about the complications? How does this affect me?"

You can have more complications than normal with gestational diabetes as part of your pregnancy. Learning more about them and what can happen helps you cope with them and make better choices.

1. A larger than normal baby is a complication you may have to address. I discussed in the previous section about why your baby may become larger than normal based on your blood sugar levels. As a mom-to-be you may also gain too much weight with a large baby. Keeping your blood sugar levels in a normal range and tracking what you eat so you don't get high blood sugars is very important to reduce your chances of having a larger than normal baby.

2. Having a larger than normal baby puts you at risk of having a C-section. Your baby may not fit down the birth canal because of the size and risk to both he/she and you. C-sections are major surgery, take longer to recover from and cost more. And with a new baby, recovering from a C-section can be more difficult.

3. Pre-eclampsia is another complication that might arise because of gestational diabetes. I had pre-eclampsia with my son, and my blood pressure got really high and I was repeatedly traveling to the hospital to get checked. This increases stress, that in turn increases blood pressure. Women with diabetes during pregnancy tend to have high blood pressure more often. Pre-eclampsia can cause swelling in the hands and feet that will not go away, and affect your child or yourself due to the kidney damage that can be caused.

4. Developing hypoglycemic episodes is a very common complication. (Hypoglycemia is when your blood sugar level gets too low – usually less than 60 mg/dl and you start to sweat and feel faint.) Your doctor may give you medication to reduce your blood sugar to help you cope with the gestational diabetes, and taking that medication might make your blood sugar too low if you don't eat enough with it, especially insulin. If you happen to get in a hurry and don't eat but have taken your insulin shot, you might experience hypoglycemia. Keep a small amount of peanut butter and crackers in your purse to take if your blood sugar gets too low.

5. Finally, developing diabetes later in life is another of the complications associated with gestational diabetes. Women who have gestational diabetes have a 2x higher risk of developing type 2 diabetes within 10 years. Have periodic checkups after you deliver your baby so your provider can check your blood sugar levels and hemoglobin A1c for

signs of pre-diabetes or diabetes. It is recommended that you do that at least every 3 years.

Exercise, medication, and eating right are the keys to controlling your gestational diabetes well. Even after you deliver your baby and are back to a "normal" diet, you should remember to eat a balanced diet and keep exercising so you can maintain a healthy body weight.

Gestational Diabetes Treatment – Meals, Exercise, and Medications

Your number one goal for treatment of gestational diabetes is to keep your blood sugars in control. In control is generally defined as less than 95 mg/dl before meals, and less than 140 mg/dl at 1 hour after starting your meal.

You may feel just fine, but your baby is getting too much sugar and that is potentially harmful for you both. So checking your blood sugar levels is crucial to your health and your baby. You must do this to make sure your gestational diabetes is under control.

Meals and Exercise

You know you need to read labels and understand how much carbohydrate you should eat in a day. You also should understand that every woman is different and may need more or less calories to get through their day. {My personal experience was different with each pregnancy} So don't compare yourself to others, just try to manage your condition. Use the blood sugar levels your doctor recommends and keep track of what you are eating and drinking so you can diagnose the hidden sugar and carbohydrate in foods that might increase your blood sugar levels.

Exercise is key to controlling gestational diabetes. You should talk to your doctor about what level of exercise is ok, but you should see it as part of your treatment. You can walk for 15 minutes after each meal, and do some stretching to keep your body aches to a minimum. Walking after a meal helps your body use the glucose from the meal better and keep your blood sugar levels lower.

Medications

Gestational diabetes usually makes you a high-risk pregnancy, and doctors will be looking for other issues as well as your pregnancy progresses. Once you have tried diet and exercise for about 2 weeks, and it has not lowered your glucose levels enough, you may be prescribed medications.

Insulin

Insulin is the safest medication you can take for gestational diabetes. Your body already has insulin; it is just not using it well. You have to inject it, it cannot be taken in pill form (as of now). Insulin works quickly to lower your blood sugar level and is dosed based on your blood glucose level and how much carbohydrate you eat. Every woman is an individual, and your doctor or nurse educator, will work with you to find the right dosage. Insulin is safe because it does not cross the placenta, and has been used many years to treat gestational diabetes.

Part of the issue with gestational diabetes is that your placenta is releasing hormones that affect your body's ability to handle the insulin you are already producing. You may need more insulin at meals, and you have to continue to check your blood sugars every day if you are on insulin.

Oral Agents

Glyburide is the main oral agent used in pregnancy. The reason doctors use oral agents is to avoid having to inject insulin at all meals. Oral agents can cross the placenta and are classified as a pregnancy category risk of B at a minimum. Other medications that are used are metformin and glucophage. Metformin can affect your kidneys, and increase problems if you have pre-eclampsia. It works by decreasing your body's production of glucose and improve the use of insulin your body is already making. Glyburide works to stimulate insulin release, and increase insulin sensitivity in the body. It allows your body to use the insulin it already has better.

Making the Choice

As always, it is a personal decision to make with your doctor's advice. Some studies have shown that glyburide and insulin show similar outcomes when used in gestational diabetes. Medication will not eliminate your meal planning or exercise, it just makes it work better. You will have to do all of those things to get the best outcome. Treatment is not easy, and involves food, exercise, and possibly medication if needed to be most effective.

What Happens After I Deliver The Baby?

You have survived the endless weeks testing your blood sugar, eating right, measuring foods, and exercising. You have delivered a healthy baby boy or girl. Now what?

For most women, the gestational diabetes resolves with the birth. Your placenta is no longer adding hormones to your body to upset your natural balance, and your blood sugars go back to normal. Your pancreas will produce enough insulin for your body and you will not have to continue on the gestational diabetes meal plan.

If your gestational diabetes does not resolve (a rare case), it is likely that you were diabetic prior to the pregnancy and the routine screening caught it. Either way, your doctor will likely have you continue to monitor your blood sugar levels for about two days as a precaution.

You won't continue to take insulin or other medications (unless it's determined you need them), but your doctor wants to see how your body processes glucose without the help of medications. You can continue with a diabetic diet after the birth, as it is a healthy option and provides the nutrients you and your baby need, especially if you are breast feeding and need additional calories.

What About My Next Pregnancy?

You may wonder if you are at a higher risk of having gestational diabetes in your next pregnancy. You are at a very high risk of becoming diabetic again in your next pregnancy. Before you become pregnant again, start following the diabetic diet to get your body used to the balanced carbohydrate and healthy eating styles. You will also have a good nutrient balance that is healthy for your next baby as well by eating a variety of foods and getting the vitamins and minerals in them.

Maintaining a healthy body weight is very important as well to your next pregnancy. If you are overweight, losing 10-15 pounds can make a huge difference in the management of your gestational diabetes in the next pregnancy.

Also, make sure you let your doctor know you had gestational diabetes with your prior pregnancy so they can test you earlier. The earlier you start to manage the insulin and blood sugars, the better the outcome with your baby. You may even want to go in prior to becoming pregnant and have your hemoglobin A1c tested to make sure your blood sugars are under control before getting pregnant to have the best possible conditions for the first weeks of your new baby's life.

What About Developing Type 2 Diabetes Later?

You also are at risk for developing type 2 diabetes later in life, so continuing to watch the amount of carbohydrate you eat and exercise to maintain or reach a healthy weight is a good idea. Continue to eat the foods you were eating during pregnancy in the right portions, and once your doctor clears you to exercise – take the baby for a walk in the stroller.

I know you will feel a huge sigh of relief once your doctor pronounces you "free" of gestational diabetes and you can continue to focus on your baby. Just don't forget that mom needs to care for herself as well to keep her as healthy as possible for the baby.

After experiencing gestational diabetes and following a meal plan as well as possibly taking medication, I am sure you will want to reduce your risk of developing type 2 diabetes later in life. Managing diabetes is not hard, but it can be complicated and multi-faceted as you may have found during your pregnancy. You can do things to reduce your risk of developing type 2 diabetes.

Methods similar to what you used in your pregnancy are the best way to reduce your risk of developing gestational diabetes. You don't have to count all the carbohydrates and check your blood sugars but you do need to eat a balanced diet. Eating the smaller meals and snacks throughout the day is an excellent way to allow your body to use the food you give it without overloading your pancreas. If you can, continue with the 3 small meals and 3 snacks to eat healthier and keep your stomach full and reduce the temptation for between meal snacks that are not so healthy for you.

Physical exercise continues to be a healthy choice. You did it during your pregnancy and you should continue with at least 30 minutes per day after your doctor releases you to exercise. It will help you burn off your calories, use your glucose better and give you more energy. You will sleep better and find your daily activities less stressful when you take a daily walk.

Finally, if you are overweight, losing some weight will reduce your risk of developing type 2 diabetes. Your weight affects a lot of your life, and you can be much healthier and live much longer through losing some weight. Losing just 10% of your body weight can be a significant change that will keep you from being as insulin resistant and make exercising even easier. Talk to you doctor about a healthy weight and your options for losing weight.

If you become diabetic, you can check out our website for more meal plans and patterns at http://www.healthydietmenusforyou.com

14 Weeks Of Dinner Meals With Grocery Lists

The next pages are the meat of the program you need. You will find 14 sets of individual weeks of dinner meals – entrée, starches, and vegetables. All with nutritional information and all controlled for your special needs as a person with gestational diabetes. This plan is jam-packed with over 90 of the best tasting gestational diabetes friendly recipes you will find anywhere.

You will know exactly what foods to buy, how to improve you diet by knowing what options are best for you, and avoid the usual boring diabetes recipes that have no taste. You need good tasting food to get through the next few months of your pregnancy.

These meals are designed to keep your blood sugar levels as balanced as possible through correct portioning and timing of meals. Also, these are meals your entire family can eat – no special foods just for you. You will have the peace of mind of knowing you can use these recipes and they are healthy for every facet of your life – and you can continue to use them after you deliver your baby.

Each meal has 60 gm of carbohydrate or less for you to keep your diabetes under control. If you are not eating 60 gm of carbohydrates, you can eliminate whatever amount of carbohydrates you need to since it has the nutritional information right there in the meal plan. You get side dishes that are matched to the meal, and won't push you over on your carbohydrate count.

So, on the next pages, you will have each week of recipes and then a grocery list for that week set out by meal. The goal of this plan is to make it so that you can take a week and go to the grocery store without much planning time and more you time! You won't have to dig for recipes and find foods that you love just to see that they are not good for you. My theory is that all foods can fit – so you will find a huge variety of foods as well as excellent recipes and meals for your whole gang.

14 Weeks Of Dinner Meals With Grocery Lists

How To Use Your Gestational Diabetes Meal Plan

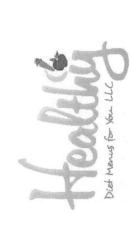

Diet Menus for You, LLC

Menu Plans are not too complicated but a bit of explanation might help! You have the weekly meal plan, and you see that it's long, about 7-17 pages. Don't let it overwhelm you. The aim is to make it as clear and simple as possible for your use. We have the meal plan and grocery listing separately so you can use the section you need.

The Meal Plan Pages – Plans are broken down into sections for your ease of use - each weekly meal plan has 7 meals which contain from 1 - 4 recipes. Always an entree and usually some side dishes.

At the top right of the page, you will see the name of the diet that the meal plan is for. Those items are not shown in the picture.

Next, you will see the name of the meal - Meal 1, Meal 2, etc. and the first recipe which is always considered the entree. You will see the name of the recipe, and the ingredients as well as the instructions listed. The names for the ingredients are kind of vague, but that is so that you can find the items in your stores. I realize that you may not have every brand so when I planned your menu, I created meals that were flexible. When you are looking at this list, it should be descriptive of the types of items you will need.

With each recipe, you will also have information on how many servings it is supposed to provide. This way ,you know that the recipe is made for 4. If you only need enough for 2, you could cut the recipe in half. In this case, it's a broccoli side dish, and has 6 servings, so you can measure out what is supposed to be on the plate for that recipe. It helps you know what you are making and eating so you can plan your meals easily.

Meal Plan

www.healthydietmen...

Healthy
Diet Menus for You, LLC

Meal:	Chicken Marsala DM 1400	
Recipe		**Ingredients**
Chicken Marsala	16 ounces	Chicken, Breast Boneless
Serves: 4	4 cup	Vegetable, Mushrooms, slices, raw
Serving Size: 4 ounce chicken breast, plus sauce	0.25 Teaspoo	Herb, Garlic, Raw
	1 Tablespoon	Flour, White bleached enriched
Meal plan has recipes listed with serving sizes, ingredients, and instructions. Recipes are listed by meal with all sides as separate recipes.	1.666 cup	Soup, Chicken Broth Low Sodium
	0.25 tsp	Salt
	0.25 tsp	Spice, Black Pepper
	2 Oz	Wine, dessert, sweet - marsala

Ingr...

Coat a large nons...
spray. Over med...
breasts for 6 min...
pan and set aside...
cooking spray, an...
Add mushrooms a...
the liquid is evapo...
well to coat the m...
more minute. Ac...
incorporate the flo...
to high. Let simm...
pepper. Serve sa...

Nutritionals

Calories	391.4	Sodium:	636.8	Protein:	36	Phos	417.
		Fat:	16.4	Carbs:	25.9	Chol:	84.7	Pot:	508.6
		Sat Fat: 6.338		Fiber:	6.044		
				Sugar:	3.761		

Nutritional information is complete for every recipe so you know what you are eating in each portion.

Instructions

1. Arrange onion slices on a plate. Drizzle vinegar over onion slices. Heat a large grill pan over medium heat. Coat pan with cooking spray. Add onion to pan; cover and cook 3 minutes on each side. Remove from pan; cover and keep warm.

2. Heat pan over medium-high heat. Coat pan with cooking spray. Divide beef into 4 equal portions, shaping each into a 1/2-inch-thick patty. Sprinkle patties evenly with salt and pepper. Add patties to pan; cook 3 minutes on

How To Use Your Gestational Diabetes Meal Plan

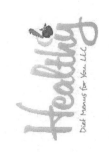

Roasted Broccoli with Almonds

5 Cup	Vegetable, Broccoli Florets, Raw
1 Tablespoon	Oil, Vegetable or Olive
0.25 tsp	Salt
0.25 tsp	Spice, Black Pepper
0.25 Cup	Nuts, Almond Sliced

Cut broccoli
broccoli in a
broccoli with
Bake 14 min

Example of a side dish recipe

Serves: 6

Serving Size: 3/4 Cup

Finally, you have the nutritional information section by recipe that provides you with information on a **PER SERVING** basis for the recipe above it. While the total amount of the recipe is what you make, and you have the information on the number of portions it makes – a recipe is included based on being right for that diet based on how much it contains per serving. In the case of the gestational diabetes diet, it is important to know how many calories but also how many grams of carbohydrate are in a serving so if you are counting how many grams of carbohydrate you can have, it's all right there. Your dietitian may have told you how many grams of carbohydrate, protein, sodium and other nutrients to eat per meal. I add up the amounts of each nutrient for the entire meal to get your correct amount. CHO = Carbohydrates. All nutrients show up just in case you need to track another

Grocery List

The grocery list is fairly straightforward so that you can use it several different ways. It has the name of the diet and the week on the top of the page. It is sorted by grocery aisle area - breads, meats, frozen, canned, etc. This helps you with your shopping so that all of the items you need in one section of the store are together. You can go around your kitchen area or pantry before going to the grocery store, cross off what you already have, and get a weeks worth of dinners (and any leftovers for lunch the next day) quickly and easily saving you time. We provide a grocery list for you listed by meal.

Please let me know if you have any further questions or suggestions about how to make the meal planning system best work for you! After all, that is who it's for!

Grocery List

Chicken Marsala

Quantity		Grocery Item
0.25	tsp	Salt
0.25	tsp	Spice, Black Pepper
1	Tablespoons	Flour, White bleached enriched
1.666	cup	Soup, Chicken Broth Low Sodium
0.25	Teaspoon	Herb, Garlic, Raw
4	cup	Vegetable, Mushrooms, slices,
16	ounces	Chicken, Breast Boneless
2	Oz	Wine, dessert, sweet marsala

Example of a grocery list shown by meal, so you can choose to only make that meal for the week or send someone for just those items.

Creamy Herbed Mashed Potatoes

Quantity		Grocery Item
0.5	tsp	Spice, Black Pepper

Week 1 Meals and Grocery Lists

Banana Oat Pancakes with Strawberries

Blackened Tuna Steaks with Coconut Rice, Tossed Pear and Almond Salad, and Roasted Broccoli with Almonds

Crispy Cod with Brussels Sprouts and Bacon, Rice and Beans and Ratatouille

Meatless Skillet Lasagna with Lemon Spinach, Corn on the Cob and Roasted Asparagus

Pork Chops with Cranberry Glaze with Roasted Acorn Squash and Rosemary Roasted Potatoes

Seafood Risotto with Red Apple Coleslaw and Italian Green Beans

Vegetable and Bean Chili with Bacon Potato Salad and Oven Fries

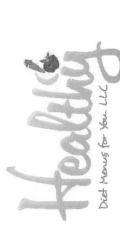

Healthy
Diet Menus for You. LLC

Meal Plan

www.healthydietmenusforyou.com

Diet: *Gestational Diabetic - 2400*

Meal: *Banana Oat Pancakes GDM*

Recipe		Ingredients	Instructions	Nutritionals					
Banana Oat Pancakes	11 ounces	Milk, Buttermilk Lowfat	In a large bowl, combine oats in buttermilk. Let stand until oat soften. Mix in mashed bananas, eggs and vanilla. Gradually stir in baking mix. Coat a griddle or nonstick skillet with cooking spray. Use one 4th cup batter for each pancake and cook pancake until browned on bottom and some bubbles begin to break around edges. Turn pancake over. Cook until browned on bottom and firm to touch in center. Repeat procedure until all pancakes are gone. Serve pancakes with sugar-free syrup.	Calories 272.9	Sodium: 525.5	Protein: 10.6	Phos 362.1	
Serves: 5	1.5 1	Fruit, Banana		Fat: 4.804	Carbs: 46.9	Chol:		Pot: 414.6
	2 Each	Egg, Whole		Sat Fat: 1.699	Fiber: 4.212			
Serving Size: 2 pancakes	1.5 Cup	Bisquick, Heart Smart			Sugar: 10.1			
	1 Teaspoon	Flavoring, Vanilla Extract						

Recipe		Ingredients	Instructions	Nutritionals					
Strawberries	9 Cup	Fruit, Strawberries, halves/slices, raw	Remove tops and wash prior to serving.	Calories 73	Sodium: 2.2	Protein: 1.5	Phos 54.7	
Serves: 6				Fat: 0.6	Carbs: 17.5	Chol: 0		Pot: 348.8
Serving Size: 1.5 Cups of Strawberries				Sat Fat: 0	Fiber: 4.5			
					Sugar: 11.1			

Meal: *Tuna Steaks GDM*

Recipe		Ingredients	Instructions	Nutritionals					
Blackened Tuna Steaks	3 teaspoon	Spice, Paprika	In a small bowl, combine paprika time, black pepper, garlic and chili powder, as well as cayenne pepper and mix well to incorporate. Dredge 1 side of each tuna steak in blackening spice. Coat a large nonstick skillet with cooking spray. Add tuna steaks spice side down to pan over medium-high heat. Cook on both sides for 45 min. or until done.	Calories 132.9	Sodium: 49.6	Protein: 27	Phos 227.4	
Serves: 4	1 Teaspoon	Herb, Thyme Ground		Fat: 1.487	Carbs: 2.07	Chol: 51		Pot: 569.9
	0.5 tsp	Spice, Black Pepper		Sat Fat: 0.342	Fiber: 1.142			
Serving Size: 4 ounce steak	1 Teaspoon	Herb, Garlic, Raw			Sugar: 0.263			
	1 teaspoon	Spice, Chili Powder						
	16 Ounces	Fish, Tuna, Fresh						
	0.5 Teaspoon	Spice, Pepper, Cayenne						

Coconut Rice

Serves: 4
Serving Size: 1/2 cup

Ingredients

Amount	Ingredient
10 oz	Water
0.25 tsp	Salt
4 Ounces	Milk, Coconut, canned
8 Ounces	Grain, Rice, Basmati, raw

Instructions

Combine basmati rice, water, coconut milk and salt in a small saucepan. Bring to a boil. Cover, reduce heat and simmer 16 min. or until liquid is absorbed.

Nutritionals

Calories	224.5	Sodium:	153.5	Protein:	3.868	Phos	80.3
Fat:	6.331	Carbs:	37.8	Chol:	0	Pot:	116.1
Sat Fat:	5.427	Fiber:	0.601				
		Sugar:	0.056				

Tossed Pear and Almond Salad

Serves: 6
Serving Size: Salad

Ingredients

Amount	Ingredient
2 Fruit	Fruit, Pear Raw
6 Cup	Lettuce, Raw Iceberg
0.25 Cup	Nuts, Almond Sliced
6 Tablespoon	Salad Dressing, Vinaigrette

Instructions

Toss Salad together and divide into 6 portions

Nutritionals

Calories	127	Sodium:	222	Protein:	2	Phos	46
Fat:	7	Carbs:	16	Chol:	0	Pot:	191
Sat Fat:	1	Fiber:	3				
		Sugar:	7				

Roasted Broccoli with Almonds

Serves: 6
Serving Size: 3/4 Cup

Ingredients

Amount	Ingredient
5 Cup	Vegetable, Broccoli Florets, Raw
1 Tablespoon	Oil, Vegetable or Olive
0.25 tsp	Salt
0.25 tsp	Spice, Black Pepper
0.25 Cup	Nuts, Almond Sliced

Instructions

Cut broccoli off stem if necessary. Place broccoli in a sprayed baking dish. Drizzle broccoli with olive oil, garlic, salt and pepper. Bake 14 minutes at 450°F. Sprinkle with almonds and divide into 6 servings.

Nutritionals

Calories	123	Sodium:	164	Protein:	7	Phos	162
Fat:	6	Carbs:	15	Chol:	0	Pot:	685
Sat Fat:	1	Fiber:	6				
		Sugar:	4				

Meal: Crispy Cod GDM

Crispy Cod

Serves: 4
Serving Size: 4 ounce file

Ingredients

Amount	Ingredient
1.5 Cup	Cereal, Cornflakes
1 Teaspoon	Herb, Garlic, Raw
1 Teaspoon	Spice, Onion Powder
0.5 tsp	Salt
1 Each	Egg, Whole
2 Each	Egg White
1 Teaspoon	Sauce, Pepper, Tabasco
0.13 Cup	Flour, Wheat, White, All Purpose, unbleached, enriched
16 oz	Fish, Cod, Pacific, Raw

Instructions

Preheat oven to 350°. Coat a shallow baking pan with cooking spray. In a medium bowl, crush corn flakes into crumbs, and combine cornflake crumbs, garlic and onion, salt. In a separate bowl, lightly beat egg and egg whites. Add hot pepper sauce and mix well. Place flour in a separate bowl. Dip each cod fillet in flour, then egg mixture, then cornflake mixture, coating well. Place fillets in baking pan. Spray fillets lightly with cooking spray and bake 18 to 20 min.

Nutritionals

Calories	170.1	Sodium:	478.8	Protein:	24.7	Phos	268.5
Fat:	2.13	Carbs:	12.1	Chol:	101.6	Pot:	534.9
Sat Fat:	0.558	Fiber:	0.509				
		Sugar:	1.149				

Recipe 1

Brussel Sprouts and Bacon

Serves: 4

Serving Size: 4 ounces

Ingredients	
0.5 tsp	Salt
1 tsp	Spice, Black Pepper
4 Slices	Pork Bacon, Cured or Smoked, lower sodium, slices
2 Teaspoon	Herb, Garlic, Raw
1 teaspoon	Spice, Red Pepper
0.06 Cup	Nuts, Almond Sliced
1 Pounds	Vegetable, Brussels Sprouts, raw

Instructions

Cut the brussels sprouts in half and trim bottoms. Heat a large skillet or saute pan over medium heat. Add the bacon and cook until crispy, about 5 minutes. Remove to a plate lined with paper towels. Discard all but 1 tablespoon of the rendered bacon fat. Add the garlic, pepper flakes, brussels sprouts and salt to the skillet. Saute until the sprouts are lightly browned on the outside and tender - but still firm - throughout. Approx 10-12 minutes. Add the almonds and bacon (crumbled) and saute for another minute or two. Season with salt and pepper.

Nutritionals

Calories 121	Sodium: 402.1	Protein: 7.2	Phos 127
Fat: 6.2	Carbs: 12	Chol: 6.8	Pot: 528.2
Sat Fat: 1.6	Fiber: 5		
	Sugar: 2.7		

Recipe 2

Rice and Beans Side

Serves: 4

Serving Size: 1/2 cup

Ingredients	
1 Cup	Grain, Rice, Brown, Long grain
1 Cup	Beans, Black, Canned
0.25 Cup	Herb, Cilantro Raw
0.25 tsp	Spice, Cumin, Ground
0.25 teaspoo	Spice, Chili Powder

Instructions

Cook long-grain brown rice according to package directions. Combine cooked rice, 1 cup rinsed and drained canned black beans, 1 tablespoon chopped fresh cilantro, 1/4 teaspoon salt, 1/4 teaspoon ground cumin, and 1/4 teaspoon chili powder.

Nutritionals

Calories 221.8	Sodium: 97.6	Protein: 6.859	Phos 201.6
Fat: 1.619	Carbs: 44.9	Chol: 0	Pot: 274.6
Sat Fat: 0.33	Fiber: 3.909		
	Sugar: 0.722		

Recipe 3

Ratatouille

Serves: 6

Serving Size: 1 Cup

Ingredients	
3 Teaspoon	Oil, Olive
2 Teaspoon	Herb, Garlic, Raw
1 Each	Vegetable, Eggplant
1.5 Cup	Vegetable, Zucchini, slices
1 Cup	Vegetable, Pepper, Green
0.5 tsp	Salt
0.25 tsp	Spice, Black Pepper
8 ounces	Vegetable, Tomato, Red Canned, No Added Salt

Instructions

Add oil to a large nonstick skillet over medium to high heat. Add garlic and sauté for 30 seconds. Add remaining ingredients and cook 10 to 15 min., stirring occasionally, until vegetables are tender.

Nutritionals

Calories 41.4	Sodium: 201.3	Protein: 1.074	Phos 28.3
Fat: 2.468	Carbs: 4.775	Chol: 0	Pot: 228.7
Sat Fat: 0.362	Fiber: 1.612		
	Sugar: 2.585		

Meatless Skillet Lasagna
Serves: 9
Serving Size: 1 cup

Ingredients
Amount	Ingredient
10 Ounces	Pasta, Farfalle, enriched, dry
3 Cup	Sauce, Pasta, ready-to-serve
1 Cup	Cheese, Ricotta, Part Skim Milk
1 Cup	Cheese, Mozzarella Part Skim
2 Ounces	Cheese, Parmesan, dry grated - Romano, grated
1 Tablespoon	Herb, Parsley, dried
4 Each	Veggie Burger

Instructions
Cook pasta according to package directions, omitting salt. Drain. In a deep nonstick skillet or wok, cooked veggie meat for 3 to 4 min. until done. Add pasta sauce and heat. In a medium bowl, combine remaining ingredients and mix well. Add cheese mixture to the sauce and mix well until thoroughly heated. Add cooked pasta the sauce and toss to coat.

Nutritionals
Calories 325.6	Sodium: 700.7	Protein: 18.1	Phos 298.
Fat: 10.7	Carbs: 40.1	Chol: 19.3	Pot: 529.8
Sat Fat: 4.189	Fiber: 5.204		
	Sugar: 8.443		

Lemon Spinach
Serves: 4
Serving Size: 1/2 cup

Ingredients
Amount	Ingredient
4 Oz	Beverage, Alcoholic, Wine, Table, Dry White
2 ounces	Lemon Juice, Bottled
0.75 Teaspoo	Herb, Garlic, Raw
1.25 Ounces	Vegetable, Spinach, raw, torn

Instructions
In pan, stir in wine and lemon juice, cook 1 minute. Add garlic, and cook 1 minute. Add spinach, tossing 1 minute or until the spinach wilts.

Nutritionals
Calories 44.4	Sodium: 58.7	Protein: 2.2	Phos 43.6
Fat: 0.298	Carbs: 4.279	Chol: 0	Pot: 429.3
Sat Fat: 0.048	Fiber: 1.621		
	Sugar: 0.691		

Corn On The Cob
Serves: 6
Serving Size: 1 ear of corn

Ingredients
Amount	Ingredient
6 Each	Vegetable, Corn on Cob, sm/med, ckd w/o fat or salt

Instructions
Shuck and clean corn. Boil until tender, about 4-6 minutes.

Nutritionals
Calories 82.7	Sodium: 1.5	Protein: 2.5	Phos 78.8
Fat: 0.9	Carbs: 19.2	Chol: 0	Pot: 190.6
Sat Fat: 0.1	Fiber: 2.8		
	Sugar: 0		

Roasted Asparagus
Serves: 6
Serving Size: 4 oz

Ingredients
Amount	Ingredient
24 Ounces	Vegetable, Asparagus Fresh
0.5 teaspoon	Spice, Garlic Powder
0.5 Teaspoon	Spice, Lemon Pepper

Instructions
Place asparagus in a sprayed baking dish and coat with olive oil spray. Sprinkle with garlic powder and lemon pepper. Bake for 8 minutes at 450° F or until done.

Nutritionals
Calories 29	Sodium: 9	Protein: 3	Phos 63
Fat: 0.4	Carbs: 5	Chol: 5	Pot: 185
Sat Fat: 0	Fiber: 2		
	Sugar: 0		

Meal: *Pork Chops Cranberry Glz GDM*

Pork Chops with Cranberry Glaze

Serves: 4

Serving Size: 4-5 ounce pork chop

Nutritionals

Calories 275.4	Sodium: 237.4	Protein: 31.7	Phos: 328.7
Fat: 6.55	Carbs: 20.4	Chol: 97.8	Pot: 603.6
Sat Fat: 1.736	Fiber: 1.105		
	Sugar: 16.3		

Ingredients

20 ounces	Pork, Center Rib Chop
1 Teaspoon	Herb, Garlic, Raw
0.25 tsp	Salt
0.5 tsp	Spice, Black Pepper
1 Teaspoon	Oil, Olive
0.5 ounces	Honey
8 Tablespoon	Vinegar, balsamic
3 oz	Water
0.333 Cups	Fruit, Cranberries, dried - Craisins
8 Ounces	Vegetable, Onions, Red, Sliced

Instructions

Stephen pork chops well with garlic, salt and pepper. Add oil to a large nonstick skillet over medium to high heat. Sauté chops for 6 to 8 min. or until browned, turning once. Remove from pan and keep chops warm. Spray pan with cooking spray. Add onions and cook for 5 to 6 min. or until they begin to caramelize. Stir in honey, balsamic vinegar, water and cranberries and simmer for 5 to 7 min. or until. Cranberries are soft and sauce takes honey glaze consistency. Pour cranberry sauce over pork chops and serve.

Roasted Acorn Squash

Serves: 8

Serving Size: 1/8 recipe

Nutritionals

Calories 100.8	Sodium: 72.5	Protein: 1.822	Phos: 81.8
Fat: 1.354	Carbs: 23.7	Chol: 0	Pot: 787.9
Sat Fat: 0.204	Fiber: 3.419		
	Sugar: 0		

Ingredients

0.5 tsp	Salt
0.25 tsp	Spice, Black Pepper
2 Teaspoon	Oil, Olive
32 Ounces	Vegetable, Squash, Acorn, peeled, raw

Instructions

Preheat oven to 400°. Cut them off of each squash and cut in half lengthwise. Scoop out seeds; rinse and dry each squash, half. Spray all sides of squash halves with cooking spray. Season inside of each half with salt and pepper. Place cut side down on a nonstick cooking spray coated baking sheet. Bake for 45 min.. Scoop squash meat out into a medium bowl; discard skins. Add olive oil and beat with a sturdy whisk until fluffy.

Rosemary Roasted Potatoes

Serves: 6

Serving Size: 3/4 cup Potatoes

Nutritionals

Calories 132.8	Sodium: 12.3	Protein: 3.094	Phos 85.4
Fat: 2.581	Carbs: 25.5	Chol: 0	Pot: 642
Sat Fat: 0.407	Fiber: 3.056		
	Sugar: 1.443		

Ingredients

5 each	Vegetable, Potato
1 Tablespoon	Oil, Vegetable or Olive
0.75 Teaspoo	Herb, Garlic, Raw
3 teaspoon	Herb, Rosemary, Dried
2 teaspoon	Spice, Paprika

Instructions

Wash and dice potatoes into bite-sized pieces. Place into a large bowl or Ziplock bag; toss with olive oil. Sprinkle garlic, rosemary, paprika (optional), and pepper over potatoes and shake to coat. Layer potatoes in a single layer on a baking sheet coated with cooking spray. Bake at 400 F for 30 minutes or until slightly browned. Serves 5.

Meal: *Seafood Risotto GDM*

Recipe	Ingredients	Instructions	Nutritionals					

Seafood Risotto

Serves: 9

Serving Size: 1 cup

1 Tablespoon	Vegetable, Onions, chopped, raw	
2.5 Cup	Rice, White Medium Grain	
3.5 cup	Soup, Chicken Broth Low Sodium	
28 oz	Water	
6 Teaspoon	Oil, Olive	
16 Ounces	Shellfish, Scallops, raw	
16 Ounces	Shrimp, peeled and deveined	
4 Oz	Beverage, Alcoholic, Wine, Table, Dry White	
0.5 tsp	Salt	
0.25 tsp	Spice, Black Pepper	
2 Ounces	Cheese, parmesan, reduced fat	

Instructions: Coat a large soup pot generously with cooking spray. Over medium to high heat, sauté onions for 3 to 4 min. or until they turned clear. Stir in Rice, and sauté for one more minute. Stir in chicken broth and water and bring to a boil. Reduce heat to a simmer and stir constantly with a large wooden spoon for 20 min. Cover and remove from heat. Add oil to a large nonstick skillet over medium to high heat. Add scallops and shrimp and sauté for 2 min. Add wine and cook until wine is reduced by half. Fold seafood, salt, pepper and cheese gently into risotto.

Nutritionals:
Calories	333.7	Sodium:	358.9	Protein:	25.3	Phos	344.?
Fat:	3.883	Carbs:	45	Chol:	95.7	Pot:	444.6
Sat Fat:	1.025	Fiber:	1.177				
		Sugar:	0.459				

Recipe	Ingredients	Instructions	Nutritionals					

Red Apple Coleslaw

Serves: 4

Serving Size: 3/4 cup

0.5 Cup	Mayonnaise, reduced kcal, cholest free/Hellmann	
3 Teaspoon	Vinegar, Red Wine	
1 Each	Sugar Substitute Packet, Equal	
1 Teaspoon	Spice, Celery Seed	
2 Cup	Vegetable, Cabbage Heads, Red, raw	
1 Cup	Vegetable, Onions, Young Green, raw	
1 Each	Fruit, Apple w/skin, raw	
0.5 tsp	Spice, Black Pepper	

Instructions: In a large bowl, whisk the mayo, vinegar, sweetener, and celery seeds together. Add the shredded cabbage, scallions, and grated apple. Season with pepper. Toss to thoroughly combine ingredients. Chill, covered, until cold about 2 hours. Serves 4.

Nutritionals:
Calories	149.2	Sodium:	217.1	Protein:	1.4	Phos	39.9
Fat:	10.3	Carbs:	15.2	Chol:	10.5	Pot:	237.5
Sat Fat:	1.6	Fiber:	2.8				
		Sugar:	8.6				

Recipe: Italian Green Beans

Serves: 6
Serving Size: 1/2 cup

Ingredients

Amount	Ingredient
3 Teaspoon	Oil, Olive
1 Cup	Vegetable, Onions
2 Teaspoon	Herb, Garlic, Raw
1 Can	Vegetable, Tomato Diced Canned
0.25 Teaspoo	Herb, Oregano, Ground
0.25 Teaspoo	Herb, Basil, Ground
16 Ounces	Vegetable, Beans, Italian, Frozen

Instructions

Steam green beans until tender crisp. Set aside. Heat olive oil in a medium nonstick skillet over medium-high heat. Sauté onions until clear. Add garlic; sauté 30 seconds. Add tomatoes, basil, and oregano, and simmer for 15 to 20 min. for tomato mixture over steamed green beans and mix well.

Nutritionals

Calories 67.1	Sodium: 217.2	Protein: 2.111	Phos 46.7
Fat: 2.519	Carbs: 10.9	Chol: 0	Pot: 315.5
Sat Fat: 0.37	Fiber: 3.596		
	Sugar: 3.97		

Meal: Vegetable Bean Chili GDM

Recipe: Vegetable and Bean Chili

Serves: 8
Serving Size: 1 cup

Ingredients

Amount	Ingredient
0.5 Cup	Vegetable, Onions
3 Teaspoon	Oil, Olive
2 Cup	Vegetable, Carrots
1 Cup	Vegetable, Zucchini, slices
2 Teaspoon	Herb, Garlic, Raw
2 Cup	Beans, Black, Canned
2 Cup	Beans, Kidney, canned/Rinsed
1.85 Cup	Sauce, Tomato, no salt added
32 ounces	Vegetable, Tomato, Red Canned, No Added Salt
3 teaspoon	Spice, Chili Powder
0.5 Cup	Vegetable, Pepper, Green

Instructions

Heat oil in a large soup pot over medium-high heat. Add onion and carrots, and sauté 5 min. Drain and rinse beans prior to use. Add green pepper and, zucchini and sauté another 2 min. Add garlic and sauté for 30 seconds. Add chili powder, and all remaining ingredients; bring to a boil. Cover, reduce heat, and simmer 30 to 35 min. or until the vegetables are tender.

Nutritionals

Calories 209	Sodium: 322.1	Protein: 10.3	Phos 189.5
Fat: 2.802	Carbs: 38.5	Chol: 0	Pot: 987.5
Sat Fat: 0.436	Fiber: 10.4		
	Sugar: 10		

Recipe: Bacon Potato Salad

Serves: 6
Serving Size: 1/2 cup

Ingredients

Amount	Ingredient
2 Slices	Beef, Bacon, lean, ckd
4 each	Vegetable, Potato
0.25 Cup	Mayonnaise, reduced kcal, cholest free/Hellmann
0.33 Tablesp	Dijon Mustard

Instructions

Fry bacon, drain and pat grease off. Crumble. Peel potatoes, cook until tender - about 40 minutes at a low boil, and cube/slice them. Toss the warm potatoes with mayo, mustard, salt and pepper. Add bacon and serve.

Nutritionals

Calories 131.3	Sodium: 124.9	Protein: 2.5	Phos 47.9
Fat: 3.3	Carbs: 23	Chol: 0.82	Pot: 280.2
Sat Fat: 0.5	Fiber: 2		
	Sugar: 0.9		

Recipe	Ingredients		Instructions	Nutritionals			
Oven Fries	3 each	Vegetable, Potato	Cut potatoes into strips like fries. Beat egg whites and toss with fries. Sprinkle with Mrs. Dash type seasoning. Bake for 30 minutes at 400°F or until done.	Calories 75	Sodium: 45	Protein: 3.3	Phos 55
Serves: 6	1 Teaspoon	Spice, Mrs. Dash		Fat: 0.2	Carbs: 15	Chol: 0	Pot: 406
Serving Size: 1/2 potato	3 Each	Egg White		Sat Fat: 0	Fiber: 2		
					Sugar: 1		

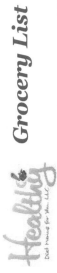

Grocery List

Banana Oat Pancakes GDM Meal

Banana Oat Pancakes

Quantity		Grocery Item
1.5	Cup	Bisquick, Heart Smart
11	ounces	Milk, Buttermilk Lowfat
1.5	1	Fruit, Banana
1	Teaspoon	Flavoring, Vanilla Extract
2	Each	Egg, Whole

Strawberries

Quantity		Grocery Item
9	Cup	Fruit, Strawberries, halves/slices, raw

Tuna Steaks GDM Meal

Blackened Tuna Steaks

Quantity		Grocery Item
1	Teaspoon	Herb, Thyme Ground
16	Ounces	Fish, Tuna, Fresh
1	Teaspoon	Herb, Garlic, Raw
3	teaspoon	Spice, Paprika
1	teaspoon	Spice, Chili Powder
0.5	tsp	Spice, Black Pepper
0.5	Teaspoon	Spice, Pepper, Cayenne

Coconut Rice

Quantity		Grocery Item
4	Ounces	Milk, Coconut, canned
8	Ounces	Grain, Rice, Basmati, raw
0.25	tsp	Salt
10	oz	Water

Tossed Pear and Almond Salad

Quantity		Grocery Item
6	Tablespoon	Salad Dressing, Vinaigrette
6	Cup	Lettuce, Raw Iceberg
2	Fruit	Fruit, Pear Raw
0.25	Cup	Nuts, Almond Sliced

Roasted Broccoli with Almonds

Quantity		Grocery Item
5	Cup	Vegetable, Broccoli Florets, Raw
0.25	tsp	Salt
1	Tablespoon	Oil, Vegetable or Olive
0.25	tsp	Spice, Black Pepper
0.25	Cup	Nuts, Almond Sliced

Crispy Cod GDM Meal

Crispy Cod

Quantity		Grocery Item
1	Teaspoon	Herb, Garlic, Raw
1	Teaspoon	Spice, Onion Powder
0.13	Cup	Flour, Wheat, White, All Purpose,
1	Each	Egg, Whole
0.5	tsp	Salt
2	Each	Egg White
16	oz	Fish, Cod, Pacific, Raw
1	Teaspoon	Sauce, Pepper, Tabasco
1.5	Cup	Cereal, Cornflakes

Brussel Sprouts and Bacon

Quantity		Grocery Item
0.06	Cup	Nuts, Almond Sliced
1	Pounds	Vegetable, Brussels Sprouts, raw
0.5	tsp	Salt
1	teaspoon	Spice, Red Pepper
2	Teaspoon	Herb, Garlic, Raw
4	Slices	Pork Bacon, Cured or Smoked, lower
1	tsp	Spice, Black Pepper

Pork Chops Cranberry Glz GDM Meal

Pork Chops with Cranberry Glaze

Quantity		Grocery Item
0.25	tsp	Salt
0.5	tsp	Spice, Black Pepper
20	ounces	Pork, Center Rib Chop
0.5	ounces	Honey
3	oz	Water
1	Teaspoon	Herb, Garlic, Raw
8	Tablespoon	Vinegar, balsamic
1	Teaspoon	Oil, Olive
0.333	Cups	Fruit, Cranberries, dried - Craisins
8	Ounces	Vegetable, Onions, Red, Sliced

Roasted Acorn Squash

Quantity		Grocery Item
2	Teaspoon	Oil, Olive
0.25	tsp	Spice, Black Pepper
0.5	tsp	Salt
32	Ounces	Vegetable, Squash, Acorn, peeled, raw

Rosemary Roasted Potatoes

Quantity		Grocery Item
2	teaspoon	Spice, Paprika
3	teaspoon	Herb, Rosemary, Dried
5	each	Vegetable, Potato
0.75	Teaspoon	Herb, Garlic, Raw
1	Tablespoon	Oil, Vegetable or Olive

Meatless Skillet Lasagna GDM Meal

Meatless Skillet Lasagna

Quantity		Grocery Item
10	Ounces	Pasta, Farfalle, enriched, dry
1	Cup	Cheese, Ricotta, Part Skim Milk
1	Cup	Cheese, Mozzarella Part Skim
4	Each	Veggie Burger
3	Cup	Sauce, Pasta, ready-to-serve
2	Ounces	Cheese, Parmesan, dry grated - Romano,
1	Tablespoon	Herb, Parsley, dried

Lemon Spinach

Quantity		Grocery Item
4	Oz	Beverage, Alcoholic, Wine, Table, Dry White
2	ounces	Lemon Juice, Bottled
1.25	Ounces	Vegetable, Spinach, raw, torn
0.75	Teaspoon	Herb, Garlic, Raw

Corn On The Cob

Quantity		Grocery Item
6	Each	Vegetable, Corn on Cob, sm/med, ckd w/o

Roasted Asparagus

Quantity		Grocery Item
0.5	Teaspoon	Spice, Lemon Pepper
24	Ounces	Vegetable, Asparagus Fresh
0.5	teaspoon	Spice, Garlic Powder

Rice and Beans Side

Quantity		Grocery Item
0.25	Cup	Herb, Cilantro Raw
1	Cup	Beans, Black, Canned
1	Cup	Grain, Rice, Brown, Long grain
0.25	teaspoon	Spice, Chili Powder
0.25	tsp	Spice, Cumin, Ground

Ratatouille

Quantity		Grocery Item
1.5	Cup	Vegetable, Zucchini, slices
3	Teaspoon	Oil, Olive
2	Teaspoon	Herb, Garlic, Raw
1	Each	Vegetable, Eggplant
1	Cup	Vegetable, Pepper, Green
0.25	tsp	Spice, Black Pepper
0.5	tsp	Salt
8	ounces	Vegetable, Tomato, Red Canned, No Added

Seafood Risotto GDM Meal

Seafood Risotto

Quantity		Grocery Item
1	Tablespoon	Vegetable, Onions, chopped, raw
4	Oz	Beverage, Alcoholic, Wine, Table, Dry White
3.5	cup	Soup, Chicken Broth Low Sodium
28	oz	Water
16	Ounces	Shrimp, peeled and deveined
2.5	Cup	Rice, White Medium Grain
16	Ounces	Shellfish, Scallops, raw
2	Ounces	Cheese, parmesan, reduced fat
0.5	tsp	Salt
0.25	tsp	Spice, Black Pepper
6	Teaspoon	Oil, Olive

Red Apple Coleslaw

Quantity		Grocery Item
1	Each	Sugar Substitute Packet, Equal
0.5	Cup	Mayonnaise, reduced kcal, cholest
0.5	tsp	Spice, Black Pepper
1	Cup	Vegetable, Onions, Young Green, raw
1	Teaspoon	Spice, Celery Seed
2	Cup	Vegetable, Cabbage Heads, Red, raw
3	Teaspoon	Vinegar, Red Wine
1	Each	Fruit, Apple w/skin, raw

Italian Green Beans

Quantity		Grocery Item
2	Teaspoon	Herb, Garlic, Raw
0.25	Teaspoon	Herb, Oregano, Ground
1	Cup	Vegetable, Onions
3	Teaspoon	Oil, Olive
16	Ounces	Vegetable, Beans, Italian, Frozen
1	Can	Vegetable, Tomato Diced Canned
0.25	Teaspoon	Herb, Basil, Ground

Vegetable Bean Chili GDM Meal

Vegetable and Bean Chili

Quantity		Grocery Item
0.5	Cup	Vegetable, Pepper, Green
0.5	Cup	Vegetable, Onions
2	Cup	Vegetable, Carrots
2	Cup	Beans, Kidney, canned/Rinsed
1.85	Cup	Sauce, Tomato, no salt added
3	teaspoon	Spice, Chili Powder
2	Teaspoon	Herb, Garlic, Raw
2	Cup	Beans, Black, Canned
1	Cup	Vegetable, Zucchini, slices
32	ounces	Vegetable, Tomato, Red Canned, No Added
3	Teaspoon	Oil, Olive

Bacon Potato Salad

Quantity		Grocery Item
0.33	Tablespoon	Dijon Mustard
2	Slices	Beef, Bacon, lean, ckd
0.25	Cup	Mayonnaise, reduced kcal, cholest
4	each	Vegetable, Potato

Oven Fries

Quantity		Grocery Item
3	Each	Egg White
3	each	Vegetable, Potato
1	Teaspoon	Spice, Mrs. Dash

Week 2 Meals and Grocery Lists

Herbed Chicken Parmesan with Creamy Mashed Potatoes and Broccoli Casserole

Baked True Lemon Chicken with Brussels Sprouts and Bacon and Bulgur Salad

Honey Garlic Pork Chops with Skinny Mashed Potatoes, Pear Feta Salad, and Ratatouille

Baked Asparagus Omelet with Rosemary Roasted Potatoes and Pears

Baked Beef Pot Pie with Ratatouille and Oranges

Grilled Turkey and Ham Sandwich with Oven Fries, Creamy Lemon Coleslaw, and Italian Green Beans

Lime Butter Catfish with Rice and Noodle Pilaf, Steamed Carrots and Down Home Baked Beans

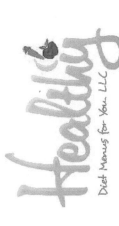

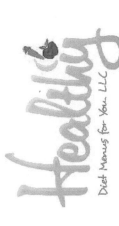Healthy
Diet Menus for You, LLC

Meal Plan

www.healthydietmenusforyou.com

Diet: *Gestational Diabetic - 2400*

Meal: *Herbed Chicken Parmesan GDM*

Recipe	Ingredients		Instructions	Nutritionals			
Herbed Chicken Parmesa	0.33 Cup	Cheese, Grated Parmesan, Reduced Fat	Preheat broiler. Combine 2 tablespoons of parmesan, breadcrumbs, parsley, basil, and 1/8 tsp of salt in a shallow dish. Place egg white in a shallow dish. Dip each chicken tender in egg white; dredge in the breadcrumb mixture. Melt butter in a large nonstick skillet over medium high heat. Add chicken; cook 3 minutes on each side or until done. Set aside. Combine 1/8 tsp salt, pasta sauce, vinegar, and pepper in a microwave safe bowl. Cover with plastic wrap; ven. Microwave sauce mixture at high 2 minutes or until thoroughly heated. Pour the sauce over chicken in pan. Sprinkle evenly with the remaining parmesan and provolone cheese. Wrap the handle of pan with foil, and broil 2 minutes or until the cheese melts.	Calories 447.3	Sodium: 1462	Protein: 24	Phos 407.5
Serves: 4	0.25 Cup	Breadcrumbs, Plain, Grated, Dry		Fat: 25.3	Carbs: 31.2	Chol: 65	Pot: 686.3
	1 Tablespoon	Herb, Parsley, dried		Sat Fat: 7.9	Fiber: 3		
Serving Size: 4 oz chicker w/sauce	0.5 Teaspoon	Herb, Basil, Ground			Sugar: 8.2		
	0.25 tsp	Salt					
	1 Each	Egg White					
	16 Ounces	Chicken, Breast Tenders Boneless					
	1 tablespoon	Butter, Light w/no added salt					
	1.5 Cup	Sauce, Spaghetti, meatless - pizza sauce					
	0.66 Tablesp	Vinegar, balsamic					
	0.25 tsp	Spice, Black Pepper					
	1.5 oz	Cheese, Provolone Shredded					

Recipe	Ingredients		Instructions	Nutritionals			
Creamy Herbed Mashed Potatoes	4 Cup	Vegetable, Potato, Flesh only, diced, raw	Peel and cube potatoes. Place potato in a saucepan; cover with water. Bring to a boil; cover, reduce heat, and simmer 10 minutes or until tender. Drain. Return potato to pan. Add milk and remaining ingredients; mash with a potato masher to desired consistency.	Calories 147.1	Sodium: 215.1	Protein: 3.1	Phos 73
Serves: 6	4 fluid ounces	Milk, Nonfat/Skim		Fat: 4.6	Carbs: 23.8	Chol: 11	Pot: 422.7
	1 Tablespoon	Cream, Sour, Reduced Fat		Sat Fat: 2.8	Fiber: 2.1		
Serving Size: 3/4 Cup	3 tablespoon	Butter, Light w/no added salt			Sugar: 2.3		
	3 Tablespoon	Herb, Chives, raw					
	4 Springs	Herb, Parsley, Raw, Fresh					
	0.5 tsp	Salt					
	0.5 tsp	Spice, Black Pepper					

47

Recipe: Broccoli Casserole

Serves: 8
Serving Size: 1/2 cup

Nutritionals

Calories 53.3	Sodium: 300	Protein: 3.796	Phos 135.?
Fat: 2.291	Carbs: 5.245	Chol: 7.318	Pot: 231.2
Sat Fat: 1.228	Fiber: 0.179		
	Sugar: 1.884		

Ingredients

Amount	Ingredient
4 Cup	Vegetable, Broccoli Florets, Raw
4 fluid ounces	Milk, Nonfat/Skim
0.125 tsp	Spice, Black Pepper
0.5 Cup	Cheese, Cheddar reduced fat
6 Ounces	Soup, Cream of Celery, Fat Free

Instructions

Preheat oven to 350°. In a large bowl, combine all ingredients. Pour into a medium casserole dish and bake for 30 min.

Meal: Baked Lemon Chicken GDM

Recipe: Baked True Lemon Chicken

Serves: 4
Serving Size: 4 oz chicken breast

Nutritionals

Calories 267.8	Sodium: 203.7	Protein: 26.5	Phos 267.?
Fat: 10.9	Carbs: 14.2	Chol: 87.5	Pot: 485.8
Sat Fat: 5.5	Fiber: 0.8		
	Sugar: 0.8		

Ingredients

Amount	Ingredient
4 Packet	True Lemon packet
16 ounces	Chicken, Breast Boneless
0.5 teaspoon	Salt, Kosher
0.5 tsp	Spice, Black Pepper
0.5 Stick	Butter, Light, Stick, Salted - Land O Lakes
8 Tablespoon	Flour, White bleached enriched
0.5 Cup	Vegetable, Onions
1 Teaspoon	Herb, Garlic, Raw

Instructions

Pound the chicken breasts. Dredge with flour. Melt the butter in the baking pan. Coat chicken on all sides with flour. Bake the chicken at 375°F brushing with pan drippings during the cooking. Cook for 30 minutes. Make the true lemon baste: While chicken is cooking, in a small bowl, mix true lemon, minced onion, garlic and salt and pepper. Add a third cup of water if mixture is too dry. Use to brush chicken during cooking several times. Serves 4.

Recipe: Brussel Sprouts and Bacon

Serves: 4
Serving Size: 4 ounces

Nutritionals

Calories 121	Sodium: 402.1	Protein: 7.2	Phos 127
Fat: 6.2	Carbs: 12	Chol: 6.8	Pot: 528.2
Sat Fat: 1.6	Fiber: 5		
	Sugar: 2.7		

Ingredients

Amount	Ingredient
0.5 tsp	Salt
1 tsp	Spice, Black Pepper
4 Slices	Pork Bacon, Cured or Smoked, lower sodium, slices
2 Teaspoon	Herb, Garlic, Raw
1 teaspoon	Spice, Red Pepper
0.06 Cup	Nuts, Almond Sliced
1 Pounds	Vegetable, Brussels Sprouts, raw

Instructions

Cut the brussels sprouts in half and trim bottoms. Heat a large skillet or saute pan over medium heat. Add the bacon and cook until crispy, about 5 minutes. Remove to a plate lined with paper towels. Discard all but 1 tablespoon of the rendered bacon fat. Add the garlic, pepper flakes, brussels sprouts and salt to the skillet. Saute until the sprouts are lightly browned on the outside and tender - but still firm - throughout. Approx 10-12 minutes. Add the almonds and bacon (crumbled) and saute for another minute or two. Season with salt and pepper.

Recipe	Ingredients		Instructions	Nutritionals			
Warm Bulgur Salad **Serves: 4** **Serving Size: 1 cup**	3 Cup	Bulgar	Combine 3 cups hot cooked bulgur and 5 ounces baby spinach; cover and let stand 15 minutes or until spinach wilts. Stir in 1 cup halved cherry tomatoes, 3 tablespoons fresh lemon juice, 2 tablespoons extra-virgin olive oil, 1/2 teaspoon salt, and 1/4 teaspoon black pepper. Sprinkle with 1/4 cup (1 ounce) crumbled feta cheese.	Calories 169.9	Sodium: 292.9	Protein: 4.988	Phos 79.7
	0.75 Ounces	Vegetable, Spinach, raw, torn		Fat: 7.986	Carbs: 22.2	Chol: 3.154	Pot: 366.6
	1 Cup	Vegetable, Tomato, Red, Cherry		Sat Fat: 1.541	Fiber: 5.848		
	1 ounces	Lemon Juice, Bottled				Sugar: 1.559	
	2 Tablespoon	Oil, Vegetable or Olive					
	0.25 tsp	Spice, Black Pepper					
	0.15 Cup	Cheese, Feta					

Meal: *Honey Garlic Pork Chop GDM*

Recipe	Ingredients		Instructions	Nutritionals			
Honey Garlic Pork Chops **Serves: 6** **Serving Size: 3 oz pork chop**	18 ounces	Pork, Center Rib Chop	Cook chops over medium heat about 8 minutes or until done. Remove chops and keep warm. In pan, combine remaining ingredients and cook for 3-4 minutes; stirring until heated. Serve over chops.	Calories 233	Sodium: 258	Protein: 26	Phos 217
	2 ounces	Honey		Fat: 8.6	Carbs: 13	Chol: 69	Pot: 387
	2 Tablespoon	Soy Sauce, Low Sodium		Sat Fat: 3.1	Fiber: 0		
	1 tsp	Garlic, Minced				Sugar: 12	
	2 ounces	Lemon Juice, Bottled					

Recipe	Ingredients		Instructions	Nutritionals			
Skinny Mashed Potatoes **Serves: 6** **Serving Size: 1/2 cup (4 oz)**	0.75 cup	Soup, Chicken Broth Low Sodium	Peel and dice potatoes. Boil until tender, drain and add broth and garlic powder. Mash until smooth. Divide into 6 servings.	Calories 125	Sodium: 16	Protein: 3	Phos 66
	5 each	Vegetable, Potato		Fat: 0.3	Carbs: 28	Chol: 0	Pot: 485
	0.5 teaspoon	Spice, Garlic Powder		Sat Fat: 0	Fiber: 2.5		
						Sugar: 1.2	

Recipe	Ingredients		Instructions	Nutritionals			
Pear Feta Salad **Serves: 6** **Serving Size: 1 cup salad mixed**	6 Cups	Vegetables, Mixed salad greens, raw	Core and slice pears. Toss salad with dressing and top with pears and feta cheese.	Calories 131.7	Sodium: 391.5	Protein: 3.3	Phos 75.8
	3 Fruit	Fruit, Pear Raw		Fat: 6	Carbs: 18.4	Chol: 6	Pot: 338.7
	0.5 Cup	Cheese, Feta		Sat Fat: 2.2	Fiber:		
	12 Tablespoo	Salad Dressing, Dijon Vinaigrette, light/Wishbone				Sugar: 10.7	

Recipe		Ingredients		Instructions	Nutritionals			
Ratatouille	3 Teaspoon	Oil, Olive		Add oil to a large nonstick skillet over medium to high heat. Add garlic and sauté for 30 seconds. Add remaining ingredients and cook 10 to 15 min., stirring occasionally, until vegetables are tender.	Calories 41.4	Sodium: 201.3	Protein: 1.074	Phos 28.3
Serves: 6	2 Teaspoon	Herb, Garlic, Raw			Fat: 2.468	Carbs: 2.468	Chol: 0	Pot: 228.7
Serving Size: 1 Cup	1 Each	Vegetable, Eggplant			Sat Fat: 0.362	Fiber: 1.612		
	1.5 Cup	Vegetable, Zucchini, slices				Sugar: 2.585		
	1 Cup	Vegetable, Pepper, Green						
	0.5 tsp	Salt						
	0.25 tsp	Spice, Black Pepper						
	8 ounces	Vegetable, Tomato, Red Canned, No Added Salt						

Meal: *Baked Asparagus Omelette GDM*

Recipe		Ingredients		Instructions	Nutritionals			
Baked Asparagus Omelet	16 Ounces	Vegetable, Asparagus Fresh		Microwave asparagus in 1/2 cup water for 2-3 minutes or until crispy-tender. Drain and arrange in bottom of pie pan that has been sprayed with pan spray. Sprinkle cheese and chopped onions evenly on top. Combine egg substitute, eggs, half & half, salt and pepper. Pour over asparagus slowly. Bake for 40 minutes at 350'	Calories 157	Sodium: 425	Protein: 13.8	Phos 277
Serves: 6	1 Cup	Cheese, Mozzarella Part Skim			Fat: 7.8	Carbs: 8.9	Chol: 118	Pot: 354
Serving Size: 1/6 pie	0.25 Cup	Vegetable, Green Onion			Sat Fat: 3.3	Fiber: 1.7		
	0.5 Cup	Egg Substitute				Sugar: 2.5		
	1 Each	Egg, Whole						
	0.5 tsp	Salt						
	2 tsp	Spice, Black Pepper						
	1 cup	Fat Free Half and Half Cream						

Recipe		Ingredients		Instructions	Nutritionals			
Rosemary Roasted Potatoes	5 each	Vegetable, Potato		Wash and dice potatoes into bite-sized pieces. Place into a large bowl or Ziplock bag; toss with olive oil. Sprinkle garlic, rosemary, paprika (optional), and pepper over potatoes and shake to coat. Layer potatoes in a single layer on a baking sheet coated with cooking spray. Bake at 400 F for 30 minutes or until slightly browned. Serves 5.	Calories 132.8	Sodium: 12.3	Protein: 3.094	Phos 85.4
Serves: 6	1 Tablespoon	Oil, Vegetable or Olive			Fat: 2.581	Carbs: 25.5	Chol: 0	Pot: 642
Serving Size: 3/4 cup Potatoes	0.75 Teaspoo	Herb, Garlic, Raw			Sat Fat: 0.407	Fiber: 3.056		
	3 teaspoon	Herb, Rosemary, Dried				Sugar: 1.443		
	2 teaspoon	Spice, Paprika						

Recipe		Instructions	Nutritionals			
Pear		Piece of fruit	Calories 115.5	Sodium: 0	Protein: 1.3	Phos 30.2
	6 Fruit	Fruit, Pear Raw	Fat: 0.6	Carbs: 29.3	Chol: 0	Pot: 332.8
Serves: 6			Sat Fat: 0	Fiber: 9.9		
Serving Size: 1 medium pear				Sugar: 19.4		

Meal: *Beef Pot Pie GDM*

Recipe		Instructions	Nutritionals			
Baked Beef Pot Pie		Steam vegetables until just tender and drain. Brown beef and onion together and drain. Melt light butter in a large skillet and blend in flour until smooth. Add broth and bring to a low boil and stir until thickened. Add seasonings, vegetables and beef and cook for 5-7 minutes. Combine self rising flour and milk, stir until just mixed, pour evenly over pie. Bake for 10 minutes at 425°F or until done.	Calories 311	Sodium: 385	Protein: 24	Phos 390
	16 Ounces	Vegetable, Mixed Frozen				
	16 ounces	Beef, Ground (95% lean)	Fat: 8.2	Carbs: 33	Chol: 55	Pot: 580
	0.5 Cup	Vegetable, Onions				
	3 tablespoon	Butter, Light w/no added salt	Sat Fat: 4	Fiber: 4.5		
	4 Tablespoon	Flour, White bleached enriched				
	1 Cup	Flour, White Self Rise		Sugar: 5		
Serves: 6	2 cup	Soup, Chicken Broth Low Sodium				
Serving Size: 1/6 of pan	1 fluid ounces	Milk, Nonfat/Skim				
	0.5 Teaspoon	Herb, Thyme Ground				
	0.5 teaspoon	Spice, Nutmeg Ground				
	0.25 tsp	Spice, Black Pepper				

Recipe		Instructions	Nutritionals			
Ratatouille		Add oil to a large nonstick skillet over medium to high heat. Add garlic and sauté for 30 seconds. Add remaining ingredients and cook 10 to 15 min., stirring occasionally, until vegetables are tender.	Calories 41.4	Sodium: 201.3	Protein: 1.074	Phos 28.3
	3 Teaspoon	Oil, Olive				
	2 Teaspoon	Herb, Garlic, Raw	Fat: 2.468	Carbs: 4.775	Chol: 0	Pot: 228.7
	1 Each	Vegetable, Eggplant				
	1.5 Cup	Vegetable, Zucchini, slices	Sat Fat: 0.362	Fiber: 1.612		
	1 Cup	Vegetable, Pepper, Green				
Serves: 6	0.5 tsp	Salt		Sugar: 2.585		
Serving Size: 1 Cup	0.25 tsp	Spice, Black Pepper				
	8 ounces	Vegetable, Tomato, Red Canned, No Added Salt				

Orange

Serves: 6
Serving Size: 1 Peeled Orange

Ingredients	
6 1	Fruit, Orange, All Varieties, peeled, raw

Instructions: Piece of fruit.

Nutritionals: Calories 86.5 · Fat: 0.2 · Sat Fat: 0 · Protein: 1.7 · Carbs: 21.6 · Fiber: 4.4 · Sugar: 17.2 · Phos 25.8 · Sodium: 0 · Chol: 0 · Pot: 333

Meal: Turkey and Ham Sandwich GDM

Grilled Turkey and Ham Sandwich

Serves: 4
Serving Size: 1 sandwich

Amount	Ingredients
1 tablespoon	Salad Dressing, Mayo, LT/Kraft
1 Tablespoon	Mustard, Dijon
8 Each	Bread, White, reduced kcal
2 ounces	Lunch Meat, Ham, Low Sodium
3 Ounces	Lunch Meat, Turkey, Low Sodium
1 Cup	Vegetable, Tomato Red Raw
4 Slice	Cheese, natural, Cheddar, reduced fat

Instructions:
1. Combine mayonnaise and mustard in a small bowl. Spread about 1 teaspoon mayonnaise mixture over 1 side of each of 4 bread slices. Top each slice with 1 turkey slice, 1 ham slice, 1 cheese slice, and 2 tomato slices. Top with remaining bread slices.

2. Heat a large nonstick skillet over medium heat. Coat pan with cooking spray. Add sandwiches to pan; cook 4 minutes or until lightly browned. Turn sandwiches over; cook 2 minutes or until cheese melts.

Nutritionals: Calories 268.3 · Fat: 8.767 · Sat Fat: 1.897 · Protein: 16.8 · Carbs: 30.1 · Fiber: 3.689 · Sugar: 4.453 · Phos 265.6 · Sodium: 975.1 · Chol: 30.6 · Pot: 287

Oven Fries

Serves: 6
Serving Size: 1/2 potato

Amount	Ingredients
3 each	Vegetable, Potato
1 Teaspoon	Spice, Mrs. Dash
3 Each	Egg White

Instructions: Cut potatoes into strips like fries. Beat egg whites and toss with fries. Sprinkle with Mrs. Dash type seasoning. Bake for 30 minutes at 400F or until done.

Nutritionals: Calories 75 · Fat: 0.2 · Sat Fat: 0 · Protein: 3.3 · Carbs: 15 · Fiber: 2 · Sugar: 1 · Phos 55 · Sodium: 45 · Chol: 0 · Pot: 406

Creamy Lemon Coleslaw

Serves: 6
Serving Size: 1/6 of container

Amount	Ingredients
1 Each	Vegetable, Cabbage Head
6 Each	Sugar Substitute Packet, Equal
0.125 Cup	Vegetable, Onions
0.5 teaspoon	Salt, Kosher
6 Tablespoon	Miracle Whip Light
2 Packet	True Lemon packet

Instructions: Shred cabbage and chop onions. Combine all ingredients in a bowl, and toss lightly. Refrigerate if not used immediately.

Nutritionals: Calories 81 · Fat: 3 · Sat Fat: 0.5 · Protein: 1.7 · Carbs: 12 · Fiber: 3 · Sugar: 5.5 · Phos 34 · Sodium: 158 · Chol: 4 · Pot: 211

Italian Green Beans

Serves: 6
Serving Size: 1/2 cup

Ingredients

Amount	Ingredient
3 Teaspoon	Oil, Olive
1 Cup	Vegetable, Onions
2 Teaspoon	Herb, Garlic, Raw
1 Can	Vegetable, Tomato Diced Canned
0.25 Teaspoo	Herb, Oregano, Ground
0.25 Teaspoo	Herb, Basil, Ground
16 Ounces	Vegetable, Beans, Italian, Frozen

Instructions

Steam green beans until tender crisp. Set aside. Heat olive oil in a medium nonstick skillet over medium-high heat. Sauté onions until clear. Add garlic; sauté 30 seconds. Add tomatoes, basil, and oregano, and simmer for 15 to 20 min. for tomato mixture over steamed green beans and mix well.

Nutritionals

Calories 67.1	Sodium: 217.2	Protein: 2.111	Phos 46.7
Fat: 2.519	Carbs: 10.9	Chol: 0	Pot: 315.5
Sat Fat: 0.37	Fiber: 3.596		
	Sugar: 3.97		

Meal: *Lime Butter Catfish GDM*

Lime Butter Catfish

Serves: 6
Serving Size: 4 oz

Ingredients

Amount	Ingredient
24 Ounces	Fish, Catfish Boneless
5 tablespoon	Butter, Light w/no added salt
0.25 tsp	Spice, Black Pepper
2 Each	Fruit, Lime
0.75 Cup	Vegetable, Onions

Instructions

Chop onions and make zest from the lime peel. Season filets with pepper; saute in 1 teaspoon light butter per filet in a large pan over medium-high heat. Saute for 3 minutes on each side or until fish flakes easily. Let 3 tablespoons butter soften/melt and add lime zest and minced onions. Squeeze lime over filets; top each filet with lime/butter mixture.

Nutritionals

Calories 310	Sodium: 651	Protein: 23	Phos 304
Fat: 22	Carbs: 4	Chol: 79	Pot: 491
Sat Fat: 7	Fiber: 1		
	Sugar: 1		

Rice and Noodle Pilaf

Serves: 6
Serving Size: 2/3 cup

Ingredients

Amount	Ingredient
2 tablespoon	Butter, Light w/no added salt
0.3 Cup	Pasta, Spaghetti
1 Cup	Rice, Medium Brown
16 oz	Water
0.25 tsp	Salt
0.25 tsp	Spice, Black Pepper

Instructions

Break spaghetti noodles into small sections about 1-2 inches long. Melt the butter in a large saucepan over medium heat, and add spaghetti.
Sauté spaghetti for 5 minutes or until lightly browned. Add the rice, stirring to coat. Stir in the boiling water, salt, and pepper, and bring to a boil. Cover; reduce heat, and simmer for 20 minutes or until the liquid is absorbed. Remove pilaf from heat, and let stand for 10 minutes. Fluff with a fork.

Nutritionals

Calories 188.2	Sodium: 103.8	Protein: 4.4	Phos 131.1
Fat: 3.4	Carbs: 34.5	Chol: 4.5	Pot: 105.3
Sat Fat: 1.6	Fiber: 1.5		
	Sugar: 0.6		

Steamed Carrots

Serves: 6
Serving Size: 1/2 cup

Ingredients

Amount	Ingredient
3 Cup	Vegetable, Carrots
1 Teaspoon	Spice, Mrs. Dash

Instructions

Steam carrots until tender, season with Mrs. Dash

Nutritionals

Calories 33	Sodium: 2	Protein: 1	Phos 22
Fat: 0	Carbs: 0	Chol: 0	Pot: 165
Sat Fat: 0	Fiber: 3		
	Sugar: 0		

Recipe	Ingredients	Instructions	Nutritionals			
Down Home Baked Bean.	8 Tablespoon Sauce, BBQ	In a small saucepan over high heat, combine the barbeque sauce with the dry mustard, onion, bacon bits, beans and kale. Bring to a boil, reduce the heat to low, and simmer the beans for 10 minutes, or until the kale is tender, stirring occasionally. The sauce should thicken slightly and the beans should be very tender.	Calories 131	Sodium: 285	Protein: 6.03	Phos 114
Serves: 4	0.25 Teaspoo Spice, Dry Mustard		Fat: 1.5	Carbs: 23.7	Chol: 4.5	Pot: 276
Serving Size: 1/2 cup	0.33 Cup Vegetable, Onions		Sat Fat: 0.3	Fiber: 4.2		
	1 tablespoon Bacon Bits			Sugar: 12.1		
	1 Cup Beans, Cannellini White, canned					
	1 Cup Vegetable, Kale, raw					

54

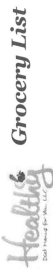

Grocery List

Herbed Chicken Parmesan GDM Meal

Herbed Chicken Parmesan

Quantity		Grocery Item
0.33	Cup	Cheese, Grated Parmesan, Reduced Fat
0.25	Cup	Breadcrumbs, Plain, Grated, Dry
1.5	oz	Cheese, Provolone Shredded
1	Tablespoon	Herb, Parsley, dried
0.66	Tablespoon	Vinegar, balsamic
1	Each	Egg White
0.5	Teaspoon	Herb, Basil, Ground
1	tablespoon	Butter, Light w/no added salt
0.25	tsp	Spice, Black Pepper
0.25	tsp	Salt
16	Ounces	Chicken, Breast Tenders Boneless
1.5	Cup	Sauce, Spaghetti, meatless - pizza sauce

Creamy Herbed Mashed Potatoes

Quantity		Grocery Item
4	Springs	Herb, Parsley, Raw, Fresh
1	Tablespoons	Cream, Sour, Reduced Fat
3	tablespoon	Butter, Light w/no added salt
0.5	tsp	Spice, Black Pepper
0.5	tsp	Salt
3	Tablespoon	Herb, Chives, raw
4	Cup	Vegetable, Potato, Flesh only, diced, raw
4	fluid ounces	Milk, Nonfat/Skim

Broccoli Casserole

Quantity		Grocery Item
0.125	tsp	Spice, Black Pepper
6	Ounces	Soup, Cream of Celery, Fat Free
4	fluid ounces	Milk, Nonfat/Skim
0.5	Cup	Cheese, Cheddar reduced fat
4	Cup	Vegetable, Broccoli Florets, Raw

Baked Lemon Chicken GDM Meal

Baked True Lemon Chicken

Quantity		Grocery Item
0.5	Cup	Vegetable, Onions
0.5	Stick	Butter, Light, Stick, Salted - Land O Lakes
8	Tablespoons	Flour, White bleached enriched
1	Teaspoon	Herb, Garlic, Raw
16	ounces	Chicken, Breast Boneless
0.5	tsp	Spice, Black Pepper
4	Packet	True Lemon packet
0.5	teaspoon	Salt, Kosher

Brussel Sprouts and Bacon

Quantity		Grocery Item
1	teaspoon	Spice, Red Pepper
0.5	tsp	Salt
0.06	Cup	Nuts, Almond Sliced
1	Pounds	Vegetable, Brussels Sprouts, raw
4	Slices	Pork Bacon, Cured or Smoked, lower
1	tsp	Spice, Black Pepper
2	Teaspoon	Herb, Garlic, Raw

Baked Asparagus Omelette GDM
Meal

Baked Asparagus Omelet

Quantity		Grocery Item
16	Ounces	Vegetable, Asparagus Fresh
1	Cup	Cheese, Mozzarella Part Skim
0.25	Cup	Vegetable, Green Onion
1	cup	Fat Free Half and Half Cream
0.5	Cup	Egg Substitute
2	tsp	Spice, Black Pepper
1	Each	Egg, Whole
0.5	tsp	Salt

Rosemary Roasted Potatoes

Quantity		Grocery Item
1	Tablespoon	Oil, Vegetable or Olive
5	each	Vegetable, Potato
3	teaspoon	Herb, Rosemary, Dried
2	teaspoon	Spice, Paprika
0.75	Teaspoon	Herb, Garlic, Raw

Pear

Quantity		Grocery Item
6	Fruit	Fruit, Pear Raw

Pear Feta Salad

Quantity		Grocery Item
6	Cups	Vegetables, Mixed salad greens, raw
3	Fruit	Fruit, Pear Raw
0.5	Cup	Cheese, Feta
12	Tablespoons	Salad Dressing, Dijon Vinaigrette,

Ratatouille

Quantity		Grocery Item
1	Cup	Vegetable, Pepper, Green
2	Teaspoon	Herb, Garlic, Raw
0.5	tsp	Salt
0.25	tsp	Spice, Black Pepper
3	Teaspoon	Oil, Olive
1	Each	Vegetable, Eggplant
8	ounces	Vegetable, Tomato, Red Canned, No Added
1.5	Cup	Vegetable, Zucchini, slices

Warm Bulgur Salad

Quantity		Grocery Item
0.15	Cup	Cheese, Feta
2	Tablespoon	Oil, Vegetable or Olive
0.75	Ounces	Vegetable, Spinach, raw, torn
0.25	tsp	Spice, Black Pepper
1	Cup	Vegetable, Tomato, Red, Cherry
1	ounces	Lemon Juice, Bottled
3	Cup	Bulgar

Honey Garlic Pork Chop GDM
Meal

Honey Garlic Pork Chops

Quantity		Grocery Item
1	tsp	Garlic, Minced
18	ounces	Pork, Center Rib Chop
2	ounces	Lemon Juice, Bottled
2	Tablespoon	Soy Sauce, Low Sodium
2	ounces	Honey

Skinny Mashed Potatoes

Quantity		Grocery Item
0.5	teaspoon	Spice, Garlic Powder
5	each	Vegetable, Potato
0.75	cup	Soup, Chicken Broth Low Sodium

Italian Green Beans

Quantity		Grocery Item
1	Can	Vegetable, Tomato Diced Canned
2	Teaspoon	Herb, Garlic, Raw
3	Teaspoon	Oil, Olive
0.25	Teaspoon	Herb, Basil, Ground
0.25	Teaspoon	Herb, Oregano, Ground
1	Cup	Vegetable, Onions
16	Ounces	Vegetable, Beans, Italian, Frozen

Lime Butter Catfish GDM Meal

Lime Butter Catfish

Quantity		Grocery Item
0.25	tsp	Spice, Black Pepper
5	tablespoon	Butter, Light w/no added salt
0.75	Cup	Vegetable, Onions
24	Ounces	Fish, Catfish Boneless
2	Each	Fruit, Lime

Rice and Noodle Pilaf

Quantity		Grocery Item
0.3	Cup	Pasta, Spaghetti
1	Cup	Rice, Medium Brown
2	tablespoon	Butter, Light w/no added salt
16	oz	Water
0.25	tsp	Spice, Black Pepper
0.25	tsp	Salt

Turkey and Ham Sandwich GDM Meal

Grilled Turkey and Ham Sandwich

Quantity		Grocery Item
1	Cup	Vegetable, Tomato Red Raw
4	Slice	Cheese, natural, Cheddar, reduced fat
3	Ounces	Lunch Meat, Turkey, Low Sodium
1	Tablespoon	Mustard, Dijon
8	Each	Bread, White, reduced kcal
1	tablespoon	Salad Dressing, Mayo, LT/Kraft
2	ounces	Lunch Meat, Ham, Low Sodium

Oven Fries

Quantity		Grocery Item
1	Teaspoon	Spice, Mrs. Dash
3	each	Vegetable, Potato
3	Each	Egg White

Creamy Lemon Coleslaw

Quantity		Grocery Item
6	Each	Sugar Substitute Packet, Equal
2	Packet	True Lemon packet
0.125	Cup	Vegetable, Onions
1	Each	Vegetable, Cabbage Head
6	Tablespoon	Miracle Whip Light
0.5	teaspoon	Salt, Kosher

Beef Pot Pie GDM Meal

Baked Beef Pot Pie

Quantity		Grocery Item
0.5	Cup	Vegetable, Onions
16	Ounces	Vegetable, Mixed Frozen
0.5	Teaspoon	Herb, Thyme Ground
2	cup	Soup, Chicken Broth Low Sodium
16	ounces	Beef, Ground (95% lean)
0.25	tsp	Spice, Black Pepper
4	Tablespoons	Flour, White bleached enriched
0.5	teaspoon	Spice, Nutmeg Ground
1	fluid ounces	Milk, Nonfat/Skim
3	tablespoon	Butter, Light w/no added salt
1	Cup	Flour, White Self Rise

Ratatouille

Quantity		Grocery Item
1	Each	Vegetable, Eggplant
2	Teaspoon	Herb, Garlic, Raw
1.5	Cup	Vegetable, Zucchini, slices
8	ounces	Vegetable, Tomato, Red Canned, No Added
3	Teaspoon	Oil, Olive
0.5	tsp	Salt
0.25	tsp	Spice, Black Pepper
1	Cup	Vegetable, Pepper, Green

Orange

Quantity	Grocery Item
1	Fruit, Orange, All Varieties, peeled, raw

Steamed Carrots

Quantity		Grocery Item
3	Cup	Vegetable, Carrots
1	Teaspoon	Spice, Mrs. Dash

Down Home Baked Beans

Quantity		Grocery Item
1	tablespoon	Bacon Bits
0.33	Cup	Vegetable, Onions
8	Tablespoon	Sauce, BBQ
1	Cup	Beans, Cannellini White, canned
0.25	Teaspoon	Spice, Dry Mustard
1	Cup	Vegetable, Kale, raw

Week 3 Meals and Grocery Lists

Grilled Flank Steak with Avocado and Tomato Salsa, Coconut Rice and Italian Green Beans

Pecan Crusted Tilapia with Creamy Herbed Mashed Potatoes and Pears

Almost Fried True Lemon Chicken with Rice and Noodle Pilaf and Corn on the Cob

Southwest Turkey Burgers with Bacon Potato Salad and Strawberries

Chicken Cordon Bleu with Brussels Sprouts and Bacon, Rosemary Roasted Potatoes and Bananas

Baked Ziti and Veggies with Ratatouille and Rice and Noodle Pilaf

Spiced Pork Chops with Apple Topping with Asparagus, Creamy Herbed Mashed Potatoes and Braised Red Cabbage

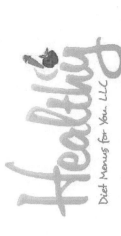

Meal Plan

www.healthydietmenusforyou.com

Meal: *Grilled Flank Steak GDM*

Recipe			Ingredients	Instructions	Nutritionals					

Grilled Flank Steak w/Avocado and Tomato Salsa

0.667	Tables	Oil, Vegetable or Olive		Calories 253	Sodium: 84	Protein: 26	Phos 315
1	tsp	Spice, Black Pepper		Fat: 11	Carbs: 12	Chol: 48	Pot: 564
0.5	Cup	Vegetable, Tomato Red Raw		Sat Fat: 3.5	Fiber: 2.6		
0.5	Cup	Vegetable, Tomato Yellow Raw			Sugar: 1		

Serves: 6

0.5	Cup	Fruit, Avocado
1	Tablespoon	Vegetable, Onions, Red
1	Tablespoon	Lime Juice
2	Tablespoon	Herb, Tarragon Fresh
24	Ounces	Beef, Flank Lean Trimmed
0.5	teaspoon	Salt, Kosher
12	Each	Tortilla, Corn

Serving Size: 3oz steak/2Tblsp salsa

Instructions:

Prepare grill to medium-high heat. Dice avocado, tomatoes and onions. Combine avocado, tomato, onion, lime juice, tarragon, olive oil, kosher salt and 1/4 tsp pepper. Sprinkle steak with remaining pepper. Place steak on grill rack coated with cooking spray. Grill for 5-6 minutes on each side or until desired doneness. Remove and let stand for 5 minutes. Cut steak across the grain into thin slices. Serve with salsa and 2 tortillas. Makes 6 servings: 2 tortillas, 3 oz steak, 2 tablespoon salsa.

Recipe			Ingredients	Instructions	Nutritionals					

Coconut Rice

10	oz	Water		Calories 224.5	Sodium: 153.5	Protein: 3.868	Phos 80.3
0.25	tsp	Salt		Fat: 6.331	Carbs: 37.8	Chol: 0	Pot: 116.1
4	Ounces	Milk, Coconut, canned		Sat Fat: 5.427	Fiber: 0.601		
8	Ounces	Grain, Rice, Basmati, raw			Sugar: 0.056		

Serves: 4

Serving Size: 1/2 cup

Instructions:

Combine basmati rice, water, coconut milk and salt in a small saucepan. Bring to a boil. Cover, reduce heat and simmer 16 min. or until liquid is absorbed.

Recipe		Ingredients	Instructions	Nutritionals			
Italian Green Beans			Steam green beans until tender crisp. Set aside. Heat olive oil in a medium nonstick skillet over medium-high heat. Sauté onions until clear. Add garlic; sauté 30 seconds. Add tomatoes, basil, and oregano, and simmer for 15 to 20 min. for tomato mixture over steamed green beans and mix well.	Calories 67.1	Sodium: 217.2	Protein: 2.111	Phos 46.7
Serves: 6				Fat: 2.519	Carbs: 10.9	Chol: 0	Pot: 315.5
Serving Size: 1/2 cup				Sat Fat: 0.37	Fiber: 3.596		
					Sugar: 3.97		
	3 Teaspoon	Oil, Olive					
	1 Cup	Vegetable, Onions					
	2 Teaspoon	Herb, Garlic, Raw					
	1 Can	Vegetable, Tomato Diced Canned					
	0.25 Teaspoo	Herb, Oregano, Ground					
	0.25 Teaspoo	Herb, Basil, Ground					
	16 Ounces	Vegetable, Beans, Italian, Frozen					

Meal: *Pecan Crusted Tilapia GDM*

Recipe		Ingredients	Instructions	Nutritionals			
Pecan Crusted Tilapia			Combine the breadcrumbs, pecans, salt, garlic powder and black pepper in a shallow dish. Combine the buttermilk and hot sauce in a medium bowl. Place flour in another shallow dish. Dredge fillet first in flour, then dip in buttermilk mixture, and finally dredge in breadcrumb mixture. Repeat for all fillets. Now heat 1.5 teaspoons oil in a large nonstick skillet over medium high heat. Add 2 fillets, cook 3 minutes on each side or until fish flakes easily when tested with a fork. Repeat procedure with remaining oil and fillets. Serve with lemon wedges. Makes 4 servings.	Calories 347.1	Sodium: 967	Protein: 36.7	Phos: 347.4
Serves: 4				Fat: 13.9	Carbs: 21.3	Chol: 81.3	Pot: 642.8
Serving Size: 6 oz of fish				Sat Fat: 3	Fiber: 2.5		
					Sugar: 2.5		
	0.5 Cup	Breadcrumbs, Plain, Grated, Dry					
	0.125 Cup	Nuts, Pecans, dried					
	0.5 tsp	Salt					
	0.25 teaspoo	Spice, Garlic Powder					
	0.25 tsp	Spice, Black Pepper					
	4 ounces	Milk, Buttermilk Lowfat					
	0.5 Tablespo	Sauce, Hot Pepper					
	4 Tablespoon	Flour, White bleached enriched					
	24 Oz	Fish, Tilapia, baked or broiled					
	1 Tablespoon	Oil, Vegetable or Olive					
	1 Each	Fruit, Lemon w/peel, raw					

Recipe		Ingredients	Instructions	Nutritionals			
Creamy Herbed Mashed Potatoes			Peel and cube potatoes. Place potato in a saucepan; cover with water. Bring to a boil; cover, reduce heat, and simmer 10 minutes or until tender. Drain. Return potato to pan. Add milk and remaining ingredients; mash with a potato masher to desired consistency.	Calories 147.1	Sodium: 215.1	Protein: 3.1	Phos 73
Serves: 6				Fat: 4.6	Carbs: 23.8	Chol: 11	Pot: 422.7
Serving Size: 3/4 Cup				Sat Fat: 2.8	Fiber: 2.1		
					Sugar: 2.3		
	4 Cup	Vegetable, Potato, Flesh only, diced, raw					
	4 fluid ounces	Milk, Nonfat/Skim					
	1 Tablespoon	Cream, Sour, Reduced Fat					
	3 tablespoon	Butter, Light w/no added salt					
	3 Tablespoon	Herb, Chives, raw					
	4 Springs	Herb, Parsley, Raw, Fresh					
	0.5 tsp	Salt					
	0.5 tsp	Spice, Black Pepper					

Recipe

	Ingredients	Instructions	Nutritionals				
Pear		Piece of fruit	Calories 115.5	Sodium: 0	Protein: 1.3	Phos 30.2	Pot: 332.8
6 Fruit	Fruit, Pear Raw		Fat: 0.6	Carbs: 29.3	Chol: 0		
Serves: 6			Sat Fat: 0	Fiber: 9.9			
Serving Size: 1 medium pear				Sugar: 19.4			

Meal: *Almost Fried Chicken GDM*

Recipe

	Ingredients	Instructions	Nutritionals				
Almost Fried True Lemon Chicken		Preheat your oven to 400°F. Prepare pan by placing foil in it and spraying with non stick spray. Whisk egg whites with 1 packet true lemon and cayenne in mixing bowl. Pound chicken breast to about an inch thickness to quicken cooking time. Add chicken to mixture and turn to coat all sides. In a wide, shallow dish, combine bread crumbs, salt and pepper and blend well. Remove chicken pieces from egg mixture and press into bread crumbs; coating all sides with crumbs. Place chicken on a clean platter, cover and refrigerate for 1 hour. Remove from the refrigerator, and place chicken pieces in a single layer in a prepared baking dish and bake for 15 minutes. Carefully turn chicken pieces and bake for an additional 10 minutes or until cooked through and golden. Arrange chicken on a serving platter and drizzle with lemon juice.	Calories 193.5	Sodium: 266.7	Protein: 27.8	Phos 264.7	Pot: 489.5
2 Each	Egg White		Fat: 3.7	Carbs: 10.6	Chol: 72.6		
4 Packet	True Lemon packet		Sat Fat: 0.8	Fiber: 0.7			
0.5 teaspoon	Spice, Red Pepper			Sugar: 1.1			
16 ounces	Chicken, Breast Boneless						
0.5 Cup	Breadcrumbs, Plain, Grated, Dry						
0.5 teaspoon	Salt, Kosher						
0.5 tsp	Spice, Black Pepper						
1 ounces	Lemon Juice, Bottled						
Serves: 4							
Serving Size: 4 oz. chicken breast							

Recipe

	Ingredients	Instructions	Nutritionals				
Rice and Noodle Pilaf		Break spaghetti noodles into small sections about 1-2 inches long. Melt the butter in a large saucepan over medium heat, and add spaghetti. Sauté spaghetti for 5 minutes or until lightly browned. Add the rice, salt, and pepper, and bring to a boil. Cover; reduce heat, and simmer for 20 minutes or until the liquid is absorbed. Remove pilaf from heat, and let stand for 10 minutes. Fluff with a fork.	Calories 188.2	Sodium: 103.8	Protein: 4.4	Phos 131.1	Pot: 105.3
2 tablespoon	Butter, Light w/no added salt		Fat: 3.4	Carbs: 34.5	Chol: 4.5		
0.3 Cup	Pasta, Spaghetti		Sat Fat: 1.6	Fiber: 1.5			
1 Cup	Rice, Medium Brown			Sugar: 0.6			
16 oz	Water						
0.25 tsp	Salt						
0.25 tsp	Spice, Black Pepper						
Serves: 6							
Serving Size: 2/3 cup							

Corn On The Cob

Serves: 6

Serving Size: 1 ear of corn

Recipe	Ingredients	Instructions	Nutritionals			
Corn On The Cob	6 Each — Vegetable, Corn on Cob, sm/med, ckd w/o fat or salt	Shuck and clean corn. Boil until tender, about 4-6 minutes.	Calories 82.7	Sodium: 1.5	Protein: 2.5	Phos 78.8
			Fat: 0.9	Carbs: 19.2	Chol: 0	Pot: 190.6
			Sat Fat: 0.1	Fiber: 2.8		
				Sugar: 0		

Meal: *Southwest Turkey Burger GDM*

Southwest Turkey Burger

Serves: 6

Serving Size: 4 oz

Recipe	Ingredients	Instructions	Nutritionals			
Southwest Turkey Burger	8 Tablespoon — Sauce, BBQ	Mix turkey, barbeque sauce and chopped chilies together, shape into 6 patties. Broil in oven or cook in non stick pan for 10-14 minutes until done. Turn once while cooking. Top each with cheese slices and cook until cheese melts. Place each patty on a sandwich thin. Serve with condiments of choice and add calories per item nutritional panel.	Calories 393.3	Sodium: 807.5	Protein: 30.2	Phos 408
	1.5 Pound — Turkey, Ground Raw		Fat: 17	Carbs: 28.5	Chol: 109.3	Pot: 432.5
	4 oz — Vegetable, Green Chilies, Canned		Sat Fat: 6.6	Fiber: 5.3		
	6 Slice — Cheese, processed, Pepper Jack			Sugar: 2.7		
	6 Each — Bread, Sandwich Thin, Multigrain					
	0.5 Cup — Crackers, saltine, fat free, low sodium - Nabisco Fat Free Premium Crackers					

Strawberries

Serves: 6

Serving Size: 1.5 Cups of Strawberries

Recipe	Ingredients	Instructions	Nutritionals			
Strawberries	9 Cup — Fruit, Strawberries, halves/slices, raw	Remove tops and wash prior to serving.	Calories 73	Sodium: 2.2	Protein: 1.5	Phos 54.7
			Fat: 0.6	Carbs: 17.5	Chol: 0	Pot: 348.8
			Sat Fat: 0	Fiber: 4.5		
				Sugar: 11.1		

Bacon Potato Salad

Serves: 6

Serving Size: 1/2 cup

Recipe	Ingredients	Instructions	Nutritionals			
Bacon Potato Salad	2 Slices — Beef, Bacon, lean, ckd	Fry bacon, drain and pat grease off. Crumble. Peel potatoes, cook until tender - about 40 minutes at a low boil, and cube/slice them. Toss the warm potatoes with mayo, mustard, salt and pepper. Add bacon and serve.	Calories 131.3	Sodium: 124.9	Protein: 2.5	Phos 47.9
	4 each — Vegetable, Potato		Fat: 3.3	Carbs: 23	Chol: 0.82	Pot: 280.2
	0.25 Cup — Mayonnaise, reduced kcal, cholest free/Hellmann		Sat Fat: 0.5	Fiber: 2		
	0.33 Tablesp — Dijon Mustard			Sugar: 0.9		

Meal: *Chicken Cordon Bleu GDM*

Chicken Cordon Bleu

Serves: 4

Serving Size: 1 Rolled Chicken Breast

Nutritionals

Calories 320.2	Sodium: 924	Protein: 43.4	Phos 464.4
Fat: 10.2	Carbs: 11.4	Chol: 126.2	Pot: 753
Sat Fat: 4.001	Fiber: 1.029		
	Sugar: 10.27		

Ingredients

0.25 cup	Soup, Chicken Broth Low Sodium
1.5 tablespoo	Butter, Light w/no added salt
0.5 cup	Breadcrumbs, Seasoned
0.5 Ounces	Cheese, Parmesan, dry grated - Romano, grated
1 teaspoon	Spice, Paprika
24 ounces	Chicken, Breast Boneless
0.25 tsp	Salt
0.25 Teaspoo	Herb, Oregano, Ground
0.25 tsp	Spice, Black Pepper
4 ounces	Ham, prosciutto
0.1 Cup	Cheese, Mozzarella Part Skim
0.25 Teaspoo	Herb, Garlic, Raw

Instructions

Preheat oven to 350°.

Place broth in a small microwave-safe bowl; microwave at high 15 seconds or until warm. Stir in butter and garlic. Combine breadcrumbs, Parmesan, and paprika in a medium shallow bowl; set aside.

Place each chicken breast half between 2 sheets of heavy-duty plastic wrap, and pound each to 1/4-inch thickness using a meat mallet or rolling pin. Sprinkle both sides of chicken with salt, oregano, and pepper. Top each breast half with 1 slice of prosciutto and 1 tablespoon mozzarella. Roll up each breast half jelly-roll fashion. Dip each roll in chicken broth mixture; dredge in breadcrumb mixture. Place rolls, seam side down, in an 8-inch square baking dish coated with cooking spray. Pour remaining broth mixture over chicken. Bake at 350° for 28 minutes or until juices run clear and tops are golden.

Brussel Sprouts and Baco

Serves: 4

Serving Size: 4 ounces

Nutritionals

Calories 121	Sodium: 402.1	Protein: 7.2	Phos 127
Fat: 6.2	Carbs: 12	Chol: 6.8	Pot: 528.2
Sat Fat: 1.6	Fiber: 5		
	Sugar: 2.7		

Ingredients

0.5 tsp	Salt
1 tsp	Spice, Black Pepper
4 Slices	Pork Bacon, Cured or Smoked, lower sodium, slices
2 Teaspoon	Herb, Garlic, Raw
1 teaspoon	Spice, Red Pepper
0.06 Cup	Nuts, Almond Sliced
1 Pounds	Vegetable, Brussels Sprouts, raw

Instructions

Cut the brussels sprouts in half and trim bottoms. Heat a large skillet or saute pan over medium heat. Add the bacon and cook until crispy, about 5 minutes. Remove to a plate lined with paper towels. Discard all but 1 tablespoon of the rendered bacon fat. Add the garlic, pepper flakes, brussels sprouts and salt to the skillet. Saute until the sprouts are lightly browned on the outside and tender - but still firm - throughout. Approx 10-12 minutes. Add the almonds and bacon (crumbled) and saute for another minute or two. Season with salt and pepper.

Rosemary Roasted Potatoes

Serves: 6

Serving Size: 3/4 cup Potatoes

Nutritionals

Calories 132.8	Sodium: 12.3	Protein: 3.094	Phos 85.4
Fat: 2.581	Carbs: 25.5	Chol: 0	Pot: 642
Sat Fat: 0.407	Fiber: 3.056		
	Sugar: 1.443		

Ingredients

5 each	Vegetable, Potato
1 Tablespoon	Oil, Vegetable or Olive
0.75 Teaspoo	Herb, Garlic, Raw
3 teaspoon	Herb, Rosemary, Dried
2 teaspoon	Spice, Paprika

Instructions

Wash and dice potatoes into bite-sized pieces. Place into a large bowl or Ziplock bag; toss with olive oil. Sprinkle garlic, rosemary, paprika (optional), and pepper over potatoes and shake to coat. Layer potatoes in a single layer on a baking sheet coated with cooking spray. Bake at 400 F for 30 minutes or until slightly browned. Serves 5.

Recipe

Banana

Serves: 6

Serving Size: 1 banana

Ingredients	Instructions	Nutritionals			
		Calories 105	Sodium: 1.1	Protein: 1.2	Phos 26
6 1 Fruit, Banana	Piece of fruit	Fat: 0.3	Carbs: 27	Chol: 0	Pot: 422.4
		Sat Fat: 0.1	Fiber: 3		
			Sugar: 14.4		

Meal: Baked Ziti GDM

Recipe

Baked Ziti And Veggies

Serves: 4

Serving Size: 1.5 Cups

Ingredients	Instructions	Nutritionals			
3 Teaspoon Oil, Olive	1. Cook pasta according to package directions, omitting salt and fat; drain.	Calories 345	Sodium: 649.1	Protein: 17.6	Phos 314.7
2 Cup Vegetable, Tomato Red Raw	2. Preheat oven to 400°.	Fat: 15.2	Carbs: 35.8	Chol: 72.9	Pot: 620.5
2 Cup Vegetable, Squash, summer, yellow, raw	3. Heat a large skillet over medium-high heat. Add oil to pan. Add squash, zucchini, and onion; sauté 5 minutes. Add tomato and garlic; sauté 3 minutes. Remove from heat; stir in pasta, 1/2 cup mozzarella, herbs, 1/2 teaspoon salt, and pepper.	Sat Fat: 5.258	Fiber: 4.435		
1 Cup Vegetable, Zucchini, slices			Sugar: 6.047		
4 Ounces Pasta, Ziti					
0.5 Cup Vegetable, Onions	4. Combine ricotta, and egg. Stir into pasta mixture. Spoon into an 8-inch square glass or ceramic baking dish coated with cooking spray; sprinkle with remaining mozzarella. Bake at 400° for 15 minutes or until bubbly and browned.				
0.5 Teaspoon Herb, Garlic, Raw					
1 Cup Cheese, Mozzarella Part Skim					
3 Teaspoon Herb, Basil, Ground					
1 Teaspoon Herb, Oregano, Ground					
0.5 tsp Salt					
0.25 teaspoo Spice, Red Pepper					
0.25 Cup Cheese, Ricotta, Part Skim Milk					
1 Each Egg, Whole					

Recipe

Ratatouille

Serves: 6

Serving Size: 1 Cup

Ingredients	Instructions	Nutritionals			
3 Teaspoon Oil, Olive	Add oil to a large nonstick skillet over medium to high heat. Add garlic and sauté for 30 seconds. Add remaining ingredients and cook 10 to 15 min., stirring occasionally, until vegetables are tender.	Calories 41.4	Sodium: 201.3	Protein: 1.074	Phos 28.3
2 Teaspoon Herb, Garlic, Raw		Fat: 2.468	Carbs: 4.775	Chol: 0	Pot: 228.7
1 Each Vegetable, Eggplant		Sat Fat: 0.362	Fiber: 1.612		
1.5 Cup Vegetable, Zucchini, slices			Sugar: 2.585		
1 Cup Vegetable, Pepper, Green					
0.5 tsp Salt					
0.25 tsp Spice, Black Pepper					
8 ounces Vegetable, Tomato, Red Canned, No Added Salt					

Rice and Noodle Pilaf

Serves: 6
Serving Size: 2/3 cup

Ingredients		Instructions	Nutritionals	
2 tablespoon	Butter, Light w/no added salt	Break spaghetti noodles into small sections about 1-2 inches long. Melt the butter in a large saucepan over medium heat, and add spaghetti. Sauté spaghetti for 5 minutes or until lightly browned. Add the rice, stirring to coat. Stir in the boiling water, salt, and pepper, and bring to a boil. Cover; reduce heat, and simmer for 20 minutes or until the liquid is absorbed. Remove pilaf from heat, and let stand for 10 minutes. Fluff with a fork.	Calories 188.2	Sodium: 103.8	Protein: 4.4	Phos 131.1
0.3 Cup	Pasta, Spaghetti		Fat: 3.4	Carbs: 34.5	Chol: 4.5	Pot: 105.3
1 Cup	Rice, Medium Brown		Sat Fat: 1.6	Fiber: 1.5		
16 oz	Water			Sugar: 0.6		
0.25 tsp	Salt					
0.25 tsp	Spice, Black Pepper					

Meal: Spiced Pork Chop GDM

Spiced Pork Chops With Apple Topping

Serves: 4
Serving Size: 4 ounce chop +1/3 cup top

Ingredients		Instructions	Nutritionals	
1 tablespoon	Butter, Light w/no added salt	1. To prepare topping, melt butter in a nonstick skillet over medium-high heat. Add chopped apple; sauté 4 minutes or until lightly browned. Add cranberries, Brown sugar, vinegar, ginger, 1/4 teaspoon salt, mustard, and all spice; bring to a boil. Reduce heat, and simmer 8 minutes or until apples are tender; stir occasionally.	Calories 296.4	Sodium: 362.1	Protein: 24.5	Phos 304.?
0.33 Cups	Fruit, Cranberries, dried - Craisins		Fat: 4.726	Carbs: 40.4	Chol: 77.1	Pot: 633.2
5 Each	Fruit, Apple, peeled, raw, medium		Sat Fat: 1.954	Fiber: 2.736		
3 Tablespoon	Vinegar, Cider			Sugar: 33.8		
2 teaspoons	Herb, Ginger Root, peeled, sliced, raw	2. To prepare pork, while chutney simmers, heat a grill pan over medium-high heat. Combine chili powder, 1/4 teaspoon salt, garlic powder, coriander, black pepper and sprinkle over pork. Coat grill pan with cooking spray. Add pork to pan; cook 4 minutes on each side or until done. Serve with chutney.				
12 Teaspoon	Sugar, Brown					
0.5 tsp	Salt					
0.25 teaspoo	Spice, Mustard Powder					
0.75 teaspoo	Spice, Chili Powder					
0.125 Teaspo	Spice, Allspice, ground					
0.5 teaspoon	Spice, Garlic Powder					
0.25 tsp	Spice, Black Pepper					
0.5 Teaspoon	Spice, Coriander, ground					
16 ounces	Pork, Tenderloin Lean					

Asparagus

Serves: 6
Serving Size: 1/2 Cup

Ingredients		Instructions	Nutritionals	
54 Ounces	Vegetable, Asparagus Fresh	Wash and clean asparagus by cutting off hard ends of stalk. Steam for 10 minutes in steamer or cook in 1 in water in microwaveable bowl for 5-7 minutes until desired tenderness.	Calories 21.5	Sodium: 1.8	Protein: 2.3	Phos 48.3
			Fat: 0.2	Carbs: 3.7	Chol: 0	Pot: 143.2
			Sat Fat: 0	Fiber: 1.5		
				Sugar: 0		

Creamy Herbed Mashed Potatoes

Serves: 6

Serving Size: 3/4 Cup

Ingredients	
4 Cup	Vegetable, Potato, Flesh only, diced, raw
4 fluid ounces	Milk, Nonfat/Skim
1 Tablespoon	Cream, Sour, Reduced Fat
3 tablespoon	Butter, Light w/no added salt
3 Tablespoon	Herb, Chives, raw
4 Springs	Herb, Parsley, Raw, Fresh
0.5 tsp	Salt
0.5 tsp	Spice, Black Pepper

Instructions

Peel and cube potatoes. Place potato in a saucepan; cover with water. Bring to a boil; cover, reduce heat, and simmer 10 minutes or until tender. Drain. Return potato to pan. Add milk and remaining ingredients; mash with a potato masher to desired consistency.

Nutritionals

Calories	147.1	Sodium:	215.1	Protein: 3.1	Phos 73
Fat:	4.6	Carbs:	23.8	Chol: 11	Pot: 422.7
Sat Fat:	2.8	Fiber:	2.1		
		Sugar:	2.3		

Braised Red Cabbage

Serves: 4

Serving Size: 1/2 cup

Ingredients	
2 cup	Soup, Chicken Broth Low Sodium
8 Tablespoon	Vinegar, Cider
6 Teaspoon	Vinegar, Red Wine
0.5 ounces	Honey
0.5 Teaspoon	Spice, Allspice, ground
4 Cup	Vegetable, Cabbage Heads, Red, raw
2 Each	Fruit, Apple, peeled, Granny Smith, medium

Instructions

In a large saucepan, bring broth, vinegar, honey, and allspice to a boil. Add cabbage and cubed apples. Reduce heat and simmer, uncovered, for 30 min.

Nutritionals

Calories	96.9	Sodium:	57.4	Protein: 3.612	Phos 67.7
Fat:	0.938	Carbs:	2.39	Chol: 0	Pot: 362.6
Sat Fat:	0.249	Fiber:	2.39		
		Sugar:	13.9		

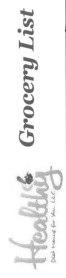

Grocery List

Diet: *Gestational Diabetic - 2400*

Grilled Flank Steak GDM Meal

Grilled Flank Steak w/Avocado and Tomato Sals

Quantity		Grocery Item
0.5	teaspoon	Salt, Kosher
24	Ounces	Beef, Flank Lean Trimmed
12	Each	Tortilla, Corn
2	Tablespoon	Herb, Tarragon Fresh
1	Tablespoon	Vegetable, Onions, Red
0.5	Cup	Vegetable, Tomato Yellow Raw
0.5	Cup	Vegetable, Tomato Red Raw
0.5	Cup	Fruit, Avocado
0.667	Tablespoon	Oil, Vegetable or Olive
1	tsp	Spice, Black Pepper
1	Tablespoon	Lime Juice

Coconut Rice

Quantity		Grocery Item
10	oz	Water
4	Ounces	Milk, Coconut, canned
0.25	tsp	Salt
8	Ounces	Grain, Rice, Basmati, raw

Italian Green Beans

Quantity		Grocery Item
0.25	Teaspoon	Herb, Oregano, Ground
1	Can	Vegetable, Tomato Diced Canned
16	Ounces	Vegetable, Beans, Italian, Frozen
1	Cup	Vegetable, Onions
3	Teaspoon	Oil, Olive
0.25	Teaspoon	Herb, Basil, Ground
2	Teaspoon	Herb, Garlic, Raw

Pecan Crusted Tilapia GDM Meal

Pecan Crusted Tilapia

Quantity		Grocery Item
4	ounces	Milk, Buttermilk Lowfat
0.25	tsp	Spice, Black Pepper
0.5	tsp	Salt
4	Tablespoons	Flour, White bleached enriched
1	Tablespoon	Oil, Vegetable or Olive
0.5	Cup	Breadcrumbs, Plain, Grated, Dry
0.5	Tablespoon	Sauce, Hot Pepper
24	Oz	Fish, Tilapia, baked or broiled
1	Each	Fruit, Lemon w/peel, raw
0.125	Cup	Nuts, Pecans, dried
0.25	teaspoon	Spice, Garlic Powder

Creamy Herbed Mashed Potatoes

Quantity		Grocery Item
4	Cup	Vegetable, Potato, Flesh only, diced, raw
0.5	tsp	Spice, Black Pepper
3	Tablespoon	Herb, Chives, raw
4	Springs	Herb, Parsley, Raw, Fresh
3	tablespoon	Butter, Light w/no added salt
4	fluid ounces	Milk, Nonfat/Skim
0.5	tsp	Salt
1	Tablespoons	Cream, Sour, Reduced Fat

Pear

Quantity		Grocery Item
6	Fruit	Fruit, Pear Raw

Almost Fried Chicken GDM Meal

Almost Fried True Lemon Chicken

Quantity		Grocery Item
0.5	teaspoon	Spice, Red Pepper
0.5	teaspoon	Salt, Kosher
0.5	Cup	Breadcrumbs, Plain, Grated, Dry
1	ounces	Lemon Juice, Bottled
2	Each	Egg White
16	ounces	Chicken, Breast Boneless
4	Packet	True Lemon packet
0.5	tsp	Spice, Black Pepper

69

Brussel Sprouts and Bacon

Quantity		Grocery Item
1	tsp	Spice, Black Pepper
4	Slices	Pork Bacon, Cured or Smoked, lower
2	Teaspoon	Herb, Garlic, Raw
1	teaspoon	Spice, Red Pepper
0.5	tsp	Salt
1	Pounds	Vegetable, Brussels Sprouts, raw
0.06	Cup	Nuts, Almond Sliced

Rosemary Roasted Potatoes

Quantity		Grocery Item
1	Tablespoon	Oil, Vegetable or Olive
5	each	Vegetable, Potato
3	teaspoon	Herb, Rosemary, Dried
2	teaspoon	Spice, Paprika
0.75	Teaspoon	Herb, Garlic, Raw

Banana

Quantity		Grocery Item
6	1	Fruit, Banana

Bacon Potato Salad

Quantity		Grocery Item
0.25	Cup	Mayonnaise, reduced kcal, cholest
4	each	Vegetable, Potato
2	Slices	Beef, Bacon, lean, ckd
0.33	Tablespoon	Dijon Mustard

Chicken Cordon Bleu GDM Meal

Chicken Cordon Bleu

Quantity		Grocery Item
0.1	Cup	Cheese, Mozzarella Part Skim
0.5	cup	Breadcrumbs, Seasoned
0.25	Teaspoon	Herb, Garlic, Raw
1	teaspoon	Spice, Paprika
4	ounces	Ham, prosciutto
24	ounces	Chicken, Breast Boneless
0.25	cup	Soup, Chicken Broth Low Sodium
1.5	tablespoon	Butter, Light w/no added salt
0.5	Ounces	Cheese, Parmesan, dry grated - Romano,
0.25	tsp	Salt
0.25	Teaspoon	Herb, Oregano, Ground
0.25	tsp	Spice, Black Pepper

Rice and Noodle Pilaf

Quantity		Grocery Item
16	oz	Water
1	Cup	Rice, Medium Brown
0.3	Cup	Pasta, Spaghetti
2	tablespoon	Butter, Light w/no added salt
0.25	tsp	Spice, Black Pepper
0.25	tsp	Salt

Corn On The Cob

Quantity		Grocery Item
6	Each	Vegetable, Corn on Cob, sm/med, ckd w/o

Southwest Turkey Burger GDM Meal

Southwest Turkey Burgers

Quantity		Grocery Item
8	Tablespoon	Sauce, BBQ
1.5	Pound	Turkey, Ground Raw
4	oz	Vegetable, Green Chilies, Canned
6	Each	Bread, Sandwich Thin, Multigrain
0.5	Cup	Crackers, saltine, fat free, low sodium -
6	Slice	Cheese, processed, Pepper Jack

Strawberries

Quantity		Grocery Item
9	Cup	Fruit, Strawberries, halves/slices, raw

Baked Ziti GDM Meal

Baked Ziti And Veggies

Quantity		Grocery Item
3	Teaspoon	Herb, Basil, Ground
2	Cup	Vegetable, Tomato Red Raw
0.5	Teaspoon	Herb, Garlic, Raw
1	Each	Egg, Whole
0.5	tsp	Salt
0.25	teaspoon	Spice, Red Pepper
0.5	Cup	Vegetable, Onions
0.25	Cup	Cheese, Ricotta, Part Skim Milk
1	Cup	Vegetable, Zucchini, slices
3	Teaspoon	Oil, Olive
4	Ounces	Pasta, Ziti
2	Cup	Vegetable, Squash, summer, yellow, raw
1	Teaspoon	Herb, Oregano, Ground
1	Cup	Cheese, Mozzarella Part Skim

Ratatouille

Quantity		Grocery Item
1	Each	Vegetable, Eggplant
8	ounces	Vegetable, Tomato, Red Canned, No Added
0.25	tsp	Spice, Black Pepper
1.5	Cup	Vegetable, Zucchini, slices
3	Teaspoon	Oil, Olive
0.5	tsp	Salt
2	Teaspoon	Herb, Garlic, Raw
1	Cup	Vegetable, Pepper, Green

Rice and Noodle Pilaf

Quantity		Grocery Item
0.3	Cup	Pasta, Spaghetti
0.25	tsp	Spice, Black Pepper
16	oz	Water
1	Cup	Rice, Medium Brown
2	tablespoon	Butter, Light w/no added salt
0.25	tsp	Salt

Spiced Pork Chop GDM Meal

Spiced Pork Chops With Apple Topping

Quantity		Grocery Item
0.5	Teaspoon	Spice, Coriander, ground
0.5	tsp	Salt
0.33	Cups	Fruit, Cranberries, dried - Craisins
5	Each	Fruit, Apple, peeled, raw, medium
2	teaspoons	Herb, Ginger Root, peeled, sliced, raw
0.25	tsp	Spice, Black Pepper
0.125	Teaspoons	Spice, Allspice, ground
1	tablespoon	Butter, Light w/no added salt
16	ounces	Pork, Tenderloin Lean
0.5	teaspoon	Spice, Garlic Powder
0.75	teaspoon	Spice, Chili Powder
0.25	teaspoons	Spice, Mustard Powder
12	Teaspoon Pac	Sugar, Brown
3	Tablespoons	Vinegar, Cider

Asparagus

Quantity		Grocery Item
54	Ounces	Vegetable, Asparagus Fresh

Creamy Herbed Mashed Potatoes

Quantity		Grocery Item
0.5	tsp	Spice, Black Pepper
4	Cup	Vegetable, Potato, Flesh only, diced, raw
4	Springs	Herb, Parsley, Raw, Fresh
1	Tablespoons	Cream, Sour, Reduced Fat
4	fluid ounces	Milk, Nonfat/Skim
0.5	tsp	Salt
3	tablespoon	Butter, Light w/no added salt
3	Tablespoon	Herb, Chives, raw

Braised Red Cabbage

Quantity		Grocery Item
0.5	Teaspoons	Spice, Allspice, ground
6	Teaspoon	Vinegar, Red Wine
4	Cup	Vegetable, Cabbage Heads, Red, raw
8	Tablespoons	Vinegar, Cider
2	cup	Soup, Chicken Broth Low Sodium
0.5	ounces	Honey
2	Each	Fruit, Apple, peeled, Granny Smith, medium

Week 4 Meals and Grocery Lists

Chicken, Cashew, and Red Pepper Stir-fry with Steamed Carrots and Pears

Grilled Balsamic Skirt Steak with Spanish Rice and Roasted Broccoli with Almonds

Ancho Pork and Hominy Stew with Red Cabbage, Bacon Potato Salad and Oranges

Garlic and Herb Oven Fried Halibut with Corn on the Cob and Garden Coleslaw with Almonds

Southwest Salad with Cucumber Salad

Creamy Stove Top Macaroni and Cheese with Asparagus and Tomato Ranch Salad

Chicken with Lemon Caper Sauce with Rosemary Roasted Potatoes, Spicy Greens and Roasted Broccoli with Almonds

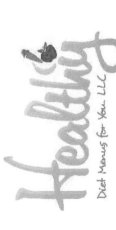

Diet Menus for You. LLC

Meal Plan

www.healthydietmenusforyou.com

Meal: *Chicken and Cashew Stirfry GDM*

Recipe		Ingredients	Instructions	Nutritionals			

Chicken, Cashew, and Red Pepper Stir-fry

Serves: 4

Serving Size: 1 Cup

		Ingredients
3.667	Teaspo	Cornstarch, hydrolyzed powder
2	tablespoon	Sauce, Bean, Soy/Wheat (Shoyu) Is
0.333	Ounces	Beverage, Alcoholic, Wine, Table, Dry Red
1	Teaspoon	Vinegar, Red Wine
1	Teaspoon	Sweet, Sugar, granulated, white
0.15	Tablesp	Sauce, Hot Pepper
16	Ounces	Chicken, Breast Tenders Boneless
0.5	Cup	Nuts, Cashew, Dry Roasted, Chopped No Salt
2	Tablespoon	Oil, Vegetable or Olive
2	Cup	Vegetable, Pepper, Sweet, Red, raw
0.25	Teaspoo	Herb, Garlic, Raw
1	Teaspoon	Spice, Ginger
0.25	Cup	Vegetable, Onions, Young Green, raw

Instructions

1. Combine 1 teaspoon cornstarch, 1 tablespoon soy sauce, dry Sherry, rice wine vinegar, sugar and hot pepper sauce in a small bowl; stir with a whisk.

2. Combine remaining 2 3/4 teaspoons cornstarch, remaining 1 tablespoon soy sauce, and chicken in a medium bowl; toss well to coat.

3. Heat a large nonstick skillet over medium-high heat. Add cashews to pan; cook 3 minutes or until lightly toasted, stirring frequently. Remove from pan.

4. Add oil to pan, swirling to coat. Add chicken mixture to pan; sauté 2 minutes or until lightly browned. Remove chicken from pan; place in a bowl. Add bell pepper to pan; sauté 2 minutes, stirring occasionally. Add garlic and ginger; cook 30 seconds. Add chicken and cornstarch mixture to pan; cook 1 minute or until sauce is slightly thick. Sprinkle with cashews and green onions.

Nutritionals

Calories 507.6	Sodium: 785.5	Protein: 20.3	Phos 349.6
Fat: 33	Carbs: 31.8	Chol: 46.5	Pot: 483.5
Sat Fat: 5.803	Fiber: 2.98		
	Sugar: 4.564		

Recipe		Ingredients	Instructions	Nutritionals			

Steamed Carrots

Serves: 6

Serving Size: 1/2 cup

		Ingredients
3	Cup	Vegetable, Carrots
1	Teaspoon	Spice, Mrs. Dash

Instructions

Steam carrots until tender, season with Mrs. Dash

Nutritionals

Calories 33	Sodium: 2	Protein: 1	Phos 22
Fat: 0	Carbs: 8	Chol: 0	Pot: 165
Sat Fat: 0	Fiber: 3		
	Sugar: 0		

Pear

Serves: 6

Serving Size: 1 medium pear

Ingredients		Instructions
6 Fruit	Fruit, Pear Raw	Piece of fruit

Nutritionals

Calories 115.5	Sodium: 0	Protein: 1.3	Phos 30.2
Fat: 0.6	Carbs: 29.3	Chol: 0	Pot: 332.8
Sat Fat: 0	Fiber: 9.9	Sugar: 19.4	

Meal: Grilled Skirt Steak GDM

Grilled Balsamic Skirt Steak

Serves: 4

Serving Size: 3 ounces

Ingredients		Instructions
4 Tablespoon	Vinegar, balsamic	1. Combine vinegar, worcestershire sauce, brown sugar and garlic in a large zip-top plastic bag. Cut steak into 4 equal pieces. Add steak, turning to coat; seal and marinate at room temperature 25 minutes, turning once. Remove steak from bag; discard marinade.
1 Tablespoon	Worcestershire Sauce	
2 Teaspoo	P Sugar, Brown	
0.25 Teaspoo	Herb, Garlic, Raw	2. Heat a large grill pan over medium-high heat. Coat pan with cooking spray. Sprinkle both sides of steak with 1/4 teaspoon salt and pepper. Add steak to pan; cook 3 minutes on each side or until desired degree of doneness. Remove steak from pan; sprinkle with remaining 1/4 teaspoon salt. Tent with foil; let stand 5 minutes. Cut steak diagonally across the grain into thin slices
0.25 tsp	Salt	
16 Ounces	Beef, Skirt Steak, trimmed to 1/4" fat	
0.25 tsp	Spice, Black Pepper	

Nutritionals

Calories 214.6	Sodium: 270.9	Protein: 22.4	Phos 240.6
Fat: 10.2	Carbs: 6.114	Chol: 55.6	Pot: 497.1
Sat Fat: 3.937	Fiber: 0.049	Sugar: 5.048	

Spanish Rice

Serves: 6

Serving Size: 1/2 Cup

Ingredients		Instructions
2 Tablespoon	Oil, Vegetable or Olive	In a large skillet, brown rice in olive oil at a medium / high heat. Add onion and garlic. Cook onion / rice mixture, stirring frequently, about 4 minutes, or until onions are softened. In a separate pan, bring chicken broth to a simmer. Add tomato chopped, oregano and salt. Add rice to broth. Bring to a simmer. Cover. Lower heat and cook 15-25 minutes, depending on the type of rice and the instructions on the rice package. Turn off heat and let sit for 5 minutes.
1 Cup	Vegetable, Onions	
1 Teaspoon	Herb, Garlic, Raw	
1.5 Cup	Grain, Rice, White, Medium grain, ckd	
3 cup	Soup, Chicken Broth Low Sodium	
1 Cup	Vegetable, Tomato Red Raw	
0.25 Teaspoo	Herb, Oregano, Ground	
0.5 tsp	Salt	

Nutritionals

Calories 248.2	Sodium: 232.7	Protein: 6.1	Phos 102
Fat: 5.5	Carbs: 43.2	Chol: 0	Pot: 246
Sat Fat: 0.9	Fiber: 1.3	Sugar: 1.7	

Roasted Broccoli with Almonds

Serves: 6
Serving Size: 3/4 Cup

Nutritionals

Calories 123	Sodium: 164	Protein: 7	Phos 162
Fat: 6	Carbs: 6	Chol: 0	Pot: 685
Sat Fat: 1	Fiber: 6		
Sugar: 4			

Ingredients

Amount	Ingredient
5 Cup	Vegetable, Broccoli Florets, Raw
1 Tablespoon	Oil, Vegetable or Olive
0.25 tsp	Salt
0.25 tsp	Spice, Black Pepper
0.25 Cup	Nuts, Almond Sliced

Instructions

Cut broccoli off stem if necessary. Place broccoli in a sprayed baking dish. Drizzle broccoli with olive oil, garlic, salt and pepper. Bake 14 minutes at 450F. Sprinkle with almonds and divide into 6 servings.

Meal: Pork and Hominy Stew GDM

Ancho Pork and Hominy Stew

Serves: 6
Serving Size: 1 1/3 cups

Nutritionals

Calories 272.2	Sodium: 703.8	Protein: 28	Phos 431.7
Fat: 7.929	Carbs: 24.8	Chol: 55.6	Pot: 1018
Sat Fat: 1.932	Fiber: 5.575		
Sugar: 6.495			

Ingredients

Amount	Ingredient
6 Teaspoon	Spice, Ancho Chile Powder
2 Teaspoon	Herb, Oregano, Ground
1 tsp	Spice, Cumin, Ground
0.5 tsp	Salt
24 ounces	Pork, Tenderloin Lean
3 Teaspoon	Oil, Olive
1.5 Cup	Vegetable, Onions
1.5 Cup	Vegetable, Pepper, Green
0.75 Teaspoo	Herb, Garlic, Raw
2.5 cup	Soup, Chicken Broth Low Sodium
12 ounces	Vegetable, Tomato, Red Canned, No Added Salt
3 Cup	Grain, Hominy, White, canned
1.5 Teaspoon	Spice, Paprika, Smoked

Instructions

1. Combine ancho chile powder, dried oregano, paprika, cumin and salt in a large bowl; set 1 1/2 teaspoons spice mixture aside. Cut pork into half-inch pieces, then add pork to remaining spice mixture in bowl, tossing well to coat.

2. Heat 2 teaspoons oil in a large Dutch oven over medium-high heat. Add pork mixture to pan; cook 5 minutes or until browned, stirring occasionally. Remove pork from pan; set aside. Add remaining 1 teaspoon oil to pan. Add onion, bell pepper, and garlic; sauté 5 minutes or until tender, stirring occasionally. Return pork to pan. Add reserved 1 1/2 teaspoons spice mixture, broth, hominy, and tomatoes; bring to a boil. Partially cover, reduce heat, and simmer 25 minutes.

Braised Red Cabbage

Serves: 4
Serving Size: 1/2 cup

Nutritionals

Calories 96.9	Sodium: 57.4	Protein: 3.612	Phos 67.7
Fat: 0.938	Carbs: 2.39	Chol: 2.39	Pot: 362.6
Sat Fat: 0.249	Fiber: 0.249		
Sugar: 13.9			

Ingredients

Amount	Ingredient
2 cup	Soup, Chicken Broth Low Sodium
8 Tablespoon	Vinegar, Cider
6 Teaspoon	Vinegar, Red Wine
0.5 ounces	Honey
0.5 Teaspoon	Spice, Allspice, ground
4 Cup	Vegetable, Cabbage Heads, Red, raw
2 Each	Fruit, Apple, peeled, Granny Smith, medium

Instructions

In a large saucepan, bring broth, vinegar, honey, and allspice to a boil. Add cabbage and cubed apples. Reduce heat and simmer, uncovered, for 30 min.

Bacon Potato Salad

Serves: 6

Serving Size: 1/2 cup

Ingredients

Amount	Ingredient
2 Slices	Beef, Bacon, lean, ckd
4 each	Vegetable, Potato
0.25 Cup	Mayonnaise, reduced kcal, cholest free/Hellmann
0.33 Tablesp	Dijon Mustard

Instructions

Fry bacon, drain and pat grease off. Crumble. Peel potatoes, cook until tender - about 40 minutes at a low boil, and cube/slice them. Toss the warm potatoes with mayo, mustard, salt and pepper. Add bacon and serve.

Nutritionals

Calories	131.3	Sodium:	124.9	Protein:	2.5	Phos	47.9
Fat:	3.3	Carbs:	23	Chol:	0.82	Pot:	280.2
Sat Fat:	0.5	Fiber:	2				
		Sugar:	0.9				

Orange

Serves: 6

Serving Size: 1 Peeled Orange

Ingredients

Amount	Ingredient
6 1	Fruit, Orange, All Varieties, peeled, raw

Instructions

Piece of fruit.

Nutritionals

Calories	86.5	Sodium:	0	Protein:	1.7	Phos	25.8
Fat:	0.2	Carbs:	21.6	Chol:	0	Pot:	333
Sat Fat:	0	Fiber:	4.4				
		Sugar:	17.2				

Meal: Oven Fried Halibut GDM

Garlic and Herb Oven Fried Halibut

Serves: 6

Serving Size: 16 ounce filet

Ingredients

Amount	Ingredient
1 cup	Breadcrumbs, Seasoned
1 Teaspoon	Herb, Basil, Ground
0.333 Tables	Herb, Parsley, dried
0.5 Teaspoon	Spice, Onion Powder
0.25 Teaspoo	Herb, Garlic, Raw
1 Each	Egg, Whole
2 Each	Egg White
2 Tablespoon	Flour, White bleached enriched
36 Ounces	Fish, Halibut, Atlantic & Pacific, raw
0.25 tsp	Spice, Black Pepper
6 Teaspoon	Oil, Olive

Instructions

Preheat oven to 450°.

Combine bread crumbs, basil, parsley, onion powder and garlic ingredients in a shallow dish. Place egg whites and egg in a shallow dish. Place flour in a shallow dish. Sprinkle fish with salt and pepper. Dredge fish in flour. Dip in egg mixture; dredge in breadcrumb mixture.

Heat 1 tablespoon oil in a large nonstick skillet over medium-high heat. Add 3 fish fillets; cook 2 1/2 minutes on each side or until browned. Place fish on a broiler pan coated with cooking spray. Repeat procedure with remaining 1 tablespoon oil and remaining fish. Bake at 450° for 6 minutes or until fish flakes easily when tested with a fork or until desired degree of doneness.

Nutritionals

Calories	332.6	Sodium:	474.4	Protein:	40.9	Phos	436.^
Fat:	10.4	Carbs:	16.4	Chol:	89.9	Pot:	858.8
Sat Fat:	1.718	Fiber:	1.23				
		Sugar:	1.326				

Corn On The Cob

Serves: 6

Serving Size: 1 ear of cor.

Ingredients

Amount	Ingredient
6 Each	Vegetable, Corn on Cob, sm/med, ckd w/o fat or salt

Instructions

Shuck and clean corn. Boil until tender, about 4-6 minutes.

Nutritionals

Calories	82.7	Sodium:	1.5	Protein:	2.5	Phos	78.8
Fat:	0.9	Carbs:	19.2	Chol:	0	Pot:	190.6
Sat Fat:	0.1	Fiber:	2.8				
		Sugar:	0				

Garden Coleslaw With Almonds

Serves: 6

Serving Size: 3/4 Cup

Nutritionals

Calories 162.8	Sodium: 69.3	Protein: 5.15	Phos 103.5
Fat: 7.843	Carbs: 21.2	Chol: 0	Pot: 479.2
Sat Fat: 0.936	Fiber: 6.47		
	Sugar: 13.9		

Ingredients

Amount	Ingredient
0.25 Cup	Nuts, Almond Sliced
1 Each	Vegetable, Cabbage Head
1 Cup	Vegetable, Carrots
6 Teaspoon	Oil, Olive
9 Teaspoon	Vinegar, rice
1 ounces	Honey
2 ounces	Yogurt, Greek Non Fat
0.4 Tablespo	Dijon Mustard
0.25 tsp	Spice, Black Pepper

Instructions

Start by toasting the almonds; put them in a small skillet, without oil, over medium heat and shake until almonds start to get golden brown. Remove and set aside.

Make slaw by shredding cabbage and dicing. Put in bowl.

Shredded carrots, add to bowl.

Make dressing by whisking together the remaining ingredients until smooth; then pour the dressing over the slaw.

Add the toasted almonds, tossing to combine. Let stand for 30 minutes, tossing several times.

To serve, spoon portions onto individual salad plates. You will have enough salad for 4 to 6 people.

Meal: Southwest Salad GDM

Southwest Salad

Serves: 4

Serving Size: 1/4 Recipe

Nutritionals

Calories 466.7	Sodium: 487.8	Protein: 34.3	Phos 483.5
Fat: 11.1	Carbs: 59	Chol: 72.4	Pot: 1105
Sat Fat: 3.372	Fiber: 17.3		
	Sugar: 3.604		

Ingredients

Amount	Ingredient
0.33 Cup	Cheese, Cheddar reduced fat
15 oz	Chickpeas, dry, canned - garbanzos
1 Cup	Vegetable, Onions
2 teaspoon	Spice, Chili Powder
0.5 tsp	Spice, Cumin, Ground
0.25 Teaspoo	Spice, Pepper, Cayenne
2 Cup	Beans, Black, Canned
1 Cup	Vegetable, Tomato Red Raw
4 Cup	Vegetable, Lettuce, Cos/Romaine, raw
0.75 Pound	Turkey, Ground Raw

Instructions

Add onion and, ground turkey to a large nonstick skillet over medium-high heat. Cook about 8 to 10 min. or until turkey is cooked through no longer pink. Add chili powder, cumin and cayenne pepper, and cook 2 more minutes. Gently stir in beans, chickpeas, and tomatoes and cook an additional 2 min. Set aside to cool slightly. Toss meat mixture would lettuce in a large bowl. Sprinkle with cheese.

Cucumber Salad

Serves: 4

Serving Size: 1/3 cup

Nutritionals

Calories 30	Sodium: 147.6	Protein: 0.647	Phos 22.5
Fat: 0.097	Carbs: 7.258	Chol: 0	Pot: 134.4
Sat Fat: 0.034	Fiber: 0.621		
	Sugar: 5.025		

Ingredients

Amount	Ingredient
1.5 Cup	Vegetable, Cucumber, peeled, raw
8 Tablespoon	Vegetable, Onions, Red
3 Teaspoon	Sweet, Sugar, granulated, white
1 Tablespoon	Vinegar, Cider
0.25 tsp	Salt

Instructions

Combine 1 thinly sliced cucumber, red onion sliced, sugar, vinegar, and salt. Chill for 15 min.

Meal: *Stovetop Mac & Cheese GDM*

Recipe: Creamy Stove Top Macaroni and Cheese

Serves: 6
Serving Size: 1.5 Cups

Ingredients

Amount	Ingredient
4 Cup	Macaroni, unenriched, dry
6 Tablespoon	Flour, White bleached enriched
1 teaspoon	Salt, Kosher
0.25 tsp	Spice, Black Pepper
18 fluid ounce	Milk, Nonfat/Skim
2 Ounces	Cheese Spread, Light Cream Cheese
0.66 Tablesp	Dijon Mustard
0.5 Tablespo	Worcestershire Sauce
0.5 Teaspoon	Herb, Garlic, Raw
1 Cup	Cheese, processed, Cheddar type, lowfat

Instructions

Cook pasta as directed on package without additional oil or salt. Drain well and set to the side. While pasta cooks, place flour, salt and pepper in a large saucepan. Add milk, stirring with a whisk until well blended. Drop cream cheese by teaspoonfuls into milk mixture; bring to a boil over medium-high heat, stirring constantly. Reduce heat; simmer 2 minutes or until thick and cream cheese melts, stirring occasionally. Stir in mustard, Worcestershire, and garlic; simmer 1 minute. Remove from heat, add cheddar cheese, stirring until cheese melts. Combine pasta and cheese sauce in a large bowl, toss well.

Nutritionals

Calories 373.4	Sodium: 257	Protein: 18.6	Phos 338.a
Fat: 4.2	Carbs: 63.5	Chol: 11.4	Pot: 348
Sat Fat: 2.1	Fiber: 2.4		
	Sugar: 6.6		

Recipe: Asparagus

Serves: 6
Serving Size: 1/2 Cup

Ingredients

Amount	Ingredient
54 Ounces	Vegetable, Asparagus Fresh

Instructions

Wash and clean asparagus by cutting off hard ends of stalk. Steam for 10 minutes in steamer or cook in 1 in water in microwaveable bowl for 5-7 minutes until desired tenderness.

Nutritionals

Calories 21.5	Sodium: 1.8	Protein: 2.3	Phos 48.3
Fat: 0.2	Carbs: 3.7	Chol: 0	Pot: 143.2
Sat Fat: 0	Fiber: 1.5		
	Sugar: 0		

Recipe: Tomato Ranch Salad

Serves: 6
Serving Size: 3/4 cup salad w/dressing

Ingredients

Amount	Ingredient
2 Cup	Vegetable, Tomato Red Raw
4.5 Cup	Vegetable, Lettuce, Iceberg, head, raw
12 Tablespoo	Salad dressing, ranch dressing, reduced fat

Instructions

Toss lettuce and tomatoes and divide into 6 portions. Top each salad with 2T lite ranch dressing.

Nutritionals

Calories 75.6	Sodium: 280	Protein: 1.2	Phos 80.8
Fat: 3.9	Carbs: 10	Chol: 4.8	Pot: 242.1
Sat Fat: 0.3	Fiber: 1.5		
	Sugar: 3.5		

Meal: Chicken with Lemon Caper Sauce GDM

Chicken with Lemon/Caper Sauce

Serves: 4

Serving Size: 1 5-6 ounce breast + 1 T sauce

Nutritionals

Calories 250.6	Sodium: 486.6	Protein: 37.6	Phos 376.4
Fat: 8.258	Carbs: 4.827	Chol: 115.6	Pot: 693.6
Sat Fat: 3.241	Fiber: 0.446		
	Sugar: 0.463		

Ingredients

24 Ounces	Chicken, Broiler or Fryer, Thigh, no skin, raw
0.25 tsp	Salt
0.25 tsp	Spice, Black Pepper
0.125 Cup	Flour, Wheat, White, All Purpose, unbleached, enriched
2 tablespoon	Butter, Light w/no added salt
0.5 cup	Soup, Chicken Broth Low Sodium
2 ounces	Lemon Juice, Bottled
2 Tablespoon	Condiment, Capers, canned
1 Tablespoon	Herb, Parsley, dried

Instructions

1. Place chicken between 2 sheets of plastic wrap; pound to an even thickness using a meat mallet or small heavy skillet. Sprinkle chicken evenly with salt and pepper. Place flour in a shallow dish; dredge chicken in flour.

2. Melt butter in a large nonstick skillet over medium-high heat. Add chicken to pan; cook 3 minutes. Turn chicken over. Add broth, juice, and capers; reduce heat to medium, and simmer 3 minutes, basting chicken occasionally with sauce. Sprinkle with parsley; cook 1 minute. Remove chicken from pan; keep warm.

3. Bring sauce to a boil; cook 2 minutes or until thick. Serve over chicken.

Rosemary Roasted Potatoes

Serves: 6

Serving Size: 3/4 cup Potatoes

Nutritionals

Calories 132.8	Sodium: 12.3	Protein: 3.094	Phos 85.4
Fat: 2.581	Carbs: 25.5	Chol: 0	Pot: 642
Sat Fat: 0.407	Fiber: 3.056		
	Sugar: 1.443		

Ingredients

5 each	Vegetable, Potato
1 Tablespoon	Oil, Vegetable or Olive
0.75 Teaspoo	Herb, Garlic, Raw
3 teaspoon	Herb, Rosemary, Dried
2 teaspoon	Spice, Paprika

Instructions

Wash and dice potatoes into bite-sized pieces. Place into a large bowl or Ziplock bag; toss with olive oil. Sprinkle garlic, rosemary, paprika (optional), and pepper over potatoes and shake to coat. Layer potatoes in a single layer on a baking sheet coated with cooking spray. Bake at 400 F for 30 minutes or until slightly browned. Serves 5.

Spicy Greens

Serves: 4

Serving Size: 1 cup

Nutritionals

Calories 97.3	Sodium: 94.7	Protein: 9.095	Phos 148
Fat: 1.249	Carbs: 17	Chol: 0	Pot: 975.7
Sat Fat: 0.262	Fiber: 8.294		
	Sugar: 5.508		

Ingredients

2 cup	Soup, Chicken Broth Low Sodium
32 Ounces	Vegetable, Mustard Greens, raw
1 Cup	Vegetable, Onions
0.5 Teaspoon	Herb, Garlic, Raw
0.25 Teaspoo	Spice, Pepper, Cayenne
0.5 tsp	Spice, Black Pepper
1 Teaspoon	Liquid Smoke

Instructions

Wash greens thoroughly. Discard tough stems and cut greens into pieces. Place greens in a large soup pot. Add chicken broth, onion, and garlic, and simmer, covered, for 30 to 45 min. or until tender. Season with cayenne pepper, black pepper and liquid smoke.

Recipe	Ingredients		Instructions	Nutritionals			
Roasted Broccoli with Almonds	5 Cup	Vegetable, Broccoli Florets, Raw	Cut broccoli off stem if necessary. Place broccoli in a sprayed baking dish. Drizzle broccoli with olive oil, garlic, salt and pepper. Bake 14 minutes at 450°F. Sprinkle with almonds and divide into 6 servings.	Calories 123	Sodium: 164	Protein: 7	Phos 162
	1 Tablespoon	Oil, Vegetable or Olive		Fat: 6	Carbs: 15	Chol: 0	Pot: 685
Serves: 6	0.25 tsp	Salt		Sat Fat: 1	Fiber: 6		
	0.25 tsp	Spice, Black Pepper			Sugar: 4		
Serving Size: 3/4 Cup	0.25 Cup	Nuts, Almond Sliced					

82

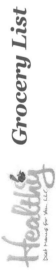

Diet: *Gestational Diabetic - 2400*

Chicken and Cashew Stirfry GDM Meal

Chicken, Cashew, and Red Pepper Stir-fry

Quantity		Grocery Item
3.667	Teaspoon	Cornstarch, hydrolyzed powder
1	Teaspoon	Spice, Ginger
1	Teaspoon	Sweet, Sugar, granulated, white
0.333	Ounces	Beverage, Alcoholic, Wine, Table, Dry Red
0.25	Cup	Vegetable, Onions, Young Green, raw
2	Cup	Vegetable, Pepper, Sweet, Red, raw
0.25	Teaspoon	Herb, Garlic, Raw
1	Teaspoon	Vinegar, Red Wine
16	Ounces	Chicken, Breast Tenders Boneless
0.15	Tablespoon	Sauce, Hot Pepper
2	Tablespoon	Oil, Vegetable or Olive
2	tablespoon	Sauce, Bean, Soy/Wheat (Shoyu) ls
0.5	Cup	Nuts, Cashew, Dry Roasted, Chopped No

Steamed Carrots

Quantity		Grocery Item
3	Cup	Vegetable, Carrots
1	Teaspoon	Spice, Mrs. Dash

Pear

Quantity		Grocery Item
6	Fruit	Fruit, Pear Raw

Grilled Skirt Steak GDM Meal

Grilled Balsamic Skirt Steak

Quantity		Grocery Item
2	Teaspoon Pac	Sugar, Brown
16	Ounces	Beef, Skirt Steak, trimmed to 1/4" fat
4	Tablespoon	Vinegar, balsamic
0.25	Teaspoon	Herb, Garlic, Raw
1	Tablespoon	Worcestershire Sauce
0.25	tsp	Salt
0.25	tsp	Spice, Black Pepper

Spanish Rice

Quantity		Grocery Item
1	Teaspoon	Herb, Garlic, Raw
0.25	Teaspoon	Herb, Oregano, Ground
1.5	Cup	Grain, Rice, White, Medium grain, ckd
2	Tablespoon	Oil, Vegetable or Olive
0.5	tsp	Salt
1	Cup	Vegetable, Onions
3	cup	Soup, Chicken Broth Low Sodium
1	Cup	Vegetable, Tomato Red Raw

Roasted Broccoli with Almonds

Quantity		Grocery Item
1	Tablespoon	Oil, Vegetable or Olive
0.25	tsp	Salt
0.25	Cup	Nuts, Almond Sliced
0.25	tsp	Spice, Black Pepper
5	Cup	Vegetable, Broccoli Florets, Raw

Pork and Hominy Stew GDM Meal

Ancho Pork and Hominy Stew

Quantity		Grocery Item
12	ounces	Vegetable, Tomato, Red Canned, No Added
1.5	Cup	Vegetable, Onions
24	ounces	Pork, Tenderloin Lean
2.5	cup	Soup, Chicken Broth Low Sodium
1.5	Teaspoon	Spice, Paprika, Smoked
0.75	Teaspoon	Herb, Garlic, Raw
1	tsp	Spice, Cumin, Ground
6	Teaspoon	Spice, Ancho Chile Powder
1.5	Cup	Vegetable, Pepper, Green
2	Teaspoon	Herb, Oregano, Ground
3	Teaspoon	Oil, Olive
0.5	tsp	Salt
3	Cup	Grain, Hominy, White, canned

Southwest Salad GDM Meal

Southwest Salad

Quantity		Grocery Item
2	teaspoon	Spice, Chili Powder
2	Cup	Beans, Black, Canned
0.5	tsp	Spice, Cumin, Ground
1	Cup	Vegetable, Onions
15	oz	Chickpeas, dry, canned - garbanzos
1	Cup	Vegetable, Tomato Red Raw
4	Cup	Vegetable, Lettuce, Cos/Romaine, raw
0.25	Teaspoon	Spice, Pepper, Cayenne
0.75	Pound	Turkey, Ground Raw
0.33	Cup	Cheese, Cheddar reduced fat

Cucumber Salad

Quantity		Grocery Item
3	Teaspoon	Sweet, Sugar, granulated, white
0.25	tsp	Salt
8	Tablespoon	Vegetable, Onions, Red
1.5	Cup	Vegetable, Cucumber, peeled, raw
1	Tablespoons	Vinegar, Cider

Oven Fried Halibut GDM Meal

Garlic and Herb Oven Fried Halibut

Quantity		Grocery Item
2	Tablespoons	Flour, White bleached enriched
1	cup	Breadcrumbs, Seasoned
0.5	Teaspoon	Spice, Onion Powder
0.25	Teaspoon	Herb, Garlic, Raw
1	Each	Egg, Whole
1	Teaspoon	Herb, Basil, Ground
0.333	Tablespoon	Herb, Parsley, dried
0.25	tsp	Spice, Black Pepper
36	Ounces	Fish, Halibut, Atlantic & Pacific, raw
6	Teaspoon	Oil, Olive
2	Each	Egg White

Corn On The Cob

Quantity		Grocery Item
6	Each	Vegetable, Corn on Cob, sm/med, ckd w/o

Garden Coleslaw With Almonds

Quantity		Grocery Item
9	Teaspoon	Vinegar, rice
1	Cup	Vegetable, Carrots
0.25	tsp	Spice, Black Pepper
1	ounces	Honey
0.4	Tablespoon	Dijon Mustard
2	ounces	Yogurt, Greek Non Fat
6	Teaspoon	Oil, Olive
1	Each	Vegetable, Cabbage Head
0.25	Cup	Nuts, Almond Sliced

Braised Red Cabbage

Quantity		Grocery Item
8	Tablespoons	Vinegar, Cider
4	Cup	Vegetable, Cabbage Heads, Red, raw
0.5	Teaspoons	Spice, Allspice, ground
0.5	ounces	Honey
6	Teaspoon	Vinegar, Red Wine
2	Each	Fruit, Apple, peeled, Granny Smith, medium
2	cup	Soup, Chicken Broth Low Sodium

Bacon Potato Salad

Quantity		Grocery Item
0.33	Tablespoon	Dijon Mustard
4	each	Vegetable, Potato
2	Slices	Beef, Bacon, lean, ckd
0.25	Cup	Mayonnaise, reduced kcal, cholest

Orange

Quantity	Grocery Item
6	1	Fruit, Orange, All Varieties, peeled, raw

Stovetop Mac & Cheese GDM Meal

Creamy Stove Top Macaroni and Cheese

Quantity		Grocery Item
2	Ounces	Cheese Spread, Light Cream Cheese
0.5	Tablespoon	Worcestershire Sauce
18	fluid ounces	Milk, Nonfat/Skim
4	Cup	Macaroni, unenriched, dry
6	Tablespoons	Flour, White bleached enriched
0.25	tsp	Spice, Black Pepper
1	teaspoon	Salt, Kosher
0.66	Tablespoon	Dijon Mustard
1	Cup	Cheese, processed, Cheddar type, lowfat
0.5	Teaspoon	Herb, Garlic, Raw

Asparagus

Quantity		Grocery Item
54	Ounces	Vegetable, Asparagus Fresh

Tomato Ranch Salad

Quantity		Grocery Item
4.5	Cup	Vegetable, Lettuce, Iceberg, head, raw
12	Tablespoon	Salad dressing, ranch dressing, reduced fat
2	Cup	Vegetable, Tomato Red Raw

Chicken with Lemon Caper Sauce GDM Meal

Chicken with Lemon/Caper Sauce

Quantity		Grocery Item
24	Ounces	Chicken, Broiler or Fryer, Thigh, no skin,
2	tablespoon	Butter, Light w/no added salt
0.125	Cup	Flour, Wheat, White, All Purpose,
2	Tablespoons	Condiment, Capers, canned
0.5	cup	Soup, Chicken Broth Low Sodium
0.25	tsp	Spice, Black Pepper
0.25	tsp	Salt
1	Tablespoon	Herb, Parsley, dried
2	ounces	Lemon Juice, Bottled

Rosemary Roasted Potatoes

Quantity		Grocery Item
2	teaspoon	Spice, Paprika
1	Tablespoon	Oil, Vegetable or Olive
5	each	Vegetable, Potato
3	teaspoon	Herb, Rosemary, Dried
0.75	Teaspoon	Herb, Garlic, Raw

Spicy Greens

Quantity		Grocery Item
0.5	Teaspoon	Herb, Garlic, Raw
1	Teaspoon	Liquid Smoke
0.25	Teaspoon	Spice, Pepper, Cayenne
1	Cup	Vegetable, Onions
2	cup	Soup, Chicken Broth Low Sodium
32	Ounces	Vegetable, Mustard Greens, raw
0.5	tsp	Spice, Black Pepper

Roasted Broccoli with Almonds

Quantity		Grocery Item
5	Cup	Vegetable, Broccoli Florets, Raw
0.25	tsp	Spice, Black Pepper
0.25	tsp	Salt
0.25	Cup	Nuts, Almond Sliced
1	Tablespoon	Oil, Vegetable or Olive

Week 5 Meals and Grocery Lists

Barbecue Chicken Burger with Roasted Asparagus and Oven Fries

Loaded Nachos with Turkey, Beans and Salsa and Garden Coleslaw with Almonds

Hamburger Stroganoff with Italian Green Beans and Tossed Pears and Almond Salad

Red Peppers Frittata with Oranges and Rosemary Roasted Potatoes

Smokey Pan Grilled Pork Chops with Couscous with Tomato and Dill, Broccoli Casserole and Macaroni Salad

Broiled Salmon with Marmalade Dijon Glaze with Coconut Rice and Ratatouille

Chicken Marsala with Creamy Herbed Mashed Potatoes, Cucumber and Tomato Salad and Pears

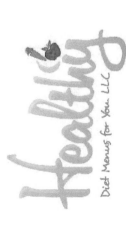
Healthy
Diet Menus for You, LLC

Meal Plan

www.healthydietmenusforyou.com

Diet: *Gestational Diabetic - 2400*

Meal: *Barbecue Chicken Burger GDM*

Recipe | Ingredients | Instructions | Nutritionals

Barbecue Chicken Burger

Qty	Unit	Ingredient
0.125	cup	Soup, Chicken Broth Low Sodium
0.75	Cup	Vegetable, Onions
0.25	Teaspoo	Herb, Garlic, Raw
14	Ounces	Chicken, Ground
5	Tablespoon	Sauce, BBQ
1	Tablespoon	Worcestershire Sauce
0.333	Tables	Dijon Mustard
1	Teaspoon	Herb, Thyme Ground
0.75	cup	Breadcrumbs, Seasoned
4	each	Bread, Roll, Hamburger, Whole Wheat

Serves: 4

Serving Size: 1 6 ounce burger

Instructions: Heat the chicken broth in a small skillet over medium heat. Add the onions and sauté until caramelized, 5 to 10 min. Add the garlic and cook for 5 min. more. Set aside to cool. In a mixing bowl combine the onion mixture with all the remaining ingredients except buns. Stir well. Form into 4 6 ounce patties. Coat a nonstick skillet with cooking spray, place over medium heat and cook burgers until no longer pink, about 5 to 6 min. per side. Serve with bun.

Nutritionals:

Calories 388.6	Sodium: 868	Protein: 24.8	Phos 278.2
Fat: 12.6	Carbs: 44.1	Chol: 85.6	Pot: 723.2
Sat Fat: 3.338	Fiber: 3.544		
	Sugar: 7.482		

Recipe | Ingredients | Instructions | Nutritionals

Roasted Asparagus

Qty	Unit	Ingredient
24	Ounces	Vegetable, Asparagus Fresh
0.5	teaspoon	Spice, Garlic Powder
0.5	Teaspoon	Spice, Lemon Pepper

Serves: 6

Serving Size: 4 oz

Instructions: Place asparagus in a sprayed baking dish and coat with olive oil spray. Sprinkle with garlic powder and lemon pepper. Bake for 8 minutes at 450° F or until done.

Nutritionals:

Calories 29	Sodium: 9	Protein: 3	Phos 63
Fat: 0.4	Carbs: 5	Chol: 0	Pot: 185
Sat Fat: 0	Fiber: 2		
	Sugar: 0		

Recipe | Ingredients | Instructions | Nutritionals

Oven Fries

Qty	Unit	Ingredient
3	each	Vegetable, Potato
1	Teaspoon	Spice, Mrs. Dash
3	Each	Egg White

Serves: 6

Serving Size: 1/2 potato

Instructions: Cut potatoes into strips like fries. Beat egg whites and toss with fries. Sprinkle with Mrs. Dash type seasoning. Bake for 30 minutes at 400°F or until done.

Nutritionals:

Calories 75	Sodium: 45	Protein: 3.3	Phos 55
Fat: 0.2	Carbs: 15	Chol: 0	Pot: 406
Sat Fat: 0	Fiber: 2		
	Sugar: 1		

Meal: *Loaded Nachos with Turkey GDM*

Recipe: Loaded Nachos with Turkey, Beans and Salsa

Serves: 6

Serving Size: 1/6th of pan

Ingredients		Instructions	Nutritionals			
1.5 Pound	Turkey, Ground Raw	Preheat oven to 425' F. Line a baking sheet with foil and spread out the tortilla chips on the sheet. Heat a large nonstick skillet on the stove over high heat. When the pan is hot, add the turkey and cook until it is just cooked through. Stir occasionally, for about 5 minutes. Stir the black beans into the turkey, and season it with the salt and pepper. Spoon the turkey mixture over the chips, and sprinkle with cheese on top. Bake for 6 minutes, or until the cheese has melted. Remove the baking sheet from the oven, and top the chips with the salsa. Drop small spoonfuls of the yogurt on top of the nachos, and scatter the cilantro on top. Serve immediately	Calories 425.3	Sodium: 843.9	Protein: 34.9	Phos 518.2
6 ounces	Tortilla chips, low fat, baked without fat		Fat: 16.7	Carbs: 34	Chol: 107.2	Pot: 548.3
1 Cup	Beans, Black, Canned		Sat Fat: 6	Fiber: 4.9		
1 teaspoon	Salt, Kosher			Sugar: 4.2		
1 tsp	Spice, Black Pepper					
0.75 Cup	Cheese, Mexican blend, reduced fat - Kraft Mexican Four Cheese made with 2% Milk					
0.75 Cup	Herb, Cilantro Raw					
1 Cup	Salsa					
6 ounces	Yogurt, Greek Non Fat					

Recipe: Garden Coleslaw With Almonds

Serves: 6

Serving Size: 3/4 Cup

Ingredients		Instructions	Nutritionals			
0.25 Cup	Nuts, Almond Sliced	Start by toasting the almonds; put them in a small skillet, without oil, over medium heat and shake until almonds start to get golden brown. Remove and set aside.	Calories 162.8	Sodium: 69.3	Protein: 5.15	Phos 103.5
1 Each	Vegetable, Cabbage Head		Fat: 7.843	Carbs: 21.2	Chol: 0	Pot: 479.2
1 Cup	Vegetable, Carrots	Make slaw by shredding cabbage and dicing. Put in bowl.	Sat Fat: 0.936	Fiber: 6.47		
6 Teaspoon	Oil, Olive	Shredded carrots, add to bowl.		Sugar: 13.9		
9 Teaspoon	Vinegar, rice	Make dressing by whisking together the remaining ingredients until smooth; then pour the dressing over the slaw.				
1 ounces	Honey	Add the toasted almonds, tossing to combine. Let stand for 30 minutes, tossing several times.				
2 ounces	Yogurt, Greek Non Fat	To serve, spoon portions onto individual salad plates. You will have enough salad for 4 to 6 people.				
0.4 Tablespo	Dijon Mustard					
0.25 tsp	Spice, Black Pepper					

90

Meal: Hamburger Stroganoff GDM

Hamburger Stroganoff
Serves: 6
Serving Size: 1/2 c stroganoff + 2/3 cup pasta

Ingredients		Instructions	Nutritionals			
1 Cup	Noodles, Egg, enriched, dry	1. Cook pasta according to package directions, omitting salt and fat. Drain and rinse under cold water; drain.	Calories 345	Sodium: 446	Protein: 25.5	Phos 313
0.333 Tables	Oil, Vegetable or Olive		Fat: 10.6	Carbs: 36.2	Chol: 88	Pot: 548
16 ounces	Beef, Ground (95% lean)	2. Heat oil in a large nonstick skillet over medium-high heat. Add beef to pan; cook 4 minutes or until browned, stirring to crumble. Add onion, garlic, and mushrooms to pan; cook 4 minutes or until most of liquid evaporates, stirring frequently. Sprinkle with flour; cook 1 minute, stirring constantly. Stir in broth; bring to a boil. Reduce heat, and simmer 1 minute or until slightly thick. Stir in salt and pepper.	Sat Fat: 4.799	Fiber: 2.771		
1 Cup	Vegetable, Onions			Sugar: 2.909		
0.25 Teaspoo	Herb, Garlic, Raw					
8 Ounces	Vegetable, Mushrooms Canned					
0.2 Cup	Flour, Wheat, White, All Purpose, unbleached, enriched					
1 Cup	Soup, Beef broth, canned, low sodium					
0.5 tsp	Salt					
0.125 tsp	Spice, Black Pepper	3. Remove from heat. Stir in sour cream and sherry. Serve over pasta. Sprinkle with parsley.				
0.5 Ounces	Wine, table, red - dry sherry					
1 Tablespoon	Herb, Parsley, dried					
12 Tablespoo	Cream, Sour, Reduced Fat					

Italian Green Beans
Serves: 6
Serving Size: 1/2 cup

Ingredients		Instructions	Nutritionals			
3 Teaspoon	Oil, Olive	Steam green beans until tender crisp. Set aside. Heat olive oil in a medium nonstick skillet over medium-high heat. Sauté onions until clear. Add garlic; sauté 30 seconds. Add tomatoes, basil, and oregano, and simmer for 15 to 20 min. for tomato mixture over steamed green beans and mix well.	Calories 67.1	Sodium: 217.2	Protein: 2.111	Phos 46.7
1 Cup	Vegetable, Onions		Fat: 2.519	Carbs: 10.9	Chol: 0	Pot: 315.5
2 Teaspoon	Herb, Garlic, Raw		Sat Fat: 0.37	Fiber: 3.596		
1 Can	Vegetable, Tomato Diced Canned			Sugar: 3.97		
0.25 Teaspoo	Herb, Oregano, Ground					
0.25 Teaspoo	Herb, Basil, Ground					
16 Ounces	Vegetable, Beans, Italian, Frozen					

Tossed Pear and Almond Salad
Serves: 6
Serving Size: Salad

Ingredients		Instructions	Nutritionals			
2 Fruit	Fruit, Pear Raw	Toss Salad together and divide into 6 portions	Calories 127	Sodium: 222	Protein: 2	Phos 46
6 Cup	Lettuce, Raw Iceberg		Fat: 7	Carbs: 7	Chol: 0	Pot: 191
0.25 Cup	Nuts, Almond Sliced		Sat Fat: 1	Fiber: 1		
6 Tablespoon	Salad Dressing, Vinaigrette			Sugar: 7		

Meal: *Red Pepper Frittata GDM*

Red Pepper Frittata
Serves: 4
Serving Size: 1 wedge

Ingredients		Nutritionals			
		Calories 191.8	Sodium: 607.1	Protein: 14	Phos 177.?
4 oz	Water	Fat: 6.072	Carbs: 20.9	Chol: 164.7	Pot: 325.6
0.75 tsp	Salt	Sat Fat: 2.532	Fiber: 2.382		
1 tsp	Spice, Black Pepper		Sugar: 5.85		
4 Each	Egg White				
3 Each	Egg, Whole				
2 Cup	Vegetable, Pepper, Sweet, Red, raw				
0.5 Cup	Vegetable, Onions				
0.5 Teaspoon	Herb, Garlic, Raw				
2.15 Ounce	Cheese, Monterey, lowfat - Monterey Jack Cheese				
0.333 Cup	Grain, Couscous				

Instructions

Preheat oven to 350°.

Bring 1/2 cup water to boil in a small saucepan; gradually stir in couscous. Remove from heat; cover and let stand 5 minutes. Fluff with a fork.

Combine 1 tablespoon water, salt, black pepper, egg whites, and eggs in a medium bowl, stirring with a whisk.

Heat a 10-inch ovenproof nonstick skillet coated with cooking spray over medium-high heat. Add bell pepper, onion, and garlic; sauté 5 minutes. Stir in couscous and egg mixture; cook over medium heat 5 minutes or until almost set. Sprinkle with cheese. Bake at 350° for 10 minutes or until set. Let stand 5 minutes before serving.

Orange
Serves: 6
Serving Size: 1 Peeled Orange

Ingredients		Nutritionals			
		Calories 86.5	Sodium: 0	Protein: 1.7	Phos 25.8
6 1	Fruit, Orange, All Varieties, peeled, raw	Fat: 0.2	Carbs: 21.6	Chol: 0	Pot: 333
		Sat Fat: 0	Fiber: 4.4		
			Sugar: 17.2		

Instructions

Piece of fruit.

Rosemary Roasted Potatoes
Serves: 6
Serving Size: 3/4 cup Potatoes

Ingredients		Nutritionals			
		Calories 132.8	Sodium: 12.3	Protein: 3.094	Phos 85.4
5 each	Vegetable, Potato	Fat: 2.581	Carbs: 25.5	Chol: 0	Pot: 642
1 Tablespoon	Oil, Vegetable or Olive	Sat Fat: 0.407	Fiber: 3.056		
0.75 Teaspoo	Herb, Garlic, Raw		Sugar: 1.443		
3 teaspoon	Herb, Rosemary, Dried				
2 teaspoon	Spice, Paprika				

Instructions

Wash and dice potatoes into bite-sized pieces. Place into a large bowl or Ziplock bag; toss with olive oil. Sprinkle garlic, rosemary, paprika (optional), and pepper over potatoes and shake to coat. Layer potatoes in a single layer on a baking sheet coated with cooking spray. Bake at 400 F for 30 minutes or until slightly browned. Serves 5.

Meal: Smoky Grilled Pork Chops GDM

Smoky Pan Grilled Pork Chops

Serves: 4
Serving Size: 1 4 ounce chop

Ingredients		Instructions
3 tsp	Spice, Cumin, Ground	1. Combine ground cumin, sugar, paprika, salt, and pepper; rub evenly over pork.
3 Teaspoon P	Sugar, Brown	
1 teaspoon	Spice, Paprika	2. Heat a grill pan over medium-high heat. Coat pan with cooking spray. Add pork to pan; cook 5 minutes on each side or until done.
0.25 tsp	Salt	
0.25 tsp	Spice, Black Pepper	
16 ounces	Pork, Center Rib Chop	

Nutritionals

Calories	205.4	Sodium:	577.4	Protein:	21.6	Phos 9.61
Fat:	11.3	Carbs:	4.201	Chol:	59	Pot: 391.9
Sat Fat:	4.118	Fiber:	0.389			
		Sugar:	2.589			

Couscous with Tomato and Dill

Serves: 4
Serving Size: 1/2 cup

Ingredients		Instructions
3 Teaspoon	Oil, Olive	Heat a small saucepan over medium-high heat. Add olive oil to pan. Stir in couscous; sauté 1 minute. Add chicken broth and salt; bring to a boil. Cover, remove from heat, and let stand 5 minutes. Fluff with a fork. Stir in tomatoes, onion, and dill.
0.5 Cup	Grain, Couscous	
0.5 cup	Soup, Chicken Broth Low Sodium	
0.25 tsp	Salt	
0.5 Cup	Vegetable, Tomato, Red, Cherry	
5 Tablespoon	Vegetable, Onions, Red	
3 Teaspoon	Herb, Dill Weed	

Nutritionals

Calories	125.3	Sodium:	159.5	Protein:	3.788	Phos 57.3
Fat:	3.774	Carbs:	19.2	Chol:	0	Pot: 146.1
Sat Fat:	0.556	Fiber:	1.58			
		Sugar:	0.953			

Broccoli Casserole

Serves: 8
Serving Size: 1/2 cup

Ingredients		Instructions
4 Cup	Vegetable, Broccoli Florets, Raw	Preheat oven to 350°. In a large bowl, combine all ingredients. Pour into a medium casserole dish and bake for 30 min.
4 fluid ounces	Milk, Nonfat/Skim	
0.125 tsp	Spice, Black Pepper	
0.5 Cup	Cheese, Cheddar reduced fat	
6 Ounces	Soup, Cream of Celery, Fat Free	

Nutritionals

Calories	53.3	Sodium:	300	Protein:	3.796	Phos 135.
Fat:	2.291	Carbs:	5.245	Chol:	7.318	Pot: 231.2
Sat Fat:	1.228	Fiber:	0.179			
		Sugar:	1.884			

Macaroni Salad

Serves: 4
Serving Size: 1/2 cup

Ingredients

Amount	Ingredient
0.5 Cup	Vegetable, Onions, Young Green, raw
0.5 tsp	Spice, Black Pepper
0.5 Cup	Vegetable, Pepper, Sweet, Red, raw
0.5 Cup	Vegetable, Celery Raw
0.75 Cup	Vegetable, Carrots
4.5 teaspoon	Spice, Paprika
0.666 Cup	Mayonnaise, reduced kcal, cholest free/Hellmann
0.5 Cup	Macaroni, unenriched, dry

Instructions

Bring a large pot of water to a boil. Add the shells and cook according to the package directions, 6-9 minutes. Drain. Rinse in cool water, and allow to drain completely. Set aside to cool. Combine the mayonnaise and paprika in a large bowl. Add the cooled pasta and the carrot, celery, bell pepper and green onion. Toss to combine. Season with pepper. Chill, covered, until cold - about 2 hours.

Nutritionals

Calories 163.8	Sodium: 368.6	Protein: 5.3	Phos 105.?
Fat: 2	Carbs: 34.1	Chol: 3.8	Pot: 324.9
Sat Fat: 0.4	Fiber: 5.7		
	Sugar: 6.7		

Meal: *Broiled Salmon GDM*

Broiled Salmon with Marmalade Dijon Glaze

Serves: 4
Serving Size: 5-6 oz fillet

Ingredients

Amount	Ingredient
0.5 cup	Marmalade, sweet, orange
1 Tablespoon	Dijon Mustard
0.5 teaspoon	Spice, Garlic Powder
0.25 tsp	Salt
0.25 tsp	Spice, Black Pepper
0.25 Teaspoo	Spice, Ginger
24 Oz	Fish, Salmon, baked or broiled

Instructions

Preheat broiler. Combine marmalade, dijon mustard, garlic powder, salt, pepper and ginger in a small bowl, stir well. Place fish on a jelly roll pan coated with cooking spray. Brush half of marmalade mixture over fish; broil 6 minutes. Brush fish with remaining marmalade mixture; broil for 2 minutes or until fish flakes easily when tested with a fork or until desired degree of doneness.

Nutritionals

Calories 333.6	Sodium: 848.7	Protein: 33.6	Phos 390
Fat: 9.9	Carbs: 9.9	Chol: 86.9	Pot: 571.9
Sat Fat: 1.7	Fiber: 0.3		
	Sugar: 24.2		

Coconut Rice

Serves: 4
Serving Size: 1/2 cup

Ingredients

Amount	Ingredient
10 oz	Water
0.25 tsp	Salt
4 Ounces	Milk, Coconut, canned
8 Ounces	Grain, Rice, Basmati, raw

Instructions

Combine basmati rice, water, coconut milk and salt in a small saucepan. Bring to a boil. Cover, reduce heat and simmer 16 min. or until liquid is absorbed.

Nutritionals

Calories 224.5	Sodium: 153.5	Protein: 3.868	Phos 80.3
Fat: 6.331	Carbs: 37.8	Chol: 0	Pot: 116.1
Sat Fat: 5.427	Fiber: 0.601		
	Sugar: 0.056		

Recipe		Ingredients	Instructions	Nutritionals			

Recipe 1

Ratatouille

Serves: 6

Serving Size: 1 Cup

Amount	Ingredient
3 Teaspoon	Oil, Olive
2 Teaspoon	Herb, Garlic, Raw
1 Each	Vegetable, Eggplant
1.5 Cup	Vegetable, Zucchini, slices
1 Cup	Vegetable, Pepper, Green
0.5 tsp	Salt
0.25 tsp	Spice, Black Pepper
8 ounces	Vegetable, Tomato, Red Canned, No Added Salt

Instructions: Add oil to a large nonstick skillet over medium to high heat. Add garlic and sauté for 30 seconds. Add remaining ingredients and cook 10 to 15 min., stirring occasionally, until vegetables are tender.

Nutritionals:

Calories 41.4	Sodium: 201.3	Protein: 1.074	Phos 28.3
Fat: 2.468	Carbs: 4.775	Chol: 0	Pot: 228.7
Sat Fat: 0.362	Fiber: 1.612		
	Sugar: 2.585		

Meal: Chicken Marsala GDM

Recipe 2

Chicken Marsala

Serves: 4

Serving Size: 4 ounce chicken breast, plus sauce

Amount	Ingredient
16 ounces	Chicken, Breast Boneless
4 cup	Vegetable, Mushrooms, slices, raw
0.25 Teaspoo	Herb, Garlic, Raw
1 Tablespoon	Flour, White bleached enriched
1.666 cup	Soup, Chicken Broth Low Sodium
0.25 tsp	Salt
0.25 tsp	Spice, Black Pepper
2 Oz	Wine, dessert, sweet - marsala

Instructions: Coat a large nonstick skillet with cooking spray. Over medium-high heat, sauté chicken breasts for 6 min. on each side. Remove from pan and set aside. Spray pan again with cooking spray, and reduce heat to medium. Add mushrooms and garlic and sauté until all the liquid is evaporated. Add flour, stirring well to coat the mushrooms. Cook for one more minute. Add wine, stirring well to incorporate the flour. Add broth and turn heat to high. Let simmer for 5 min. Add salt and pepper. Serve sauce over chicken breasts.

Nutritionals:

Calories 199.7	Sodium: 311.7	Protein: 28.7	Phos 335
Fat: 3.816	Carbs: 8.789	Chol: 72.6	Pot: 749.8
Sat Fat: 0.864	Fiber: 0.855		
	Sugar: 2.681		

Recipe 3

Creamy Herbed Mashed Potatoes

Serves: 6

Serving Size: 3/4 Cup

Amount	Ingredient
4 Cup	Vegetable, Potato, Flesh only, diced, raw
4 fluid ounces	Milk, Nonfat/Skim
1 Tablespoon	Cream, Sour, Reduced Fat
3 tablespoon	Butter, Light w/no added salt
3 Tablespoon	Herb, Chives, raw
4 Springs	Herb, Parsley, Raw, Fresh
0.5 tsp	Salt
0.5 tsp	Spice, Black Pepper

Instructions: Peel and cube potatoes. Place potato in a saucepan; cover with water. Bring to a boil; cover, reduce heat, and simmer 10 minutes or until tender. Drain. Return potato to pan. Add milk and remaining ingredients; mash with a potato masher to desired consistency.

Nutritionals:

Calories 147.1	Sodium: 215.1	Protein: 3.1	Phos 73
Fat: 4.6	Carbs: 23.8	Chol: 11	Pot: 422.7
Sat Fat: 2.8	Fiber: 2.1		
	Sugar: 2.3		

Recipe	Ingredients		Instructions	Nutritionals			
Cucumber and Tomato Salad	2 Cup	Vegetable, Cucumber, peeled, raw	Peel and dice cucumbers. Chop or dice tomatoes. In a medium bowl, toss cucumbers and tomatoes. Drizzle oil and vinegar over vegetables and toss to coat. Season with salt and pepper.	Calories 44.6	Sodium: 237.8	Protein: 0.961	Phos 29.1
Serves: 5	3 Teaspoon	Oil, Olive		Fat: 2.933	Carbs: 4.056	Chol: 0	Pot: 246.7
Serving Size: 1/5 recipe	2 Cup	Vegetable, Tomato Red Raw		Sat Fat: 0.401	Fiber: 1.264		
	6 Teaspoon	Vinegar, Red Wine			Sugar: 2.628		
	0.5 tsp	Salt					
	0.25 tsp	Spice, Black Pepper					

Recipe	Ingredients	Instructions	Nutritionals			
Pear	6 Fruit Fruit, Pear Raw	Piece of fruit	Calories 115.5	Sodium: 0	Protein: 1.3	Phos 30.2
Serves: 6			Fat: 0.6	Carbs: 29.3	Chol: 0	Pot: 332.8
Serving Size: 1 medium pear			Sat Fat: 0	Fiber: 9.9		
				Sugar: 19.4		

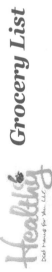

Grocery List

Hamburger Stroganoff GDM Meal

Hamburger Stroganoff

Quantity		Grocery Item
0.25	Teaspoon	Herb, Garlic, Raw
1	Cup	Vegetable, Onions
12	Tablespoons	Cream, Sour, Reduced Fat
0.5	tsp	Salt
0.125	tsp	Spice, Black Pepper
0.333	Tablespoon	Oil, Vegetable or Olive
16	ounces	Beef, Ground (95% lean)
0.2	Cup	Flour, Wheat, White, All Purpose,
1	Tablespoon	Herb, Parsley, dried
1	Cup	Soup, Beef broth, canned, low sodium
1	Cup	Noodles, Egg, enriched, dry
0.5	Ounces	Wine, table, red - dry sherry
8	Ounces	Vegetable, Mushrooms Canned

Loaded Nachos with Turkey GDM Meal

Loaded Nachos with Turkey, Beans and Salsa

Quantity		Grocery Item
1	tsp	Spice, Black Pepper
1	Cup	Beans, Black, Canned
6	ounces	Yogurt, Greek Non Fat
0.75	Cup	Cheese, Mexican blend, reduced fat -
6	ounces	Tortilla chips, low fat, baked without fat
1	Cup	Salsa
1.5	Pound	Turkey, Ground Raw
1	teaspoon	Salt, Kosher
0.75	Cup	Herb, Cilantro Raw

Garden Coleslaw With Almonds

Quantity		Grocery Item
0.4	Tablespoon	Dijon Mustard
9	Teaspoon	Vinegar, rice
2	ounces	Yogurt, Greek Non Fat
1	Each	Vegetable, Cabbage Head
1	ounces	Honey
0.25	tsp	Spice, Black Pepper
0.25	Cup	Nuts, Almond Sliced
1	Cup	Vegetable, Carrots
6	Teaspoon	Oil, Olive

Barbecue Chicken Burger GDM Meal

Barbecue Chicken Burger

Quantity		Grocery Item
1	Tablespoon	Worcestershire Sauce
0.75	Cup	Vegetable, Onions
0.333	Tablespoon	Dijon Mustard
0.75	cup	Breadcrumbs, Seasoned
1	Teaspoon	Herb, Thyme Ground
14	Ounces	Chicken, Ground
0.25	Teaspoon	Herb, Garlic, Raw
5	Tablespoon	Sauce, BBQ
4	each	Bread, Roll, Hamburger, Whole
0.125	cup	Soup, Chicken Broth Low Sodium

Roasted Asparagus

Quantity		Grocery Item
0.5	teaspoon	Spice, Garlic Powder
0.5	Teaspoon	Spice, Lemon Pepper
24	Ounces	Vegetable, Asparagus Fresh

Oven Fries

Quantity		Grocery Item
3	Each	Egg White
3	each	Vegetable, Potato
1	Teaspoon	Spice, Mrs. Dash

Broccoli Casserole

Quantity		Grocery Item
4	Cup	Vegetable, Broccoli Florets, Raw
6	Ounces	Soup, Cream of Celery, Fat Free
0.5	Cup	Cheese, Cheddar reduced fat
0.125	tsp	Spice, Black Pepper
4	fluid ounces	Milk, Nonfat/Skim

Macaroni Salad

Quantity		Grocery Item
0.5	Cup	Vegetable, Pepper, Sweet, Red, raw
4.5	teaspoon	Spice, Paprika
0.5	Cup	Vegetable, Celery Raw
0.666	Cup	Mayonnaise, reduced kcal, cholest
0.5	Cup	Vegetable, Onions, Young Green, raw
0.5	Cup	Macaroni, unenriched, dry
0.75	Cup	Vegetable, Carrots
0.5	tsp	Spice, Black Pepper

Orange

Quantity		Grocery Item
6	1	Fruit, Orange, All Varieties, peeled, raw

Rosemary Roasted Potatoes

Quantity		Grocery Item
0.75	Teaspoon	Herb, Garlic, Raw
3	teaspoon	Herb, Rosemary, Dried
1	Tablespoon	Oil, Vegetable or Olive
5	each	Vegetable, Potato
2	teaspoon	Spice, Paprika

Smoky Grilled Pork Chops GDM Meal

Smoky Pan Grilled Pork Chops

Quantity		Grocery Item
3	Teaspoon Pac	Sugar, Brown
0.25	tsp	Salt
0.25	tsp	Spice, Black Pepper
16	ounces	Pork, Center Rib Chop
3	tsp	Spice, Cumin, Ground
1	teaspoon	Spice, Paprika

Couscous with Tomato and Dill

Quantity		Grocery Item
0.25	tsp	Salt
5	Tablespoon	Vegetable, Onions, Red
3	Teaspoon	Oil, Olive
3	Teaspoon	Herb, Dill Weed
0.5	cup	Soup, Chicken Broth Low Sodium
0.5	Cup	Vegetable, Tomato, Red, Cherry
0.5	Cup	Grain, Couscous

Italian Green Beans

Quantity		Grocery Item
1	Cup	Vegetable, Onions
0.25	Teaspoon	Herb, Basil, Ground
2	Teaspoon	Herb, Garlic, Raw
0.25	Teaspoon	Herb, Oregano, Ground
3	Teaspoon	Oil, Olive
16	Ounces	Vegetable, Beans, Italian, Frozen
1	Can	Vegetable, Tomato Diced Canned

Tossed Pear and Almond Salad

Quantity		Grocery Item
2	Fruit	Fruit, Pear Raw
0.25	Cup	Nuts, Almond Sliced
6	Cup	Lettuce, Raw Iceberg
6	Tablespoon	Salad Dressing, Vinaigrette

Red Pepper Frittata GDM Meal

Red Pepper Frittata

Quantity		Grocery Item
0.333	Cup	Grain, Couscous
2.15	Ounce	Cheese, Monterey, lowfat - Monterey Jack
2	Cup	Vegetable, Pepper, Sweet, Red, raw
0.5	Teaspoon	Herb, Garlic, Raw
4	oz	Water
4	Each	Egg White
0.5	Cup	Vegetable, Onions
1	tsp	Spice, Black Pepper
0.75	tsp	Salt
3	Each	Egg, Whole

Broiled Salmon GDM Meal

Broiled Salmon with Marmalade Dijon Glaze

Quantity		Grocery Item
0.25	tsp	Spice, Black Pepper
0.25	tsp	Salt
0.5	cup	Marmalade, sweet, orange
1	Tablespoon	Dijon Mustard
0.25	Teaspoon	Spice, Ginger
24	Oz	Fish, Salmon, baked or broiled
0.5	teaspoon	Spice, Garlic Powder

Coconut Rice

Quantity		Grocery Item
10	oz	Water
4	Ounces	Milk, Coconut, canned
8	Ounces	Grain, Rice, Basmati, raw
0.25	tsp	Salt

Ratatouille

Quantity		Grocery Item
0.5	tsp	Salt
1	Each	Vegetable, Eggplant
3	Teaspoon	Oil, Olive
8	ounces	Vegetable, Tomato, Red Canned, No Added
2	Teaspoon	Herb, Garlic, Raw
0.25	tsp	Spice, Black Pepper
1.5	Cup	Vegetable, Zucchini, slices
1	Cup	Vegetable, Pepper, Green

Chicken Marsala GDM Meal

Chicken Marsala

Quantity		Grocery Item
1	Tablespoons	Flour, White bleached enriched
2	Oz	Wine, dessert, sweet - marsala
0.25	Teaspoon	Herb, Garlic, Raw
4	cup	Vegetable, Mushrooms, slices, raw
0.25	tsp	Spice, Black Pepper
0.25	tsp	Salt
16	ounces	Chicken, Breast Boneless
1.666	cup	Soup, Chicken Broth Low Sodium

Creamy Herbed Mashed Potatoes

Quantity		Grocery Item
4	Cup	Vegetable, Potato, Flesh only, diced, raw
3	tablespoon	Butter, Light w/no added salt
1	Tablespoons	Cream, Sour, Reduced Fat
4	fluid ounces	Milk, Nonfat/Skim
0.5	tsp	Spice, Black Pepper
0.5	tsp	Salt
4	Springs	Herb, Parsley, Raw, Fresh
3	Tablespoon	Herb, Chives, raw

Cucumber and Tomato Salad

Quantity		Grocery Item
0.5	tsp	Salt
0.25	tsp	Spice, Black Pepper
2	Cup	Vegetable, Tomato Red Raw
6	Teaspoon	Vinegar, Red Wine
2	Cup	Vegetable, Cucumber, peeled, raw
3	Teaspoon	Oil, Olive

Pear

Quantity		Grocery Item
6	Fruit	Fruit, Pear Raw

Week 6 Meals and Grocery Lists

Patty Melts with Grilled Onions with Rosemary Roasted Potatoes and Oranges

Cheesy Chicken Enchiladas with Corn on the Cob

Turkey Kielbasa Apple Pasta Bake with Wild Rice Pilaf and Grapes

Fish Tacos with Lime Cream Sauce with Creamy Lemon Coleslaw, Oven Fries, and Strawberries

Balsamic Plum Glazed Pork Chops with Rice and Noodle Pilaf, Roasted Acorn Squash and Steamed Carrots

Cauliflower, Broccoli with Spinach Casserole, Coconut Rice and Brussels Sprouts and Bacon

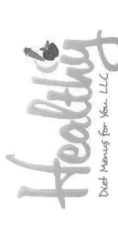

Diet Menus for You. LLC

Meal Plan

www.healthydietmenusforyou.com

Diet: *Gestational Diabetic - 2400*

Meal: *Patty Melt with Onion GDM*

Recipe		Ingredients	Instructions	Nutritionals					

Patty Melts with Grilled Onions

Serves: *4*

Serving Size: *1 sandwich*

	Ingredients
1 Tablespoon	Vinegar, balsamic
1 Cup	Vegetable, Onions, Vidalia, raw
16 ounces	Beef, Ground (95% lean)
0.25 tsp	Salt
0.25 tsp	Spice, Black Pepper
8 slice	Bread, Rye, Hi Fiber, reduced kcal
3 Tablespoon	Mustard, Dijon
1 Cup	Cheese, Mozzarella Part Skim

Instructions

1. Arrange onion slices on a plate. Drizzle vinegar over onion slices. Heat a large grill pan over medium heat. Coat pan with cooking spray. Add onion to pan; cover and cook 3 minutes on each side. Remove from pan; cover and keep warm.

2. Heat pan over medium-high heat. Coat pan with cooking spray. Divide beef into 4 equal portions, shaping each into a 1/2-inch-thick patty. Sprinkle patties evenly with salt and pepper. Add patties to pan; cook 3 minutes on each side or until done.

3. Spread about 1 teaspoon mustard blend over 4 bread slices; layer each slice with 2 tablespoons cheese, 1 patty, 2 onion slices, and 2 tablespoons cheese. Spread about 1 teaspoon mustard blend over remaining bread slices; place, mustard side down, on top of sandwiches.

4. Heat pan over medium heat. Coat pan with cooking spray. Add sandwiches to pan. Place a cast-iron or other heavy skillet on top of sandwiches; press gently to flatten. Cook 3 minutes on each side or until bread is toasted (leave cast-iron skillet on sandwiches while they cook).

Nutritionals

Calories 391.4	Sodium: 636.8	Protein: 36	Phos 417.g
Fat: 16.4	Carbs: 25.9	Chol: 84.7	Pot: 508.6
Sat Fat: 6.338	Fiber: 6.044		
	Sugar: 3.761		

Rosemary Roasted Potatoes

Serves: 6

Serving Size: 3/4 cup Potatoes

Ingredients		Instructions	Nutritionals						
5 each	Vegetable, Potato	Wash and dice potatoes into bite-sized pieces. Place into a large bowl or Ziplock bag; toss with olive oil. Sprinkle garlic, rosemary, paprika (optional), and pepper over potatoes and shake to coat. Layer potatoes in a single layer on a baking sheet coated with cooking spray. Bake at 400 F for 30 minutes or until slightly browned. Serves 5.	Calories 132.8	Sodium: 12.3	Protein: 3.094	Phos 85.4		
1 Tablespoon	Oil, Vegetable or Olive		Fat: 2.581	Carbs: 25.5	Chol: 0	Pot: 642		
0.75 Teaspoo	Herb, Garlic, Raw		Sat Fat: 0.407	Fiber: 3.056				
3 teaspoon	Herb, Rosemary, Dried			Sugar: 1.443				
2 teaspoon	Spice, Paprika							

Orange

Serves: 6

Serving Size: 1 Peeled Orange

Ingredients		Instructions	Nutritionals						
6 1	Fruit, Orange, All Varieties, peeled, raw	Piece of fruit.	Calories 86.5	Sodium: 0	Protein: 1.7	Phos 25.8		
			Fat: 0.2	Carbs: 21.6	Chol: 0	Pot: 333		
			Sat Fat: 0	Fiber: 4.4				
				Sugar: 17.2				

Meal: *Cheesy Chicken Enchilada GDM*

Cheesy Chicken Enchiladas

Serves: 8

Serving Size: 1 enchilada

Ingredients		Instructions	Nutritionals						
20 ounces	Chicken, Breast Boneless	Preheat the oven to 350'F. Cook chicken and chop or dice into bite size pieces. (2.5 cups) Combine the chicken, cheese, yogurt, butter, onion, garlic, black pepper, cream of chicken soup and chiles. Remove one cup of mixture and set aside. Heat a large skillet over medium high heat. Working with 1 tortilla at a time, put the tortilla in the pan, cook 5 seconds on each side or until toasted and soft. Remove from pan, arrange 1/2 cup chicken mixture down the center of the tortilla. Roll jelly-roll style, then place filled tortilla, seam side down in a 13 x 9 inch baking dish coated with cooking spray. Repeat procedure with remaining 7 tortillas and chicken mixture. Spread reserved chicken mixture evenly over enchiladas. Cover and bake at 350'F for 20 minutes. Uncover; sprinkle evenly with cheddar cheese and green onions, bake an additional 5 minutes or until cheese melts.	Calories 489.6	Sodium: 832.5	Protein: 38.9	Phos 537.6		
2 Cup	Cheese, Mexican blend, reduced fat - Kraft Mexican Four Cheese made with 2% Milk		Fat: 19.2	Carbs: 38.7	Chol: 100.8	Pot: 543.8		
8 Oz	Yogurt, plain, lowfat milk		Sat Fat: 9.2	Fiber: 2.1				
4 tablespoon	Butter, Light w/no added salt			Sugar: 4.3				
0.25 Cup	Vegetable, Onions							
1 tsp	Garlic, Minced							
0.25 tsp	Spice, Black Pepper							
1.25 Cup	Soup, Cream of Chicken Fat Free							
4 oz	Vegetable, Green Chilies, Canned							
8 Each	Tortilla, Flour (Wheat)							
0.5 Cup	Cheese, processed, Cheddar type, lowfat							
0.25 Cup	Vegetable, Onions, Young Green, raw							

Corn On The Cob

Recipe	Ingredients		Instructions
Corn On The Cob	6 Each	Vegetable, Corn on Cob, sm/med, ckd w/o fat or salt	Shuck and clean corn. Boil until tender, about 4-6 minutes.
Serves: 6			
Serving Size: 1 ear of corn			

Nutritionals

Calories 82.7	Sodium: 1.5	Protein: 2.5	Phos 78.8	
Fat: 0.9	Carbs: 19.2	Chol: 0	Pot: 190.6	
Sat Fat: 0.1	Fiber: 2.8			
	Sugar: 0			

Meal: *Turkey Pasta Bake GDM*

Turkey Kielbasa Apple Pasta Bake

Recipe	Ingredients		Instructions
Turkey Kielbasa Apple Pasta Bake	16 fluid ounce	Milk, Nonfat/Skim	Cook pasta and hold. Chop onions and core and chop apples. Whisk milk and flour together over medium heat. Continue to cook and stir until thickened and bubbly. Remove from heat, add cheese, salt and pepper. Stir until smooth. In a large baking dish, gently combine pasta, apples, kielbasa and cheese sauce. Cover with foil and bake 20 minutes at 350°F. Remove foil and bake for 15 more minutes. Sprinkle onions on top.
Serves: 6	0.75 cup	Cheese, Colby Jack Shredded	
Serving Size: 1/6 pan	1 cup	Noodles, Macaroni Cooked	
	2 Tablespoon	Flour, White bleached enriched	
	0.5 tsp	Salt	
	0.5 tsp	Spice, Black Pepper	
	2 cup	Fruit, Apple w/skin Granny Smith	
	8 ounce	Turkey Kielbasa Lowfat 97% Fat Free	
	0.25 Cup	Vegetable, Green Onion	

Nutritionals

Calories 160	Sodium: 617	Protein: 11	Phos 202	
Fat: 2.3	Carbs: 24	Chol: 13	Pot: 300	
Sat Fat: 1	Fiber: 1.9			
	Sugar: 8.8			

Wild Rice Pilaf

Recipe	Ingredients		Instructions
Wild Rice Pilaf	3 Teaspoon	Oil, Olive	Heat the oil in a large saucepan over medium heat. Add the mushrooms and onions, and sauté until browned, about 5 min. Add the wild rice, barley, garlic and thyme, and sauté for 1 min. longer. Add the chicken broth and salt and bring to a boil. Reduce to a simmer, cover, and cook until the liquid is absorbed, about 45 min. Let stand, covered, until ready to serve. Makes 4 cups.
Serves: 6	1 cup	Vegetable, Mushrooms, slices, raw	
Serving Size: 3/4 cup	1 Cup	Vegetable, Onions	
	0.5 Teaspoon	Herb, Garlic, Raw	
	0.5 Cup	Grain, Barley	
	1 Teaspoon	Herb, Thyme Ground	
	4 cup	Soup, Chicken Broth Low Sodium	
	0.5 Cup	Grain, Wild Rice	

Nutritionals

Calories 162.6	Sodium: 52.8	Protein: 7.812	Phos 165.9	
Fat: 3.795	Carbs: 26.5	Chol: 0	Pot: 345.5	
Sat Fat: 0.716	Fiber: 4.155			
	Sugar: 2.039			

Recipe

Recipe		Ingredients	Instructions	Nutritionals					

Grapes

Ingredients		Instructions	Nutritionals						
9 Cup	Fruit, Grapes, raw	Wash and remove stems from grapes prior to eating.	Calories 92.5	Sodium: 2.7	Protein: 0.8	Phos 13.8			
			Fat: 0.4	Carbs: 23.7	Chol: 0	Pot: 263.6			
			Sat Fat: 0.1	Fiber: 1.2					
				Sugar: 22.4					

Serves: 6

Serving Size: 1.5 cups of grapes

Meal: *Fish Tacos GDM*

Fish Tacos with Lime Cream Sauce

Ingredients		Instructions	Nutritionals		
0.25 Cup	Vegetable, Onions, Young Green, raw	To prepare crema. Grate lime rind, and squeeze lime juice into bowl. Combine the green onions, cilantro, Mayo, sour cream, lime rind and lime juice, and garlic clove in a small bowl; set aside. To prepare tacos, combine cumin, coriander, paprika, red pepper, and garlic powder in a small bowl; sprinkle spice mixture evenly over both sides of fish. Place fish on a baking sheet coated with cooking spray. Bake at 425° for 9 minutes or until fish flakes easily when tested with a fork or until desired degree of doneness. Place fish in a bowl; break into pieces with a fork. Heat tortillas according to package directions. Divide fish evenly among tortillas; top each with 1/4 cup cabbage and 1 tablespoon crema	Calories 324.3	Sodium: 241.3	Protein: 39.1	Phos 523
0.25 Cup	Herb, Cilantro Raw		Fat: 5.706	Carbs: 29.3	Chol: 69.8	Pot: 955.4
0.15 Cup	Mayonnaise, reduced kcal, cholest free/Hellmann		Sat Fat: 1.698	Fiber: 5.194		
3 Tablespoon	Cream, Sour, Reduced Fat			Sugar: 4.02		
1 Each	Fruit, Lime					
0.25 Teaspoo	Herb, Garlic, Raw					
1 tsp	Spice, Cumin, Ground					
1 Teaspoon	Spice, Coriander Seed					
0.5 teaspoon	Spice, Paprika					
0.25 teaspoo	Spice, Red Pepper					
0.125 teaspo	Spice, Garlic Powder					
24 ounces	Fish, Snapper, raw					
8 Each	Tortilla, Corn					
0.5 Each	Vegetable, Cabbage Head					

Serves: 4

Serving Size: 2 tacos

Creamy Lemon Coleslaw

Ingredients		Instructions	Nutritionals			
1 Each	Vegetable, Cabbage Head	Shred cabbage and chop onions. Combine all ingredients in a bowl, and toss lightly. Refrigerate if not used immediately.	Calories 81	Sodium: 158	Protein: 1.7	Phos 34
6 Each	Sugar Substitute Packet, Equal		Fat: 3	Carbs: 12	Chol: 4	Pot: 211
0.125 Cup	Vegetable, Onions		Sat Fat: 0.5	Fiber: 3		
0.5 teaspoon	Salt, Kosher			Sugar: 5.5		
6 Tablespoon	Miracle Whip Light					
2 Packet	True Lemon packet					

Serves: 6

Serving Size: 1/6 of container

Oven Fries

Recipe	Ingredients		Instructions	Nutritionals					
Oven Fries	3 each	Vegetable, Potato	Cut potatoes into strips like fries. Beat egg whites and toss with fries. Sprinkle with Mrs. Dash type seasoning. Bake for 30 minutes at 400°F or until done.	Calories 75	Sodium: 45	Protein: 3.3	Phos 55		
Serves: 6	1 Teaspoon	Spice, Mrs. Dash		Fat: 0.2	Carbs: 15	Chol: 0	Pot: 406		
Serving Size: 1/2 potato	3 Each	Egg White		Sat Fat: 0	Fiber: 2				
					Sugar: 1				

Strawberries

Recipe	Ingredients	Instructions	Nutritionals				
Strawberries	9 Cup	Fruit, Strawberries, halves/slices, raw	Remove tops and wash prior to serving.	Calories 73	Sodium: 2.2	Protein: 1.5	Phos 54.7
Serves: 6				Fat: 0.6	Carbs: 17.5	Chol: 0	Pot: 348.8
Serving Size: 1.5 Cups of Strawberries				Sat Fat: 0	Fiber: 4.5		
					Sugar: 11.1		

Meal: *Balsamic Glazed Pork Chop GDM*

Balsamic Plum Glazed Pork Chops

Recipe	Ingredients		Instructions	Nutritionals				
Balsamic Plum Glazed Pork Chops	0.33 tablespo	Butter, Light w/no added salt	Melt butter in a large non-stick skillet over medium high heat. Add pork to pan, cook 3 1/2 minutes on each side. Remove from pan. Coat pan with cooking spray. Add onions and garlic to pan, saute for 30 seconds. Add port and vinegar to pan; cook 30 seconds, stirring occasionally. Stir in 1/4 tsp salt and plum preserves, then cook for 30 seconds or until smooth while stirring constantly. Return pork to pan, cook 30 seconds or until desired degree of doneness while turning to coat. Sprinkle with parsley if desired.	Calories 238.7	Sodium: 575.5	Protein: 21.2	Phos 7.1	
Serves: 4	16 ounces	Pork, Center Rib Chop		Fat: 11.4	Carbs: 8.3	Chol: 59.4	Pot: 388.9	
	0.25 tsp	Salt		Sat Fat: 4.4	Fiber: 0.2			
Serving Size: 4 oz chop + glaze	0.125 Cup	Vegetable, Onions			Sugar: 2.7			
	1 Teaspoon	Herb, Garlic, Raw						
	2 Oz	Wine, dessert, sweet - port						
	2 Tablespoon	Vinegar, balsamic						
	0.33 Cup	Fruit, Plum Preserves						
	10 Springs	Herb, Parsley, Raw, Fresh						

Rice and Noodle Pilaf

Recipe	Ingredients		Instructions	Nutritionals				
Rice and Noodle Pilaf	2 tablespoon	Butter, Light w/no added salt	Break spaghetti noodles into small sections about 1-2 inches long. Melt the butter in a large saucepan over medium heat, and add spaghetti. Sauté spaghetti for 5 minutes or until lightly browned. Add the rice, stirring to coat. Stir in the boiling water, salt, and pepper, and bring to a boil. Cover; reduce heat, and simmer for 20 minutes or until the liquid is absorbed. Remove pilaf from heat, and let stand for 10 minutes. Fluff with a fork.	Calories 188.2	Sodium: 103.8	Protein: 4.4	Phos 131.1	
Serves: 6	0.3 Cup	Pasta, Spaghetti		Fat: 3.4	Carbs: 34.5	Chol: 4.5	Pot: 105.3	
	1 Cup	Rice, Medium Brown		Sat Fat: 1.6	Fiber: 1.5			
Serving Size: 2/3 cup	16 oz	Water			Sugar: 0.6			
	0.25 tsp	Salt						
	0.25 tsp	Spice, Black Pepper						

Roasted Acorn Squash

Serves: 8

Serving Size: 1/8 recipe

Ingredients		Instructions
0.5 tsp	Salt	Preheat oven to 400°. Cut them off of each squash and cut in half lengthwise. Scoop out seeds; rinse and dry each squash, half. Spray all sides of squash halves with cooking spray. Season inside of each half with salt and pepper. Place cut side down on a nonstick cooking spray coated baking sheet. Bake for 45 min.. Scoop squash meat out into a medium bowl; discard skins. Add olive oil and beat with a sturdy whisk until fluffy.
0.25 tsp	Spice, Black Pepper	
2 Teaspoon	Oil, Olive	
32 Ounces	Vegetable, Squash, Acorn, peeled, raw	

Nutritionals

Calories 100.8	Sodium: 72.5	Protein: 1.822	Phos 81.8	
Fat: 1.354	Carbs: 23.7	Chol: 0	Pot: 787.9	
Sat Fat: 0.204	Fiber: 3.419			
	Sugar: 0			

Steamed Carrots

Serves: 6

Serving Size: 1/2 cup

Ingredients		Instructions
3 Cup	Vegetable, Carrots	Steam carrots until tender, season with Mrs. Dash
1 Teaspoon	Spice, Mrs. Dash	

Nutritionals

Calories 33	Sodium: 2	Protein: 1	Phos 22
Fat: 0	Carbs: 8	Chol: 0	Pot: 165
Sat Fat: 0	Fiber: 3		
	Sugar: 0		

Meal: *Cauliflower, Broccoli and Spinach Casser*

Cauliflower, Broccoli and Spinach Casserole

Serves: 6

Serving Size: 1/6 pan

Ingredients		Instructions
0.5 Cup	Cheese, Grated Parmesan, Reduced Fat	Steam the broccoli and cauliflower for about 5 minutes. Combine flour and milk and bring to a slow boil for 1 minute. Add parmesan cheese and stir. Add spinach, nutmeg and pepper and stir. Stir all ingredients together and place in a sprayed 8x8 baking dish. Bake for 25 minutes at 250°F. Serves 6 people.
3 Cup	Vegetable, Broccoli Florets, Raw	
3 Cup	Vegetable, Cauliflower, Raw	
4 Tablespoon	Flour, White bleached enriched	
12 fluid ounce	Milk, Nonfat/Skim	
0.25 teaspoo	Spice, Nutmeg Ground	
0.25 tsp	Spice, Black Pepper	
1 Cup	Vegetable, Spinach Frozen	

Nutritionals

Calories 104	Sodium: 218	Protein: 8.3	Phos 204
Fat: 2.3	Carbs: 14.9	Chol: 8.6	Pot: 572
Sat Fat: 1.2	Fiber: 4		
	Sugar: 5.5		

Creamed Spinach

Serves: 4
Serving Size: 3 oz

Nutritionals

Calories 78.6	Sodium: 372.7	Protein: 4.8	Phos 89.5
Fat: 3.3	Carbs: 8.7	Chol: 7.6	Pot: 571.3
Sat Fat: 1.9	Fiber: 2.3		
	Sugar: 3.4		

Ingredients

Amount	Ingredient
1 tablespoon	Butter, Light w/no added salt
3 Teaspoon	Herb, Garlic, Raw
0.5 Cup	Vegetable, Onions, Young Green, raw
0.5 tsp	Salt
0.5 tsp	Spice, Black Pepper
0.25 teaspoo	Spice, Nutmeg Ground
1.25 Ounces	Vegetable, Spinach, raw, torn
1 Teaspoon	Cornstarch, hydrolyzed powder
3 ounces	Yogurt, Greek Non Fat

Instructions

Heat a large non-stick saute pan over medium heat. Add the butter to the pan, and when it has melted add the garlic and onions. Season with salt, pepper and a pinch of nutmeg. Cook, stirring often, until the onions are tender, about 4 minutes.

Raise heat to high and add half the spinach. Season it lightly with salt and pepper. Toss and stir the spinach as it cooks down. When there is enough room in the pan, add the remaining spinach. Continue to cook, stirring often, until the spinach is tender, about 3 minutes. Sprinkle the cornstarch over the spinach and stir until combined. Continue to cook the spinach until the liquid has thickened, about 1 minute. Remove the pan from heat. Add the yogurt and stir to coat the spinach. Serves 4.

Coconut Rice

Serves: 4
Serving Size: 1/2 cup

Nutriitionals

Calories 224.5	Sodium: 153.5	Protein: 3.868	Phos 80.3
Fat: 6.331	Carbs: 37.8	Chol: 0.601	Pot: 116.1
Sat Fat: 5.427	Fiber: 0		
	Sugar: 0.056		

Ingredients

Amount	Ingredient
10 oz	Water
0.25 tsp	Salt
4 Ounces	Milk, Coconut, canned
8 Ounces	Grain, Rice, Basmati, raw

Instructions

Combine basmati rice, water, coconut milk and salt in a small saucepan. Bring to a boil. Cover, reduce heat and simmer 16 min. or until liquid is absorbed.

Brussel Sprouts and Baco

Serves: 4
Serving Size: 4 ounces

Nutriitionals

Calories 121	Sodium: 402.1	Protein: 7.2	Phos 127
Fat: 6.2	Carbs: 12	Chol: 5	Pot: 528.2
Sat Fat: 1.6	Fiber: 5		
	Sugar: 2.7		

Ingredients

Amount	Ingredient
0.5 tsp	Salt
1 tsp	Spice, Black Pepper
4 Slices	Pork Bacon, Cured or Smoked, lower sodium, slices
2 Teaspoon	Herb, Garlic, Raw
1 teaspoon	Spice, Red Pepper
0.06 Cup	Nuts, Almond Sliced
1 Pounds	Vegetable, Brussels Sprouts, raw

Instructions

Cut the brussels sprouts in half and trim bottoms. Heat a large skillet or saute pan over medium heat. Add the bacon and cook until crispy, about 5 minutes. Remove to a plate lined with paper towels. Discard all but 1 tablespoon of the rendered bacon fat. Add the garlic, pepper flakes, brussels sprouts and salt to the skillet. Saute until the sprouts are lightly browned on the outside and tender - but still firm - throughout. Approx 10-12 minutes. Add the almonds and bacon (crumbled) and saute for another minute or two. Season with salt and pepper.

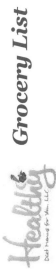

Grocery List

Patty Melt with Onion GDM Meal

Patty Melts with Grilled Onions

Quantity		Grocery Item
1	Cup	Vegetable, Onions, Vidalia, raw
1	Cup	Cheese, Mozzarella Part Skim
8	slice	Bread, Rye, Hi Fiber, reduced kcal
1	Tablespoon	Vinegar, balsamic
16	ounces	Beef, Ground (95% lean)
3	Tablespoon	Mustard, Dijon
0.25	tsp	Salt
0.25	tsp	Spice, Black Pepper

Rosemary Roasted Potatoes

Quantity		Grocery Item
1	Tablespoon	Oil, Vegetable or Olive
5	each	Vegetable, Potato
3	teaspoon	Herb, Rosemary, Dried
2	teaspoon	Spice, Paprika
0.75	Teaspoon	Herb, Garlic, Raw

Orange

Quantity	Grocery Item
6 1	Fruit, Orange, All Varieties, peeled, raw

Cheesy Chicken Enchilada GDM Meal

Cheesy Chicken Enchiladas

Quantity		Grocery Item
4	tablespoon	Butter, Light w/no added salt
0.25	tsp	Spice, Black Pepper
2	Cup	Cheese, Mexican blend, reduced fat -
0.25	Cup	Vegetable, Onions, Young Green, raw
20	ounces	Chicken, Breast Boneless
1.25	Cup	Soup, Cream of Chicken Fat Free
0.25	Cup	Vegetable, Onions
8	Oz	Yogurt, plain, lowfat milk
1	tsp	Garlic, Minced
8	Each	Tortilla, Flour (Wheat)
4	oz	Vegetable, Green Chilies, Canned
0.5	Cup	Cheese, processed, Cheddar type, lowfat

Corn On The Cob

Quantity		Grocery Item
6	Each	Vegetable, Corn on Cob, sm/med, ckd w/o

Turkey Pasta Bake GDM Meal

Turkey Kielbasa Apple Pasta Bake

Quantity		Grocery Item
16	fluid ounces	Milk, Nonfat/Skim
0.5	tsp	Spice, Black Pepper
0.5	tsp	Salt
0.25	Cup	Vegetable, Green Onion
1	cup	Noodles, Macaroni Cooked
2	Tablespoons	Flour, White bleached enriched
2	cup	Fruit, Apple w/skin Granny Smith
8	ounce	Turkey Kielbasa Lowfat 97% Fat Free
0.75	cup	Cheese, Colby Jack Shredded

Wild Rice Pilaf

Quantity		Grocery Item
0.5	Cup	Grain, Wild Rice
0.5	Cup	Grain, Barley
1	cup	Vegetable, Mushrooms, slices, raw
0.5	Teaspoon	Herb, Garlic, Raw
1	Cup	Vegetable, Onions
4	cup	Soup, Chicken Broth Low Sodium
3	Teaspoon	Oil, Olive
1	Teaspoon	Herb, Thyme Ground

Grapes

Quantity		Grocery Item
9	Cup	Fruit, Grapes, raw

111

Rice and Noodle Pilaf

Quantity		Grocery Item
16	oz	Water
2	tablespoon	Butter, Light w/no added salt
0.25	tsp	Spice, Black Pepper
0.25	tsp	Salt
1	Cup	Rice, Medium Brown
0.3	Cup	Pasta, Spaghetti

Roasted Acorn Squash

Quantity		Grocery Item
0.25	tsp	Spice, Black Pepper
32	Ounces	Vegetable, Squash, Acorn, peeled, raw
2	Teaspoon	Oil, Olive
0.5	tsp	Salt

Steamed Carrots

Quantity		Grocery Item
1	Teaspoon	Spice, Mrs. Dash
3	Cup	Vegetable, Carrots

Oven Fries

Quantity		Grocery Item
3	each	Vegetable, Potato
1	Teaspoon	Spice, Mrs. Dash
3	Each	Egg White

Strawberries

Quantity		Grocery Item
9	Cup	Fruit, Strawberries, halves/slices, raw

Balsamic Glazed Pork Chop GDM Meal

Balsamic Plum Glazed Pork Chops

Quantity		Grocery Item
0.33	Cup	Fruit, Plum Preserves
0.33	tablespoon	Butter, Light w/no added salt
0.25	tsp	Salt
2	Oz	Wine, dessert, sweet - port
0.125	Cup	Vegetable, Onions
1	Teaspoon	Herb, Garlic, Raw
2	Tablespoon	Vinegar, balsamic
16	ounces	Pork, Center Rib Chop
10	Springs	Herb, Parsley, Raw, Fresh

Fish Tacos GDM Meal

Fish Tacos with Lime Cream Sauce

Quantity		Grocery Item
1	Teaspoon	Spice, Coriander Seed
1	tsp	Spice, Cumin, Ground
0.25	Teaspoon	Herb, Garlic, Raw
1	Each	Fruit, Lime
0.5	Each	Vegetable, Cabbage Head
0.5	teaspoon	Spice, Paprika
0.125	teaspoon	Spice, Garlic Powder
0.25	teaspoon	Spice, Red Pepper
0.15	Cup	Mayonnaise, reduced kcal, cholest
3	Tablespoons	Cream, Sour, Reduced Fat
24	ounces	Fish, Snapper, raw
0.25	Cup	Vegetable, Onions, Young Green, raw
8	Each	Tortilla, Corn
0.25	Cup	Herb, Cilantro Raw

Creamy Lemon Coleslaw

Quantity		Grocery Item
6	Each	Sugar Substitute Packet, Equal
0.125	Cup	Vegetable, Onions
6	Tablespoon	Miracle Whip Light
1	Each	Vegetable, Cabbage Head
2	Packet	True Lemon packet
0.5	teaspoon	Salt, Kosher

Coconut Rice

Quantity		Grocery Item
4	Ounces	Milk, Coconut, canned
10	oz	Water
8	Ounces	Grain, Rice, Basmati, raw
0.25	tsp	Salt

Brussel Sprouts and Bacon

Quantity		Grocery Item
1	Pounds	Vegetable, Brussels Sprouts, raw
4	Slices	Pork Bacon, Cured or Smoked, lower
0.5	tsp	Salt
1	tsp	Spice, Black Pepper
2	Teaspoon	Herb, Garlic, Raw
0.06	Cup	Nuts, Almond Sliced
1	teaspoon	Spice, Red Pepper

Cauliflower, Broccoli and Spinach Casserole GDM Me

Cauliflower, Broccoli and Spinach Casserole

Quantity		Grocery Item
4	Tablespoons	Flour, White bleached enriched
0.25	tsp	Spice, Black Pepper
1	Cup	Vegetable, Spinach Frozen
12	fluid ounces	Milk, Nonfat/Skim
0.5	Cup	Cheese, Grated Parmesan, Reduced Fat
3	Cup	Vegetable, Broccoli Florets, Raw
0.25	teaspoon	Spice, Nutmeg Ground
3	Cup	Vegetable, Cauliflower, Raw

Creamed Spinach

Quantity		Grocery Item
0.5	tsp	Spice, Black Pepper
1	Teaspoon	Cornstarch, hydrolyzed powder
3	ounces	Yogurt, Greek Non Fat
1.25	Ounces	Vegetable, Spinach, raw, torn
0.5	Cup	Vegetable, Onions, Young Green, raw
3	Teaspoon	Herb, Garlic, Raw
0.25	teaspoon	Spice, Nutmeg Ground
0.5	tsp	Salt
1	tablespoon	Butter, Light w/no added salt

Week 7 Meals and Grocery Lists

Lemon-Basil Chicken with Basil Aioli with Rice and Beans Side, Broccoli Casserole and Tomato Ranch Salad

Skillet Fish Fillets with Cilantro Butter with Fried Rice, Garden Coleslaw with Almonds and Tomato Salad

Beefy Bowtie Pasta with Tomato Sauce with Brussels Sprouts with Bacon

Spiced Pork Chops with Apple Chutney with Spicy Greens and Down Home Baked Beans

Sloppy Joe's with Steamed Carrots and Creamy Lemon Coleslaw

Pasta with Tomato Basil Sauce with Lemon Spinach

Chicken Cordon Bleu with Garden Coleslaw with Almonds and Orzo with Herbs

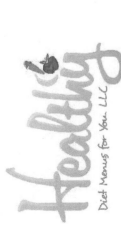

Diet Menus for You, LLC

Meal Plan

www.healthydietmenusforyou.com

Meal: *Lemon Basil Chicken GDM*

Recipe	Ingredients	Instructions	Nutritionals
Lemon-Basil Chicken with Basil Aioli	16 Tablespoo Herb, Basil, fresh	To prepare chicken, chop basil then combine fresh basil (1/2c), green onions, 2 T lemon juice, vinegar, lemon pepper, and black pepper ingredients in a large bowl. Add chicken to basil mixture, turning to coat.	Calories 215.9 Sodium: 647.9 Protein: 34.1 Phos 452.2
	0.33 Cup Vegetable, Onions, Young Green, raw		Fat: 7.4 Carbs: 3.4 Chol: 102.2 Pot: 548.6
Serves: 4	1.5 ounces Lemon Juice, Bottled		Sat Fat: 1.5 Fiber: 0.4
Serving Size: 4-5 oz chicken + 1 T Aioli	2 Tablespoon Vinegar - white wine vinegar	Heat a large nonstick skillet over medium-high heat. Coat pan with cooking spray. Add chicken to pan; cook 8 minutes on each side or until done.	Sugar: 0.8
	0.5 Teaspoon Spice, Lemon Pepper		
	0.25 tsp Spice, Black Pepper	While chicken cooks, prepare aioli. Combine 1/4 cup basil, mayonnaise, 1 T lemon juice, dijon mustard, garlic and olive oil ingredients in a small bowl, stirring with a whisk. Serve with chicken.	
	24 ounces Chicken, Breast Boneless		
	0.125 Cup Mayonnaise, reduced kcal, cholest free/Hellmann		
	0.5 Tablespo Dijon Mustard		
	1 Teaspoon Herb, Garlic, Raw		
	0.33 Tablesp Oil, Vegetable or Olive		

Recipe	Ingredients	Instructions	Nutritionals
Rice and Beans Side	1 Cup Grain, Rice, Brown, Long grain	Cook long-grain brown rice according to package directions. Combine cooked rice, 1 cup rinsed and drained canned black beans, 1 tablespoon chopped fresh cilantro, 1/4 teaspoon salt, 1/4 teaspoon ground cumin, and 1/4 teaspoon chili powder.	Calories 221.8 Sodium: 97.6 Protein: 6.859 Phos 201.6
	1 Cup Beans, Black, Canned		Fat: 1.619 Carbs: 44.9 Chol: 0 Pot: 274.6
Serves: 4	0.25 Cup Herb, Cilantro Raw		Sat Fat: 0.33 Fiber: 3.909
Serving Size: 1/2 cup	0.25 tsp Spice, Cumin, Ground		Sugar: 0.722
	0.25 teaspoo Spice, Chili Powder		

Recipe

Broccoli Casserole

Serves: 8

Serving Size: 1/2 cup

Amount	Ingredients
4 Cup	Vegetable, Broccoli Florets, Raw
4 fluid ounces	Milk, Nonfat/Skim
0.125 tsp	Spice, Black Pepper
0.5 Cup	Cheese, Cheddar reduced fat
6 Ounces	Soup, Cream of Celery, Fat Free

Instructions: Preheat oven to 350°. In a large bowl, combine all ingredients. Pour into a medium casserole dish and bake for 30 min.

Nutritionals

Calories 53.3	Sodium: 300	Protein: 3.796	Phos 135.3
Fat: 2.291	Carbs: 5.245	Chol: 7.318	Pot: 231.2
Sat Fat: 1.228	Fiber: 0.179		
	Sugar: 1.884		

Recipe

Tomato Ranch Salad

Serves: 6

Serving Size: 3/4 cup salad w/dressing

Amount	Ingredients
2 Cup	Vegetable, Tomato Red Raw
4.5 Cup	Vegetable, Lettuce, Iceberg, head, raw
12 Tablespoo	Salad dressing, ranch dressing, reduced fat

Instructions: Toss lettuce and tomatoes and divide into 6 portions. Top each salad with 2T lite ranch dressing.

Nutritionals

Calories 75.6	Sodium: 280	Protein: 1.2	Phos 80.8
Fat: 3.9	Carbs: 10	Chol: 4.8	Pot: 242.1
Sat Fat: 0.3	Fiber: 1.5		
	Sugar: 3.5		

Meal: Skillet Fish Filet GDM

Recipe

Skillet Fillets with Cilantro Butter

Serves: 4

Serving Size: 1 4oz.fillet w/2 tsp butter

Amount	Ingredients
0.25 tsp	Salt
0.25 tsp	Spice, Cumin, Ground
0.25 teaspoo	Spice, Red Pepper
24 Oz	Fish, Tilapia, baked or broiled
1 Each	Fruit, Lemon w/peel, raw
2 tablespoon	Butter, Light w/no added salt
0.25 Cup	Herb, Cilantro Raw
0.5 teaspoon	Fruit, Lemon Peel, Raw
0.25 teaspoo	Spice, Paprika

Instructions: Combine salt, cumin and red pepper; sprinkle over both sides of fish. Heat a large nonstick skillet over medium-high heat. Coat pan with cooking spray. Coat both sides of fish with cooking spray; place in pan. Cook 3 minutes on each side or until fish flakes easily when tested with a fork or until desired degree of doneness. Place fish on a serving platter; squeeze lemon quarters over fish.

Place butter and remaining ingredients in a small bowl; stir until well blended. Serve with fish.

Nutritionals

Calories 202.6	Sodium: 311.4	Protein: 34.8	Phos 298.3
Fat: 6.576	Carbs: 3.247	Chol: 91.8	Pot: 579.9
Sat Fat: 3.516	Fiber: 1.468		
	Sugar: 0.038		

Fried Rice

Serves: 8

Serving Size: 1/2 cup

Ingredients

Amount	Ingredient
1.5 Cup	Rice, white, cooked, instant
0.125 cup	Soup, Chicken Broth Low Sodium
2 Teaspoon	Vinegar, Red Wine
1 Tablespoon	Soy Sauce, Low Sodium
0.5 tsp	Salt
1 Teaspoon	Oil, Sesame Oil
0.25 tsp	Spice, Black Pepper
1 tablespoon	Oil, Canola
1 Cup	Egg Substitute
1 Cup	Vegetable, Onions, Young Green, raw
1 Cup	Vegetable, Peas, Green, Frozen

Instructions

Cook Rice according to directions on package, omitting salt and fat. Spread Rice in a shallow baking pan and separate grains with a fork. In a small bowl, whisk together broth, vinegar, soy sauce, salt, sesame oil, and black pepper. Set aside. Coat a large nonstick skillet or wok with cooking spray and heat canola oil over moderately high heat until hot. Stirfry, egg substitute until scrambled about 30 seconds. Add scallions and stirfry 1 min. Add peas and stirfry until heated through. Add Rice and stirfry, stirring frequently 2 to 3 min. or until heated throughout. Stir liquid and add to fried rice, tossing to coat evenly.

Nutritionals

Calories 194.2	Sodium: 291.4	Protein: 7.416	Phos 84.7
Fat: 3.609	Carbs: 32	Chol: 0.314	Pot: 200.8
Sat Fat: 0.534	Fiber: 2.083		
	Sugar: 1.384		

Garden Coleslaw With Almonds

Serves: 6

Serving Size: 3/4 Cup

Ingredients

Amount	Ingredient
0.25 Cup	Nuts, Almond Sliced
1 Each	Vegetable, Cabbage Head
1 Cup	Vegetable, Carrots
6 Teaspoon	Oil, Olive
9 Teaspoon	Vinegar, rice
1 ounces	Honey
2 ounces	Yogurt, Greek Non Fat
0.4 Tablespo	Dijon Mustard
0.25 tsp	Spice, Black Pepper

Instructions

Start by toasting the almonds; put them in a small skillet, without oil, over medium heat and shake until almonds start to get golden brown. Remove and set aside.

Make slaw by shredding cabbage and dicing. Put in bowl.
Shredded carrots, add to bowl.
Make dressing by whisking together the remaining ingredients until smooth; then pour the dressing over the slaw.
Add the toasted almonds, tossing to combine. Let stand for 30 minutes, tossing several times.
To serve, spoon portions onto individual salad plates. You will have enough salad for 4 to 6 people.

Nutritionals

Calories 162.8	Sodium: 69.3	Protein: 5.15	Phos 103.5
Fat: 7.843	Carbs: 21.2	Chol: 0	Pot: 479.2
Sat Fat: 0.936	Fiber: 6.47		
	Sugar: 13.9		

Tomato Ranch Salad

Serves: 6

Serving Size: 3/4 cup salad w/dressing

Ingredients

Amount	Ingredient
2 Cup	Vegetable, Tomato Red Raw
4.5 Cup	Vegetable, Lettuce, Iceberg, head, raw
12 Tablespoo	Salad dressing, ranch dressing, reduced fat

Instructions

Toss lettuce and tomatoes and divide into 6 portions. Top each salad with 2T lite ranch dressing.

Nutritionals

Calories 75.6	Sodium: 280	Protein: 1.2	Phos 80.8
Fat: 3.9	Carbs: 10	Chol: 4.8	Pot: 242.1
Sat Fat: 0.3	Fiber: 1.5		
	Sugar: 3.5		

Meal: *Beefy Bowtie Pasta GDM*

Beefy Bowtie Pasta with Tomato Sauce

Serves: 4
Serving Size: 1.5 Cup

	Nutritionals				
Calories 439.9	Sodium: 208.3	Protein: 25.3		Phos 326.q	
Fat: 11.1	Carbs: 54.9	Chol: 44.3		Pot: 718.6	
Sat Fat: 3.677	Fiber: 4.168				
	Sugar: 3.172				

Ingredients		Instructions
4 Teaspoon	Oil, Olive	1. Heat 1 teaspoon oil in a large skillet over medium-high heat. Add beef, cook 5 minutes, stirring to crumble. Remove beef from pan with a slotted spoon. Discard drippings from pan. Reduce heat to medium-low. Add 2 teaspoons oil, onion, and carrot; cook 5 minutes or until tender, stirring occasionally. Add rosemary and garlic; cook 1 minute, stirring constantly.
8 ounces	Beef, Ground (95% lean)	
0.5 Cup	Vegetable, Onions	
0.25 Cup	Vegetable, Carrots	
1 teaspoon	Herb, Rosemary, Dried	
0.5 Teaspoon	Herb, Garlic, Raw	
4 Oz	Beverage, Alcoholic, Wine, Table, Dry White	2. Return beef to pan; add wine. Increase heat to medium-high; cook for 3 minutes or until liquid almost evaporates. Add remaining pepper. Stir in tomatoes and broth; bring to a simmer. Partially cover and simmer 10 minutes, stirring occasionally.
0.125 tsp	Spice, Black Pepper	
12 ounces	Vegetable, Tomato, Red Canned, No Added Salt	
0.5 cup	Soup, Chicken Broth Low Sodium	3. While sauce simmers, cook pasta according to package directions. Drain; return pasta to pan. Stir in 1 cup sauce and remaining 1 teaspoon oil. Spoon 1 cup pasta mixture onto each of 4 plates; top each serving with 3/4 cup remaining sauce, 2 tablespoons ricotta..
8 oz	Pasta, Bow Tie	
0.5 Cup	Cheese, Ricotta, Part Skim Milk	

Brussel Sprouts and Bacon

Serves: 4
Serving Size: 4 ounces

	Nutritionals				
Calories 121.	Sodium: 402.1	Protein: 7.2		Phos 127	
Fat: 6.2	Carbs: 12	Chol: 5		Pot: 528.2	
Sat Fat: 1.6	Fiber: 5				
	Sugar: 2.7				

Ingredients		Instructions
0.5 tsp	Salt	Cut the brussels sprouts in half and trim bottoms. Heat a large skillet or saute pan over medium heat. Add the bacon and cook until crispy, about 5 minutes. Remove to a plate lined with paper towels. Discard all but 1 tablespoon of the rendered bacon fat. Add the garlic, pepper flakes, brussels sprouts and salt to the skillet. Saute until the sprouts are lightly browned on the outside and tender - but still firm - throughout. Approx 10-12 minutes. Add the almonds and bacon (crumbled) and saute for another minute or two. Season with salt and pepper.
1 tsp	Spice, Black Pepper	
4 Slices	Pork Bacon, Cured or Smoked, lower sodium, slices	
2 Teaspoon	Herb, Garlic, Raw	
1 teaspoon	Spice, Red Pepper	
0.06 Cup	Nuts, Almond Sliced	
1 Pounds	Vegetable, Brussels Sprouts, raw	

Recipe 1: Spiced Pork Chops with Apple Chutney

Serves: 4

Serving Size: 1 pork chop with 1/3 c chutney

Ingredients

Amount	Ingredient
1 tablespoon	Butter, Light w/no added salt
3 Each	Fruit, Apple, peeled, raw, medium
0.25 Cups	Fruit, Cranberries, dried - Craisins
9 Teaspoon P	Sugar, Brown
3 Tablespoon	Vinegar, Cider
2 teaspoons	Herb, Ginger Root, peeled, sliced, raw
0.25 tsp	Salt
0.5 teaspoon	Spice, Mustard Powder
0.125 Teaspo	Spice, Allspice, ground
0.5 oz	Vegetable, Green Chilies, Canned
0.5 teaspoon	Spice, Garlic Powder
0.5 Teaspoon	Spice, Coriander Seed
0.25 tsp	Spice, Black Pepper
16 Oz	Pork, Center Cut Chops, Fresh Pork
0.5 teaspoon	Salt, Kosher

Instructions

Chutney: melt butter in a non-stick skillet over medium high heat. Add apple that has been peeled and cubed. Sauté for 4 minutes or until lightly browned. Add cranberries, brown sugar, cider vinegar, ginger, salt, mustard and allspice. Bring to a boil. Reduce heat, and simmer 8 minutes or until apples are tender. Stir occasionally.

Pork: While the chutney simmers, heat a grill pan over medium-high heat. Combine chipotle and salt, garlic powder, coriander and pepper then sprinkle over pork. Coat grill pan with cooking spray. Add pork to pan; cook 4 minutes on each side or until done. Serve with chutney.

Nutritionals

Calories 317.3	Sodium: 602.9	Protein: 21.9	Phos 20.7	
Fat: 13	Carbs: 29.6	Chol: 62.4	Pot: 499.7	
Sat Fat: 5.2	Fiber: 2.1			
	Sugar: 23.6			

Recipe 2: Spicy Greens

Serves: 4

Serving Size: 1 cup

Ingredients

Amount	Ingredient
2 cup	Soup, Chicken Broth Low Sodium
32 Ounces	Vegetable, Mustard Greens, raw
1 Cup	Vegetable, Onions
0.5 Teaspoon	Herb, Garlic, Raw
0.25 Teaspoo	Spice, Pepper, Cayenne
0.5 tsp	Spice, Black Pepper
1 Teaspoon	Liquid Smoke

Instructions

Wash greens thoroughly. Discard tough stems and cut greens into pieces. Place greens in a large soup pot. Add chicken broth, onion, and garlic, and simmer, covered, for 30 to 45 min. or until tender. Season with cayenne pepper, black pepper and liquid smoke.

Nutritionals

Calories 97.3	Sodium: 94.7	Protein: 9.095	Phos 148	
Fat: 1.249	Carbs: 17	Chol: 0	Pot: 975.7	
Sat Fat: 0.262	Fiber: 8.294			
	Sugar: 5.508			

Recipe	Ingredients	Instructions	Nutritionals			
Down Home Baked Bean. **Serves: 4** **Serving Size: 1/2 cup**	8 Tablespoon Sauce, BBQ 0.25 Teaspoo Spice, Dry Mustard 0.33 Cup Vegetable, Onions 1 tablespoon Bacon Bits 1 Cup Beans, Cannellini White, canned 1 Cup Vegetable, Kale, raw	In a small saucepan over high heat, combine the barbeque sauce with the dry mustard, onion, bacon bits, beans and kale. Bring to a boil, reduce the heat to low, and simmer the beans for 10 minutes, or until the kale is tender, stirring occasionally. The sauce should thicken slightly and the beans should be very tender.	Calories 131 Fat: 1.5 Sat Fat: 0.3	Sodium 285 Carbs: 23.7 Fiber: 4.2 Sugar: 12.1	Protein: 6.03 Chol: 4.5	Phos 114 Pot: 276

Meal: Sloppy Joe's GDM

Recipe	Ingredients	Instructions	Nutritionals			
Sloppy Joe's **Serves: 6** **Serving Size: 4 oz meat + 1 bun**	2 Pound Turkey, Ground Raw 8 Oz Sauce, Chili 0.25 Cup Sugar, granulated, white 1 Cup Condiment, Tomato catsup - ketchup 4 Tablespoon Vinegar 12 teaspoon Mustard, Yellow 6 Each Roll, white, soft - hamburger bun	Cook and drain ground meat. Add chili sauce, sugar, ketchup, vinegar and mustard and heat. Serve meat over open faced buns.	Calories 468.2 Fat: 14.9 Sat Fat: 3.9	Sodium 1406 Carbs: 50.5 Fiber: 1.3 Sugar: 20.1	Protein: 32.2 Chol: 119.4	Phos 304. Pot: 710.3

Recipe	Ingredients	Instructions	Nutritionals			
Steamed Carrots **Serves: 6** **Serving Size: 1/2 cup**	3 Cup Vegetable, Carrots 1 Teaspoon Spice, Mrs. Dash	Steam carrots until tender, season with Mrs. Dash	Calories 33 Fat: 0 Sat Fat: 0	Sodium 2 Carbs: 0 Fiber: 0 Sugar: 0	Protein: 1 Chol: 0	Phos 22 Pot: 165

Recipe	Ingredients	Instructions	Nutritionals			
Creamy Lemon Coleslaw **Serves: 6** **Serving Size: 1/6 of container**	1 Each Vegetable, Cabbage Head 6 Each Sugar Substitute Packet, Equal 0.125 Cup Vegetable, Onions 0.5 teaspoon Salt, Kosher 6 Tablespoon Miracle Whip Light 2 Packet True Lemon packet	Shred cabbage and chop onions. Combine all ingredients in a bowl, and toss lightly. Refrigerate if not used immediately.	Calories 81 Fat: 3 Sat Fat: 0.5	Sodium 158 Carbs: 12 Fiber: 3 Sugar: 5.5	Protein: 1.7 Chol: 4	Phos 34 Pot: 211

Meal: *Pasta with Tomato Basil Sauce GDM*

Recipe	Ingredients		Instructions	Nutritionals			
Pasta with Tomato Basil Sauce	1.125 Cup	Macaroni, unenriched, dry	1. Cook pasta according to package directions, omitting salt and fat. Drain; place pasta in a large bowl.	Calories 430.2	Sodium: 952.5	Protein: 17.1	Phos 248.5
	2 Tablespoon	Oil, Vegetable or Olive		Fat: 12.8	Carbs: 62.2	Chol: 10.2	Pot: 449.7
Serves: 4	3 Teaspoon	Herb, Garlic, Raw	2. While pasta cooks, heat oil in a medium saucepan over medium heat. Halve tomatoes and tear basil leaves into small pieces, then add minced garlic to pan; cook 1 minute, stirring frequently. Add tomatoes and salt; cover and cook 4 minutes. Remove from heat; stir in basil and pepper. Add tomato mixture to pasta; toss well to combine. Top with cheese.	Sat Fat: 3.7	Fiber: 5.2		
	4 Cup	Vegetable, Tomato, Red, Cherry			Sugar: 1.1		
Serving Size: 1.5 c pasta - 2T cheese	0.5 tsp	Salt					
	16 Tablespoo	Herb, Basil, fresh					
	0.25 tsp	Spice, Black Pepper					
	0.5 Cup	Cheese, Grated Parmesan, Reduced Fat					

Recipe	Ingredients		Instructions	Nutritionals			
Lemon Spinach	4 Oz	Beverage, Alcoholic, Wine, Table, Dry White	In pan, stir in wine and lemon juice, cook 1 minute. Add garlic, and cook 1 minute. Add spinach, tossing 1 minute or until the spinach wilts.	Calories 44.4	Sodium: 58.7	Protein: 2.2	Phos 43.6
Serves: 4	2 ounces	Lemon Juice, Bottled		Fat: 0.298	Carbs: 4.279	Chol: 0	Pot: 429.3
Serving Size: 1/2 cup	0.75 Teaspoo	Herb, Garlic, Raw		Sat Fat: 0.048	Fiber: 1.621		
	1.25 Ounces	Vegetable, Spinach, raw, torn			Sugar: 0.691		

Meal: *Chicken Cordon Bleu GDM*

Recipe	Ingredients	Instructions	Nutritionals					

Chicken Cordon Bleu

			Calories 320.2	Sodium: 924	Protein: 43.4	Phos 464.		
			Fat:	10.2	Carbs: 11.4	Chol: 126.2	Pot: 753	
			Sat Fat: 4.001	Fiber: 1.029				
				Sugar: 10.27				

Serves: 4

Serving Size: 1 Rolled Chicken Breast

Amount	Ingredient
0.25 cup	Soup, Chicken Broth Low Sodium
1.5 tablespoo	Butter, Light w/no added salt
0.5 cup	Breadcrumbs, Seasoned
0.5 Ounces	Cheese, Parmesan, dry grated - Romano, grated
1 teaspoon	Spice, Paprika
24 ounces	Chicken, Breast Boneless
0.25 tsp	Salt
0.25 Teaspoo	Herb, Oregano, Ground
0.25 tsp	Spice, Black Pepper
4 ounces	Ham, prosciutto
0.1 Cup	Cheese, Mozzarella Part Skim
0.25 Teaspoo	Herb, Garlic, Raw

Instructions:

Preheat oven to 350°.

Place broth in a small microwave-safe bowl; microwave at high 15 seconds or until warm. Stir in butter and garlic. Combine breadcrumbs, Parmesan, and paprika in a medium shallow bowl; set aside.

Place each chicken breast half between 2 sheets of heavy-duty plastic wrap, and pound each to 1/4-inch thickness using a meat mallet or rolling pin. Sprinkle both sides of chicken with salt, oregano, and pepper. Top each breast half with 1 slice of prosciutto and 1 tablespoon mozzarella. Roll up each breast half jelly-roll fashion. Dip each roll in chicken broth mixture; dredge in breadcrumb mixture. Place rolls, seam side down, in an 8-inch square baking dish coated with cooking spray. Pour remaining broth mixture over chicken. Bake at 350° for 28 minutes or until juices run clear and tops are golden.

Recipe	Ingredients	Instructions	Nutritionals					

Garden Coleslaw With Almonds

			Calories 162.8	Sodium: 69.3	Protein: 5.15	Phos 103.		
			Fat:	7.843	Carbs: 21.2	Chol: 0	Pot: 479.2	
			Sat Fat: 0.936	Fiber: 6.47				
				Sugar: 13.9				

Serves: 6

Serving Size: 3/4 Cup

Amount	Ingredient
0.25 Cup	Nuts, Almond Sliced
1 Each	Vegetable, Cabbage Head
1 Cup	Vegetable, Carrots
6 Teaspoon	Oil, Olive
9 Teaspoon	Vinegar, rice
1 ounces	Honey
2 ounces	Yogurt, Greek Non Fat
0.4 Tablespo	Dijon Mustard
0.25 tsp	Spice, Black Pepper

Instructions:

Start by toasting the almonds; put them in a small skillet, without oil, over medium heat and shake until almonds start to get golden brown. Remove and set aside.

Make slaw by shredding cabbage and dicing. Put in bowl.

Shredded carrots, add to bowl.

Make dressing by whisking together the remaining ingredients until smooth; then pour the dressing over the slaw.

Add the toasted almonds, tossing to combine. Let stand for 30 minutes, tossing several times.

To serve, spoon portions onto individual salad plates. You will have enough salad for 4 to 6 people.

Recipe	Ingredients	Instructions	Nutritionals
Orzo with Herbs		Cook 1 cup orzo pasta according to package directions, omitting salt and fat. Drain; toss orzo with 1/4 cup chopped fresh basil, 2 tablespoons chopped fresh parsley, 1 tablespoon extra-virgin olive oil, and 1/4 teaspoon freshly ground black pepper.	Calories 171.2 Sodium: 208.2 Protein: 5.279 Phos 54.6
	2 Tablespoon Herb, Basil, fresh		Fat: 4.234 Carbs: 27.6 Chol: 0 Pot: 65.4
Serves: 4	4 Tablespoon Herb, Parsley, Raw, Chopped		Sat Fat: 0.628 Fiber: 1.777
	1 Tablespoon Oil, Vegetable or Olive		
Serving Size: 1/2 cup	0.25 tsp Spice, Black Pepper		Sugar: 0.534
	8 Ounces Macaroni, cooked, fat not added in cooking - orzo		

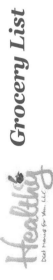

Diet: *Gestational Diabetic - 2400*

Lemon Basil Chicken GDM Meal

Lemon-Basil Chicken with Basil Aioli

Quantity		Grocery Item
1.5	ounces	Lemon Juice, Bottled
16	Tablespoon	Herb, Basil, fresh
0.25	tsp	Spice, Black Pepper
0.33	Tablespoon	Oil, Vegetable or Olive
0.5	Tablespoon	Dijon Mustard
24	ounces	Chicken, Breast Boneless
0.5	Teaspoon	Spice, Lemon Pepper
1	Teaspoon	Herb, Garlic, Raw
0.33	Cup	Vegetable, Onions, Young Green, raw
2	Tablespoons	Vinegar - white wine vinegar
0.125	Cup	Mayonnaise, reduced kcal, cholest

Rice and Beans Side

Quantity		Grocery Item
0.25	tsp	Spice, Cumin, Ground
0.25	teaspoon	Spice, Chili Powder
0.25	Cup	Herb, Cilantro Raw
1	Cup	Beans, Black, Canned
1	Cup	Grain, Rice, Brown, Long grain

Broccoli Casserole

Quantity		Grocery Item
6	Ounces	Soup, Cream of Celery, Fat Free
0.125	tsp	Spice, Black Pepper
4	Cup	Vegetable, Broccoli Florets, Raw
0.5	Cup	Cheese, Cheddar reduced fat
4	fluid ounces	Milk, Nonfat/Skim

Tomato Ranch Salad

Quantity		Grocery Item
2	Cup	Vegetable, Tomato Red Raw
4.5	Cup	Vegetable, Lettuce, Iceberg, head, raw
12	Tablespoon	Salad dressing, ranch dressing, reduced fat

Skillet Fish Filet GDM Meal

Skillet Fillets with Cilantro Butter

Quantity		Grocery Item
0.25	Cup	Herb, Cilantro Raw
1	Each	Fruit, Lemon w/peel, raw
0.25	tsp	Salt
2	tablespoon	Butter, Light w/no added salt
0.25	teaspoon	Spice, Red Pepper
24	Oz	Fish, Tilapia, baked or broiled
0.5	teaspoon	Fruit, Lemon Peel, Raw
0.25	teaspoon	Spice, Paprika
0.25	tsp	Spice, Cumin, Ground

Fried Rice

Quantity		Grocery Item
2	Teaspoon	Vinegar, Red Wine
1	Cup	Vegetable, Onions, Young Green, raw
0.5	tsp	Salt
1	tablespoon	Oil, Canola
1	Teaspoon	Oil, Sesame Oil
0.125	cup	Soup, Chicken Broth Low Sodium
1	Cup	Vegetable, Peas, Green, Frozen
0.25	tsp	Spice, Black Pepper
1	Cup	Egg Substitute
1	Tablespoon	Soy Sauce, Low Sodium
1.5	Cup	Rice, white, cooked, instant

Spiced Pork Chop GDM Meal

Spiced Pork Chops with Apple Chutney

Quantity		Grocery Item
3	Tablespoons	Vinegar, Cider
3	Each	Fruit, Apple, peeled, raw, medium
0.5	teaspoons	Spice, Mustard Powder
0.25	tsp	Salt
16	Oz	Pork, Center Cut Chops, Fresh Pork
0.25	Cups	Fruit, Cranberries, dried - Craisins
0.5	oz	Vegetable, Green Chilies, Canned
9	Teaspoon Pac	Sugar, Brown
0.5	teaspoon	Salt, Kosher
0.5	teaspoon	Spice, Garlic Powder
0.5	Teaspoon	Spice, Coriander Seed
2	teaspoons	Herb, Ginger Root, peeled, sliced, raw
0.25	tsp	Spice, Black Pepper
1	tablespoon	Butter, Light w/no added salt
0.125	Teaspoons	Spice, Allspice, ground

Spicy Greens

Quantity		Grocery Item
0.5	tsp	Spice, Black Pepper
32	Ounces	Vegetable, Mustard Greens, raw
2	cup	Soup, Chicken Broth Low Sodium
0.25	Teaspoon	Spice, Pepper, Cayenne
0.5	Teaspoon	Herb, Garlic, Raw
1	Teaspoon	Liquid Smoke
1	Cup	Vegetable, Onions

Beefy Bowtie Pasta GDM Meal

Beefy Bowtie Pasta with Tomato Sauce

Quantity		Grocery Item
0.5	cup	Soup, Chicken Broth Low Sodium
0.5	Teaspoon	Herb, Garlic, Raw
0.5	Cup	Cheese, Ricotta, Part Skim Milk
12	ounces	Vegetable, Tomato, Red Canned, No Added
4	Oz	Beverage, Alcoholic, Wine, Table, Dry White
8	ounces	Beef, Ground (95% lean)
1	teaspoon	Herb, Rosemary, Dried
4	Teaspoon	Oil, Olive
0.5	Cup	Vegetable, Onions
8	oz	Pasta, Bow Tie
0.25	Cup	Vegetable, Carrots
0.125	tsp	Spice, Black Pepper

Brussel Sprouts and Bacon

Quantity		Grocery Item
1	tsp	Spice, Black Pepper
4	Slices	Pork Bacon, Cured or Smoked, lower
1	Pounds	Vegetable, Brussels Sprouts, raw
1	teaspoon	Spice, Red Pepper
0.06	Cup	Nuts, Almond Sliced
0.5	tsp	Salt
2	Teaspoon	Herb, Garlic, Raw

Garden Coleslaw With Almonds

Quantity		Grocery Item
2	ounces	Yogurt, Greek Non Fat
1	ounces	Honey
9	Teaspoon	Vinegar, rice
1	Cup	Vegetable, Carrots
0.25	Cup	Nuts, Almond Sliced
0.4	Tablespoon	Dijon Mustard
0.25	tsp	Spice, Black Pepper
1	Each	Vegetable, Cabbage Head
6	Teaspoon	Oil, Olive

Tomato Ranch Salad

Quantity		Grocery Item
2	Cup	Vegetable, Tomato Red Raw
4.5	Cup	Vegetable, Lettuce, Iceberg, head, raw
12	Tablespoon	Salad dressing, ranch dressing, reduced fat

128

Chicken Cordon Bleu GDM Meal

Chicken Cordon Bleu

Quantity		Grocery Item
1.5	tablespoon	Butter, Light w/no added salt
0.25	Teaspoon	Herb, Oregano, Ground
0.25	Teaspoon	Herb, Garlic, Raw
1	teaspoon	Spice, Paprika
0.5	cup	Breadcrumbs, Seasoned
0.1	Cup	Cheese, Mozzarella Part Skim
0.25	tsp	Salt
0.5	Ounces	Cheese, Parmesan, dry grated - Romano,
4	ounces	Ham, prosciutto
0.25	tsp	Spice, Black Pepper
24	ounces	Chicken, Breast Boneless
0.25	cup	Soup, Chicken Broth Low Sodium

Garden Coleslaw With Almonds

Quantity		Grocery Item
2	ounces	Yogurt, Greek Non Fat
0.25	Cup	Nuts, Almond Sliced
0.25	tsp	Spice, Black Pepper
1	ounces	Honey
1	Cup	Vegetable, Carrots
6	Teaspoon	Oil, Olive
9	Teaspoon	Vinegar, rice
0.4	Tablespoon	Dijon Mustard
1	Each	Vegetable, Cabbage Head

Creamy Lemon Coleslaw

Quantity		Grocery Item
0.125	Cup	Vegetable, Onions
0.5	teaspoon	Salt, Kosher
6	Tablespoon	Miracle Whip Light
2	Packet	True Lemon packet
1	Each	Vegetable, Cabbage Head
6	Each	Sugar Substitute Packet, Equal

Pasta with Tomato Basil Sauce GDM Meal

Pasta with Tomato Basil Sauce

Quantity		Grocery Item
1.125	Cup	Macaroni, unenriched, dry
2	Tablespoon	Oil, Vegetable or Olive
0.25	tsp	Spice, Black Pepper
16	Tablespoon	Herb, Basil, fresh
4	Cup	Vegetable, Tomato, Red, Cherry
3	Teaspoon	Herb, Garlic, Raw
0.5	Cup	Cheese, Grated Parmesan, Reduced Fat
0.5	tsp	Salt

Lemon Spinach

Quantity		Grocery Item
0.75	Teaspoon	Herb, Garlic, Raw
4	Oz	Beverage, Alcoholic, Wine, Table, Dry White
1.25	Ounces	Vegetable, Spinach, raw, torn
2	ounces	Lemon Juice, Bottled

Down Home Baked Beans

Quantity		Grocery Item
0.25	Teaspoon	Spice, Dry Mustard
1	Cup	Beans, Cannellini White, canned
0.33	Cup	Vegetable, Onions
1	Cup	Vegetable, Kale, raw
8	Tablespoon	Sauce, BBQ
1	tablespoon	Bacon Bits

Sloppy Joe's GDM Meal

Sloppy Joe's

Quantity		Grocery Item
2	Pound	Turkey, Ground Raw
6	Each	Roll, white, soft - hamburger bun
4	Tablespoon	Vinegar
1	Cup	Condiment, Tomato catsup - ketchup
0.25	Cup	Sugar, granulated, white
12	teaspoon	Mustard, Yellow
8	Oz	Sauce, Chili

Steamed Carrots

Quantity		Grocery Item
1	Teaspoon	Spice, Mrs. Dash
3	Cup	Vegetable, Carrots

Orzo with Herbs

Quantity		Grocery Item
8	Ounces	Macaroni, cooked, fat not added in cooking -
0.25	tsp	Spice, Black Pepper
1	Tablespoon	Oil, Vegetable or Olive
2	Tablespoon	Herb, Basil, fresh
4	Tablespoon	Herb, Parsley, Raw, Chopped

Week 8 Meals and Grocery Lists

Chicken Tamale Casserole with Grapes

Creole Beef Steaks with Rice and Noodle Pilaf, Bananas and Cucumber Salad

Turkey Jambalaya with Couscous with Tomato and Dill

Maple Glazed Salmon with Coconut Rice, Yellow Squash and Roasted Asparagus

Bow ties with Tomatoes, Feta and Balsamic Dressing and Down Home Baked Beans

Pork Chops with Cinnamon Apples with Braised Red Cabbage, Creamy Herbed Mashed Potatoes and Italian Green Beans

Grilled Veal Chops with Rosemary Roasted Potatoes and Orzo Salad with Corn, Tomatoes and Basil

Week 8 Meals and Grocery List

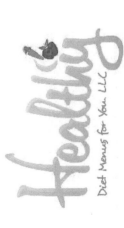

Healthy
Diet Menus for You, LLC

Meal Plan

www.healthydietmenusforyou.com

Diet: *Gestational Diabetic - 2400*

Meal: *Chicken Tamale GDM*

Recipe		Ingredients	Instructions	Nutritionals			
Chicken Tamale Casserol	0.25 Cup	Cheese, Mexican blend, reduced fat - Kraft Mexican Four Cheese made with 2% Milk	1. Preheat oven to 400˚.	Calories 385.5	Sodium: 759.3	Protein: 22.2	Phos 421.ɑ
Serves: 6	2.75 fluid oun	Milk, Nonfat/Skim	2. Combine 1/4 cup cheese, milk, egg substitute, cumin, ground red pepper, cream style corn, corn muffin mix and chilies in a large bowl, stirring just until moist. Pour mixture into a 13 x 9 inch baking dish coated with cooking spray.	Fat: 12.5	Carbs: 46.9	Chol: 33.9	Pot: 473.8
Serving Size: 1/6 PIE	0.25 Cup	Egg Substitute		Sat Fat: 3.753	Fiber: 4.051		
	1 tsp	Spice, Cumin, Ground			Sugar: 3.415		
	0.25 teaspoo	Spice, Red Pepper	3. Bake at 400° for 15 minutes or until set. Pierce entire surface liberally with a fork; pour enchilada sauce over top. Top with chicken; sprinkle with remaining 3/4 cup cheese. Bake at 400° for 15 minutes or until cheese melts. Remove from oven; let stand 5 minutes. Cut into 6 pieces; top each serving with 1 tablespoon sour cream.				
	3 Tablespoon	Vegetable, Peppers, hot, chili, adobo, chili sauce					
	1.5 Cup	Vegetable, Corn, Yellow, Sweet, canned, cream style, no added salt					
	6 Tablespoon	Cream, Sour, Reduced Fat					
	10 Ounce	Sauce, Enchilada Sauce					
	8.5 Ounces	Bread/Muffin, Corn, dry mix, unenriched					
	1.5 cup	Chicken, Lt & Dk meat, canned, meat only					

Recipe		Ingredients	Instructions	Nutritionals			
Grapes	9 Cup	Fruit, Grapes, raw	Wash and remove stems from grapes prior to eating.	Calories 92.5	Sodium: 2.7	Protein: 0.8	Phos 13.8
Serves: 6				Fat: 0.4	Carbs: 23.7	Chol: 0	Pot: 263.6
Serving Size: 1.5 cups of grapes				Sat Fat: 0.1	Fiber: 1.2		
					Sugar: 22.4		

133

Meal: *Creole Beef Steaks GDM*

Recipe		Ingredients	Instructions		Nutritionals				
Creole Beef Steaks	1 teaspoons	Spice, Mustard Powder	Combine mustard, garlic powder, ground sage, dried thyme, salt, ground cumin, ground red pepper, and black pepper. Rub evenly over steaks.		Calories 182.5	Sodium: 500.9	Protein: 25.5	Phos 244.2	
Serves: 4	1 teaspoon	Spice, Garlic Powder			Fat: 7.735	Carbs: 1.448	Chol: 76	Pot: 423.8	
	1 teaspoon	Herb, Sage, ground			Sat Fat: 2.783	Fiber: 0.489			
Serving Size: 4 ounce steak	1 Teaspoon	Herb, Thyme Ground	Heat a large nonstick skillet over medium-high heat. Coat pan with cooking spray. Add steaks to pan; cook 4 minutes on each side or until desired degree of doneness. Remove from heat; let stand 5 minutes.			Sugar: 0.093			
	0.75 tsp	Salt							
	0.5 tsp	Spice, Cumin, Ground							
	0.5 tsp	Spice, Black Pepper							
	0.5 teaspoon	Spice, Red Pepper							
	16 Ounces	Beef, tenderloin, lean							

Recipe		Ingredients	Instructions		Nutritionals				
Rice and Noodle Pilaf	2 tablespoon	Butter, Light w/no added salt	Break spaghetti noodles into small sections about 1-2 inches long. Melt the butter in a large saucepan over medium heat, and add spaghetti.		Calories 188.2	Sodium: 103.8	Protein: 4.4	Phos 131.1	
Serves: 6	0.3 Cup	Pasta, Spaghetti			Fat: 3.4	Carbs: 34.5	Chol: 4.5	Pot: 105.3	
	1 Cup	Rice, Medium Brown	Sauté spaghetti for 5 minutes or until lightly browned. Add the rice, stirring to coat. Stir in the boiling water, salt, and pepper, and bring to a boil. Cover; reduce heat, and simmer for 20 minutes or until the liquid is absorbed. Remove pilaf from heat, and let stand for 10 minutes. Fluff with a fork.		Sat Fat: 1.5	Fiber: 1.6			
Serving Size: 2/3 cup	16 oz	Water				Sugar: 0.6			
	0.25 tsp	Salt							
	0.25 tsp	Spice, Black Pepper							

Recipe		Ingredients	Instructions	Nutritionals				
Banana	6 1	Fruit, Banana	Piece of fruit	Calories 105	Sodium: 1.1	Protein: 1.2	Phos 26	
Serves: 6				Fat: 0.3	Carbs: 27	Chol: 0	Pot: 422.4	
				Sat Fat: 0.1	Fiber: 3			
Serving Size: 1 banana					Sugar: 14.4			

Recipe		Ingredients	Instructions	Nutritionals				
Cucumber Salad	1.5 Cup	Vegetable, Cucumber, peeled, raw	Combine 1 thinly sliced cucumber, red onion sliced, sugar, vinegar, and salt. Chill for 15 min.	Calories 30	Sodium: 147.6	Protein: 0.647	Phos 22.5	
Serves: 4	8 Tablespoon	Vegetable, Onions, Red		Fat: 0.097	Carbs: 7.258	Chol: 0	Pot: 134.4	
	3 Teaspoon	Sweet, Sugar, granulated, white		Sat Fat: 0.034	Fiber: 0.621			
Serving Size: 1/3 cup	1 Tablespoon	Vinegar, Cider			Sugar: 5.025			
	0.25 tsp	Salt						

Meal: *Turkey Jambalaya GDM*

Recipe		Ingredients	Instructions		Nutritionals	
Turkey Jambalaya	3 Teaspoon	Oil, Olive	Heat oil in a large Dutch oven over medium-high heat. Brown turkey and set aside. Add onion and garlic; sauté 6 minutes or until lightly browned. Stir in bell peppers, paprika, salt, oregano, red pepper, and black pepper; sauté 1 minute. Add rice; sauté 1 minute. Stir in broth and tomatoes; bring to a boil. Cover, reduce heat, and simmer 15 minutes. Add turkey and chopped sausage; cover and cook 5 minutes. Sprinkle with green onions.	Calories 450.7	Sodium: 594.9	Protein: 28.9	Phos 330.3
Serves: 6	1.5 Cup	Vegetable, Onions		Fat: 20.5	Carbs: 37.4	Chol: 108.3	Pot: 805.7
Serving Size: 1 1/4 cup	0.25 Teaspoo	Herb, Garlic, Raw		Sat Fat: 5.766	Fiber: 3.524		
	1 Cup	Vegetable, Pepper, Green			Sugar: 6.077		
	3 teaspoon	Spice, Paprika					
	1 Cup	Vegetable, Pepper, Sweet, Red, raw					
	0.5 tsp	Salt					
	0.5 Teaspoon	Herb, Oregano, Ground					
	0.5 teaspoon	Spice, Red Pepper					
	0.5 tsp	Spice, Black Pepper					
	2 cup	Soup, Chicken Broth Low Sodium					
	1 Cup	Grain, Rice, White, Long grain, Parboil, enriched, ckd					
	1.5 Pound	Turkey, Ground Raw					
	16 ounces	Vegetable, Tomato, Red Canned, No Added Salt					
	0.25 Cup	Vegetable, Onions, Young Green, raw					
	6 Ounce	Sausage, Kielbasa					

Recipe		Ingredients	Instructions		Nutritionals	
Couscous with Tomato and Dill	3 Teaspoon	Oil, Olive	Heat a small saucepan over medium-high heat. Add olive oil to pan. Stir in couscous; sauté 1 minute. Add chicken broth and salt; bring to a boil. Cover, remove from heat, and let stand 5 minutes. Fluff with a fork. Stir in tomatoes, onion, and dill.	Calories 125.3	Sodium: 159.5	Protein: 3.788	Phos 57.3
Serves: 4	0.5 cup	Grain, Couscous		Fat: 3.774	Carbs: 19.2	Chol: 0	Pot: 146.1
Serving Size: 1/2 cup	0.5 cup	Soup, Chicken Broth Low Sodium		Sat Fat: 0.556	Fiber: 1.58		
	0.25 tsp	Salt			Sugar: 0.953		
	0.5 Cup	Vegetable, Tomato, Red, Cherry					
	5 Tablespoon	Vegetable, Onions, Red					
	3 Teaspoon	Herb, Dill Weed					

Meal: *Glazed Salmon GDM*

Maple Glazed Salmon
Serves: 4
Serving Size: 6 oz Fillet

Ingredients

Amount	Ingredient
1 teaspoon	Spice, Paprika
0.5 teaspoon	Spice, Chili Powder
0.5 Teaspoon	Spice, Ancho Chile Powder
0.5 tsp	Spice, Cumin, Ground
0.5 Teaspoon	Sugar, Brown
0.5 teaspoon	Salt, Kosher
24 Oz	Fish, Salmon, baked or broiled
2 tablespoon	Syrup, Sweet Maple

Instructions

Preheat broiler. Each portion is 1 6 oz fillet, for a total of four. Combine paprika, chili powder, ground ancho chile powder, cumin, brown sugar and kosher salt; rub spice mixture evenly over flesh side of fillets. Place fish on a broiler pan coated with cooking spray; broil 6 minutes or until desired degree of doneness. Brush fillets evenly with syrup; broil 1 minute.

Nutritionals

Calories 314	Sodium: 91.1	Protein: 35.9	Phos: 365.5
Fat: 14.6	Carbs: 7.856	Chol: 104.2	Pot: 701
Sat Fat: 2.536	Fiber: 0.333		
	Sugar: 6.592		

Coconut Rice
Serves: 4
Serving Size: 1/2 cup

Ingredients

Amount	Ingredient
10 oz	Water
0.25 tsp	Salt
4 Ounces	Milk, Coconut, canned
8 Ounces	Grain, Rice, Basmati, raw

Instructions

Combine basmati rice, water, coconut milk and salt in a small saucepan. Bring to a boil. Cover, reduce heat and simmer 16 min. or until liquid is absorbed.

Nutritionals

Calories 224.5	Sodium: 153.5	Protein: 3.868	Phos 80.3
Fat: 6.331	Carbs: 37.8	Chol: 0	Pot: 116.1
Sat Fat: 5.427	Fiber: 0.601		
	Sugar: 0.056		

Yellow Squash
Serves: 6
Serving Size: 1/2 cup

Ingredients

Amount	Ingredient
1.5 Each	Vegetable, Squash, summer, yellow, raw
2 tablespoon	Butter, Light w/no added salt

Instructions

Melt margarine in a large skillet. Add sliced squash and saute until tender, about 10 minutes

Nutritionals

Calories 29.1	Sodium: 2.5	Protein: 0.7	Phos 20.1
Fat: 2.4	Carbs: 1.6	Chol: 4.5	Pot: 131.4
Sat Fat: 1.4	Fiber: 0.5		
	Sugar: 1		

Roasted Asparagus
Serves: 6
Serving Size: 4 oz

Ingredients

Amount	Ingredient
24 Ounces	Vegetable, Asparagus Fresh
0.5 teaspoon	Spice, Garlic Powder
0.5 Teaspoon	Spice, Lemon Pepper

Instructions

Place asparagus in a sprayed baking dish and coat with olive oil spray. Sprinkle with garlic powder and lemon pepper. Bake for 8 minutes at 450' F or until done.

Nutritionals

Calories 29	Sodium: 9	Protein: 3	Phos 63
Fat: 0.4	Carbs: 5	Chol: 0	Pot: 185
Sat Fat: 0	Fiber: 2		
	Sugar: 0		

Meal: *Bowtie Pasta GDM*

Recipe	Ingredients	Instructions	Nutritionals			

Bow Ties w Tomatoes, Feta and Balsamic Dressing

Serves: 4

Serving Size: 2 cups

Ingredients	
6 oz	Pasta, Bow Tie
2 Cup	Vegetable, Tomato, Red, Cherry
1 Cup	Fruit, Grapes, raw
1 Tablespoon	Herb, Basil, fresh
2 Tablespoon	Vinegar, balsamic
2 tablespoons	Vegetable, Shallots, peeled, raw
1 Tablespoon	Condiment, Capers, canned
0.33 Tablesp	Dijon Mustard
0.25 Teaspoo	Herb, Garlic, Raw
0.5 tsp	Salt
0.25 tsp	Spice, Black Pepper
1 Tablespoon	Oil, Vegetable or Olive
0.5 Cup	Cheese, Feta

Instructions

1. Cook pasta according to package directions, omitting salt and fat. Drain. Combine cooked pasta, tomatoes, grapes, and basil in a large bowl.

2. While pasta cooks, combine vinegar, shallots, garlic, pepper, salt, caper and mustard in a small bowl, stirring with a whisk. Gradually add oil to vinegar mixture, stirring constantly with a whisk. Drizzle vinaigrette over pasta mixture; toss well to coat. Add cheese; toss to combine.

Nutritionals

Calories 342.4	Sodium: 982.4	Protein: 12	Phos 195.1
Fat: 10.8	Carbs: 49.9	Chol: 25.2	Pot: 340.1
Sat Fat: 4.97	Fiber: 3.397		
	Sugar: 8.872		

Down Home Baked Bean.

Serves: 4

Serving Size: 1/2 cup

Ingredients	
8 Tablespoon	Sauce, BBQ
0.25 Teaspoo	Spice, Dry Mustard
0.33 Cup	Vegetable, Onions
1 tablespoon	Bacon Bits
1 Cup	Beans, Cannellini White, canned
1 Cup	Vegetable, Kale, raw

Instructions

In a small saucepan over high heat, combine the barbeque sauce with the dry mustard, onion, bacon bits, beans and kale. Bring to a boil, reduce the heat to low, and simmer the beans for 10 minutes, or until the kale is tender, stirring occasionally. The sauce should thicken slightly and the beans should be very tender.

Nutritionals

Calories 131	Sodium: 285	Protein: 6.03	Phos 114
Fat: 1.5	Carbs: 23.7	Chol: 4.5	Pot: 276
Sat Fat: 0.3	Fiber: 4.2		
	Sugar: 12.1		

Meal: *Pork Chop with Apples GDM*

Recipe		Ingredients	Instructions	Nutritionals				
Pork Chops with Cinnamon Apples	1 teaspoon	Herb, Sage, ground	Combine sage, salt and pepper ingredients, and sprinkle over the pork. Heat oil in a large nonstick skillet coated with cooking spray over medium heat. Add pork; cook 3 minutes on each side or until done. Remove the pork from pan. Cover and keep warm.	Calories 237.1	Sodium: 359.8	Protein: 25.4	Phos 266	
	0.5 tsp	Salt		Fat: 5.663	Carbs: 22	Chol: 79.4	Pot: 570.8	
	0.25 tsp	Spice, Black Pepper		Sat Fat: 1.743	Fiber: 3.605			
Serves: 4	16 Oz	Pork, Center Cut Chops, Fresh Pork			Sugar: 16.6			
Serving Size: 4 oz Pork Chop and 3/4 cup apple mix	0.1 Tablespo	Oil, Vegetable or Olive	Melt butter in pan over medium heat. Add apples and remaining ingredients, and cook 5 minutes or until tender, stirring frequently. Serve the apples with pork.					
	0.333 tablesp	Butter, Light w/no added salt						
	4 Each	Fruit, Apple, peeled, raw, medium						
	3 Teaspoon P	Sugar, Brown						
	0.5 ounces	Lemon Juice, Bottled						
	0.5 Teaspoon	Spice, Cinnamon, ground						

Recipe		Ingredients	Instructions	Nutritionals				
Braised Red Cabbage	2 cup	Soup, Chicken Broth Low Sodium	In a large saucepan, bring broth, vinegar, honey, and allspice to a boil. Add cabbage and cubed apples. Reduce heat and simmer, uncovered, for 30 min.	Calories 96.9	Sodium: 57.4	Protein: 3.612	Phos 67.7	
	8 Tablespoon	Vinegar, Cider		Fat: 0.938	Carbs: 2.39	Chol: 0	Pot: 362.6	
	6 Teaspoon	Vinegar, Red Wine		Sat Fat: 0.249	Fiber: 2.39			
Serves: 4	0.5 ounces	Honey			Sugar: 13.9			
Serving Size: 1/2 cup	0.5 Teaspoon	Spice, Allspice, ground						
	4 Cup	Vegetable, Cabbage Heads, Red, raw						
	2 Each	Fruit, Apple, peeled, Granny Smith, medium						

Recipe		Ingredients	Instructions	Nutritionals				
Creamy Herbed Mashed Potatoes	4 Cup	Vegetable, Potato, Flesh only, diced, raw	Peel and cube potatoes. Place potato in a saucepan; cover with water. Bring to a boil; cover, reduce heat, and simmer 10 minutes or until tender. Drain. Return potato to pan. Add milk and remaining ingredients; mash with a potato masher to desired consistency.	Calories 147.1	Sodium: 215.1	Protein: 3.1	Phos 73	
	4 fluid ounces	Milk, Nonfat/Skim		Fat: 4.6	Carbs: 23.8	Chol: 11	Pot: 422.7	
	1 Tablespoon	Cream, Sour, Reduced Fat		Sat Fat: 2.8	Fiber: 2.1			
Serves: 6	3 tablespoon	Butter, Light w/no added salt			Sugar: 2.3			
Serving Size: 3/4 Cup	3 Tablespoon	Herb, Chives, raw						
	4 Springs	Herb, Parsley, Raw, Fresh						
	0.5 tsp	Salt						
	0.5 tsp	Spice, Black Pepper						

Recipe: Italian Green Beans

Serves: 6

Serving Size: 1/2 cup

Ingredients

Amount	Ingredient
3 Teaspoon	Oil, Olive
1 Cup	Vegetable, Onions
2 Teaspoon	Herb, Garlic, Raw
1 Can	Vegetable, Tomato Diced Canned
0.25 Teaspoo	Herb, Oregano, Ground
0.25 Teaspoo	Herb, Basil, Ground
16 Ounces	Vegetable, Beans, Italian, Frozen

Instructions

Steam green beans until tender crisp. Set aside. Heat olive oil in a medium nonstick skillet over medium-high heat. Sauté onions until clear. Add garlic; sauté 30 seconds. Add tomatoes, basil, and oregano, and simmer for 15 to 20 min. for tomato mixture over steamed green beans and mix well.

Nutritionals

Calories 67.1	Sodium: 217.2	Protein: 2.111	Phos 46.7
Fat: 2.519	Carbs: 10.9	Chol: 0	Pot: 315.5
Sat Fat: 0.37	Fiber: 3.596		
	Sugar: 3.97		

Meal: Grilled Veal Chop GDM

Recipe: Grilled Veal Chops

Serves: 4

Serving Size: 4 ounce cho

Ingredients

Amount	Ingredient
0.125 Cup	Salad dressing, Italian Dressing Reduced Calorie
0.5 tsp	Salt
0.5 tsp	Spice, Black Pepper
16 Ounces	Veal, Loin, lean, raw

Instructions

Prepare an indoor or outdoor grill. Trim any visible fat from chops. Brush each side, with light Italian dressing. Season well with salt and pepper. Grill for 4 to 6 min. on each side over medium heat and serve.

Nutritionals

Calories 146.2	Sodium: 493.5	Protein: 22.9	Phos 240.?
Fat: 5.196	Carbs: 0.639	Chol: 1.542	Pot: 373.1
Sat Fat: 1.35	Fiber: 0.084		
	Sugar: 0.137		

Recipe: Rosemary Roasted Potatoes

Serves: 6

Serving Size: 3/4 cup Potatoes

Ingredients

Amount	Ingredient
5 each	Vegetable, Potato
1 Tablespoon	Oil, Vegetable or Olive
0.75 Teaspoo	Herb, Garlic, Raw
3 teaspoon	Herb, Rosemary, Dried
2 teaspoon	Spice, Paprika

Instructions

Wash and dice potatoes into bite-sized pieces. Place into a large bowl or Ziplock bag; toss with olive oil. Sprinkle garlic, rosemary, paprika (optional), and pepper over potatoes and shake to coat. Layer potatoes in a single layer on a baking sheet coated with cooking spray. Bake at 400 F for 30 minutes or until slightly browned. Serves 5.

Nutritionals

Calories 132.8	Sodium: 12.3	Protein: 3.094	Phos 85.4
Fat: 2.581	Carbs: 25.5	Chol: 0	Pot: 642
Sat Fat: 0.407	Fiber: 3.056		
	Sugar: 1.443		

Recipe	Ingredients		Instructions	Nutritionals					
Orzo Salad with Corn, Tomato and Basil	4 Packet	True Lemon packet	Combine true lemon, olive oil, red wine vinegar, salt, black pepper and garlic in a jar. Cover tightly and shake. Refrigerate. To make the salad, in a large pot, cook pasta according to package directions. Rinse and drain, place in a large bowl. Spoon half of dressing over pasta. Toss to coat. Cool to room temperature. Add remaining dressing, corn, tomato, onion, basil and olives; toss gently. Refrigerate for 1 hour or more.	Calories 277	Sodium: 324	Protein: 8.2	Phos 139
	2 Tablespoon	Oil, Vegetable or Olive		Fat: 7.4	Carbs: 48	Chol: 0	Pot: 437
Serves: 6	1 teaspoon	Salt, Kosher		Sat Fat: 1	Fiber: 5.6		
Serving Size: 2/3 cup	0.5 tsp	Spice, Black Pepper			Sugar: 3		
	4 tsp	Garlic, Minced					
	0.5 Cup	Vegetable, Onions					
	2 Teaspoon	Herb, Basil, Ground					
	3 Cup	Vegetable, Tomato Red Raw					
	2 Teaspoon	Vinegar, Red Wine					
	1.5 Cup	Pasta, Orzo Dry					
	2 Cup	Vegetable, Corn Frozen					
	0.5 Cup	Vegetable, Black Olive Sliced					

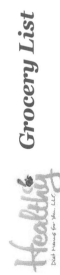
Chicken Tamale GDM Meal

Chicken Tamale Casserole

Quantity		Grocery Item
1.5	Cup	Vegetable, Corn, Yellow, Sweet, canned,
8.5	Ounces	Bread/Muffin, Corn, dry mix, unenriched
1.5	cup	Chicken, Lt & Dk meat, canned, meat only
3	Tablespoon	Vegetable, Peppers, hot, chili, adobo, chili
0.25	Cup	Egg Substitute
6	Tablespoons	Cream, Sour, Reduced Fat
0.25	Cup	Cheese, Mexican blend, reduced fat -
0.25	teaspoon	Spice, Red Pepper
2.75	fluid ounces	Milk, Nonfat/Skim
10	Ounce	Sauce, Enchilada Sauce
1	tsp	Spice, Cumin, Ground

Grapes

Quantity		Grocery Item
9	Cup	Fruit, Grapes, raw

Creole Beef Steaks GDM Meal

Creole Beef Steaks

Quantity		Grocery Item
0.75	tsp	Salt
1	Teaspoon	Herb, Thyme Ground
0.5	teaspoon	Spice, Red Pepper
0.5	tsp	Spice, Black Pepper
0.5	tsp	Spice, Cumin, Ground
1	teaspoon	Spice, Garlic Powder
1	teaspoons	Spice, Mustard Powder
16	Ounces	Beef, tenderloin, lean
1	teaspoon	Herb, Sage, ground

Rice and Noodle Pilaf

Quantity		Grocery Item
0.25	tsp	Salt
0.25	tsp	Spice, Black Pepper
2	tablespoon	Butter, Light w/no added salt
1	Cup	Rice, Medium Brown
16	oz	Water
0.3	Cup	Pasta, Spaghetti

Banana

Quantity		Grocery Item
6	1	Fruit, Banana

Cucumber Salad

Quantity		Grocery Item
1	Tablespoons	Vinegar, Cider
1.5	Cup	Vegetable, Cucumber, peeled, raw
8	Tablespoon	Vegetable, Onions, Red
3	Teaspoon	Sweet, Sugar, granulated, white
0.25	tsp	Salt

Turkey Jambalaya GDM Meal

Turkey Jambalaya

Quantity		Grocery Item
1	Cup	Grain, Rice, White, Long grain, Parboil,
0.5	teaspoon	Spice, Red Pepper
3	Teaspoon	Oil, Olive
6	Ounce	Sausage, Kielbasa
1.5	Pound	Turkey, Ground Raw
1.5	Cup	Vegetable, Onions
16	ounces	Vegetable, Tomato, Red Canned, No Added
2	cup	Soup, Chicken Broth Low Sodium
1	Cup	Vegetable, Pepper, Green
3	teaspoon	Spice, Paprika
1	Cup	Vegetable, Pepper, Sweet, Red, raw
0.25	Cup	Vegetable, Onions, Young Green, raw
0.25	Teaspoon	Herb, Garlic, Raw
0.5	Teaspoon	Herb, Oregano, Ground
0.5	tsp	Salt
0.5	tsp	Spice, Black Pepper

Couscous with Tomato and Dill

Quantity		Grocery Item
0.5	Cup	Vegetable, Tomato, Red, Cherry
0.5	Cup	Grain, Couscous
3	Teaspoon	Herb, Dill Weed
0.25	tsp	Salt
5	Tablespoon	Vegetable, Onions, Red
3	Teaspoon	Oil, Olive
0.5	cup	Soup, Chicken Broth Low Sodium

Glazed Salmon GDM Meal

Maple Glazed Salmon

Quantity		Grocery Item
0.5	teaspoon	Salt, Kosher
24	Oz	Fish, Salmon, baked or broiled
2	tablespoon	Syrup, Sweet Maple
0.5	teaspoon	Spice, Chili Powder
1	teaspoon	Spice, Paprika
0.5	tsp	Spice, Cumin, Ground
0.5	Teaspoon Pac	Sugar, Brown
0.5	Teaspoon	Spice, Ancho Chile Powder

Coconut Rice

Quantity		Grocery Item
0.25	tsp	Salt
10	oz	Water
4	Ounces	Milk, Coconut, canned
8	Ounces	Grain, Rice, Basmati, raw

Yellow Squash

Quantity		Grocery Item
2	tablespoon	Butter, Light w/no added salt
1.5	Each	Vegetable, Squash, summer, yellow, raw

Roasted Asparagus

Quantity		Grocery Item
0.5	teaspoon	Spice, Garlic Powder
0.5	Teaspoon	Spice, Lemon Pepper
24	Ounces	Vegetable, Asparagus Fresh

Bowtie Pasta GDM Meal

Bow Ties w Tomatoes, Feta and Balsamic Dress

Quantity		Grocery Item
2	Tablespoon	Vinegar, balsamic
2	Cup	Vegetable, Tomato, Red, Cherry
0.5	tsp	Salt
6	oz	Pasta, Bow Tie
1	Cup	Fruit, Grapes, raw
2	tablespoons	Vegetable, Shallots, peeled, raw
0.33	Tablespoon	Dijon Mustard
1	Tablespoon	Oil, Vegetable or Olive
0.5	Cup	Cheese, Feta
1	Tablespoons	Condiment, Capers, canned
1	Tablespoon	Herb, Basil, fresh
0.25	Teaspoon	Herb, Garlic, Raw
0.25	tsp	Spice, Black Pepper

Down Home Baked Beans

Quantity		Grocery Item
1	Cup	Vegetable, Kale, raw
1	Cup	Beans, Cannellini White, canned
8	Tablespoon	Sauce, BBQ
0.33	Cup	Vegetable, Onions
1	tablespoon	Bacon Bits
0.25	Teaspoon	Spice, Dry Mustard

Pork Chop with Apples GDM Meal

Pork Chops with Cinnamon Apples

Quantity		Grocery Item
4	Each	Fruit, Apple, peeled, raw, medium
0.5	tsp	Salt
0.25	tsp	Spice, Black Pepper
0.5	ounces	Lemon Juice, Bottled
0.333	tablespoon	Butter, Light w/no added salt
1	teaspoon	Herb, Sage, ground
16	Oz	Pork, Center Cut Chops, Fresh Pork
3	Teaspoon Pac	Sugar, Brown
0.5	Teaspoon	Spice, Cinnamon, ground
0.1	Tablespoon	Oil, Vegetable or Olive

Braised Red Cabbage

Quantity		Grocery Item
0.5	Teaspoons	Spice, Allspice, ground
2	cup	Soup, Chicken Broth Low Sodium
4	Cup	Vegetable, Cabbage Heads, Red, raw
6	Teaspoon	Vinegar, Red Wine
0.5	ounces	Honey
8	Tablespoons	Vinegar, Cider
2	Each	Fruit, Apple, peeled, Granny Smith, medium

Creamy Herbed Mashed Potatoes

Quantity		Grocery Item
4	Springs	Herb, Parsley, Raw, Fresh
0.5	tsp	Salt
1	Tablespoons	Cream, Sour, Reduced Fat
3	Tablespoon	Herb, Chives, raw
4	Cup	Vegetable, Potato, Flesh only, diced, raw
3	tablespoon	Butter, Light w/no added salt
0.5	tsp	Spice, Black Pepper
4	fluid ounces	Milk, Nonfat/Skim

Italian Green Beans

Quantity		Grocery Item
0.25	Teaspoon	Herb, Oregano, Ground
1	Can	Vegetable, Tomato Diced Canned
2	Teaspoon	Herb, Garlic, Raw
3	Teaspoon	Oil, Olive
16	Ounces	Vegetable, Beans, Italian, Frozen
0.25	Teaspoon	Herb, Basil, Ground
1	Cup	Vegetable, Onions

Grilled Veal Chop GDM Meal

Grilled Veal Chops

Quantity		Grocery Item
16	Ounces	Veal, Loin, lean, raw
0.5	tsp	Spice, Black Pepper
0.125	Cup	Salad dressing, Italian Dressing Reduced
0.5	tsp	Salt

Rosemary Roasted Potatoes

Quantity		Grocery Item
0.75	Teaspoon	Herb, Garlic, Raw
1	Tablespoon	Oil, Vegetable or Olive
2	teaspoon	Spice, Paprika
3	teaspoon	Herb, Rosemary, Dried
5	each	Vegetable, Potato

Orzo Salad with Corn, Tomato and Basil

Quantity		Grocery Item
0.5	Cup	Vegetable, Black Olive Sliced
2	Cup	Vegetable, Corn Frozen
1.5	Cup	Pasta, Orzo Dry
2	Teaspoon	Vinegar, Red Wine
4	Packet	True Lemon packet
2	Teaspoon	Herb, Basil, Ground
1	teaspoon	Salt, Kosher
0.5	Cup	Vegetable, Onions
4	tsp	Garlic, Minced
0.5	tsp	Spice, Black Pepper
3	Cup	Vegetable, Tomato Red Raw
2	Tablespoon	Oil, Vegetable or Olive

Week 9 Meals and Grocery Lists

Chicken and Bowtie Pasta Salad with Cucumber and Tomato Salad and Oven Fries

Marinated London Broil with Micro-Baked Potatoes and Roasted Broccoli with Almonds

Fried Rice with Cauliflower Florets with Lemon Mustard Butter

Arugula, Tuna, and White Bean Salad with Oranges and Rosemary Roasted Potatoes

Chicken Milanese with Couscous with Tomato and Dill, Corn on the Cob, and Broccoli Casserole

Coconut Curried Pork Stir Fry with Rice with Lemon Spinach and Asparagus

Prosciutto and Gruyere Stromboli with Cucumber Salad and Oven Fries

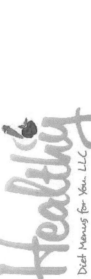

Meal Plan

www.healthydietmenusforyou.com

Meal: *Chicken and Bowtie Pasta GDM*

Recipe		Ingredients	Instructions	Nutritionals				
Chicken and Bowtie Pasta Salad	24 oz	Pasta, Bow Tie	Cook pasta according to package directions, omitting salt and fat; drain. Cool completely. Cut grapes in half.	Calories 415.4	Sodium: 529.3	Protein: 24.6	Phos	228.7
	2 ounces	Lemon Juice, Bottled		Fat: 15.3	Carbs: 45.1	Chol: 34.2	Pot:	405.4
Serves: 6	0.333 Cup	Fruit Juice, Orange, chilled	Combine orange juice, lemon juice, olive oil, mustard, sugar, salt, black pepper and Rice vinegar in a large bowl, stirring with a whisk to combine. Add pasta, chicken, grapes, celery, red onion, walnuts, chives, and parsley; toss gently to combine.	Sat Fat: 2.73	Fiber: 2.841			
	6 Teaspoon	Oil, Olive						
	3 teaspoon	Mustard, Yellow			Sugar: 10.7			
Serving Size: 1 2/3 cup	2 Teaspoon	Sweet, Sugar, granulated, white						
	1 tsp	Salt						
	0.5 tsp	Spice, Black Pepper						
	1.5 Teaspoon	Vinegar, rice						
	2 cup	Chicken, Lt & Dk meat, canned, meat only						
	1.5 Cup	Fruit, Grapes, raw						
	1 Cup	Vegetable, Celery Raw						
	5 Tablespoon	Vegetable, Onions, Red						
	0.333 cup	Nuts, Walnut						
	1 Tablespoon	Herb, Parsley, dried						
	1 Tablespoon	Herb, Chives, freeze-dried						

Cucumber and Tomato Salad

Serves: 5
Serving Size: 1/5 recipe

Ingredients	
2 Cup	Vegetable, Cucumber, peeled, raw
3 Teaspoon	Oil, Olive
2 Cup	Vegetable, Tomato Red Raw
6 Teaspoon	Vinegar, Red Wine
0.5 tsp	Salt
0.25 tsp	Spice, Black Pepper

Instructions: Peel and dice cucumbers. Chop or dice tomatoes. In a medium bowl, toss cucumbers and tomatoes. Drizzle oil and vinegar over vegetables and toss to coat. Season with salt and pepper.

Nutritionals

Calories 44.6	Sodium: 237.8	Protein: 0.961	Phos 29.1
Fat: 2.933	Carbs: 4.056	Chol: 0	Pot: 246.7
Sat Fat: 0.401	Fiber: 1.264		
	Sugar: 2.628		

Oven Fries

Serves: 6
Serving Size: 1/2 potato

Ingredients	
3 each	Vegetable, Potato
1 Teaspoon	Spice, Mrs. Dash
3 Each	Egg White

Instructions: Cut potatoes into strips like fries. Beat egg whites and toss with fries. Sprinkle with Mrs. Dash type seasoning. Bake for 30 minutes at 400'F or until done.

Nutritionals

Calories 75	Sodium: 45	Protein: 3.3	Phos 55
Fat: 0.2	Carbs: 6.5	Chol: 15	Pot: 406
Sat Fat: 0	Fiber: 2		
	Sugar: 1		

Meal: London Broil GDM

Marinated London Broil

Serves: 6
Serving Size: 2.6 oz meat

Ingredients	
8 Tablespoon	Vinegar, balsamic
3 Teaspoon	P Sugar, Brown
1 teaspoon	Herb, Rosemary, Dried
0.25 tsp	Spice, Black Pepper
0.25 tsp	Salt
16 Oz	Beef Steak, London Broil, lean only, broil or bkd

Instructions: Combine all of the items in a zippered bag. Mix well and refrigerate for 20 minutes or longer. Grill or broil for 4-6 minutes on each side or until done. Let stand 5 minutes before slicing into 6 servings.

Nutritionals

Calories 187	Sodium: 268.6	Protein: 23.6	Phos 185.2
Fat: 6.5	Carbs: 6	Chol: 64.3	Pot: 356.1
Sat Fat: 2.4	Fiber: 0		
	Sugar: 5.4		

Micro-Baked Potatoes

Serves: 6
Serving Size: 1 potatoe + 2T Butter

Ingredients	
6 Each	Vegetable, Potato, Flesh only, microwaved w/skin, no salt
12 tablespoo	Butter, Light w/no added salt

Instructions: Pierce potatoes and coat with olive oil. Microwave on high 4 minutes. Turn each potato over, cook another 4 minutes. Turn all potatoes again. Cook another 3 minutes. They are done wehn a knife can slice through them easily. Remove from microwave. Cut open and serve with 2 T butter.

Nutritionals

Calories 283.7	Sodium: 20.1	Protein: 4.1	Phos 178.7
Fat: 14.3	Carbs: 36.3	Chol: 27.1	Pot: 659.3
Sat Fat: 8.8	Fiber: 2.4		
	Sugar: 0		

Recipe: Roasted Broccoli with Almonds

Nutritionals

Calories 123	Sodium: 164	Protein: 7	Phos: 162
Fat: 6	Carbs: 6	Chol: 0	Pot: 685
Sat Fat: 1	Fiber: 6		
	Sugar: 4		

Ingredients

Amount	Ingredient
5 Cup	Vegetable, Broccoli Florets, Raw
1 Tablespoon	Oil, Vegetable or Olive
0.25 tsp	Salt
0.25 tsp	Spice, Black Pepper
0.25 Cup	Nuts, Almond Sliced

Serves: 6

Serving Size: 3/4 Cup

Instructions

Cut broccoli off stem if necessary. Place broccoli in a sprayed baking dish. Drizzle broccoli with olive oil, garlic, salt and pepper. Bake 14 minutes at 450°F. Sprinkle with almonds and divide into 6 servings.

Meal: Fried Rice GDM

Recipe: Fried Rice

Nutritionals

Calories 425	Sodium: 556.4	Protein: 13.8	Phos: 381.6
Fat: 10.4	Carbs: 69.5	Chol: 141	Pot: 394.4
Sat Fat: 1.886	Fiber: 5.637		
	Sugar: 4.027		

Ingredients

Amount	Ingredient
2 tablespoon	Oil, Canola
4 Each	Egg, Whole
0.25 tsp	Spice, Black Pepper
1.75 Cup	Vegetable, Onions, Young Green, raw
1 Teaspoon	Spice, Ginger
0.5 Teaspoon	Herb, Garlic, Raw
2.5 Cup	Grain, Rice, Brown, Long grain
4 Tablespoon	Soy Sauce, Low Sodium
0.25 tsp	Salt
2 Cup	Vegetable, Peas, Green, Frozen
0.15 Cup	Herb, Cilantro Raw

Serves: 6

Serving Size: 1 cup

Instructions

Fully cook rice. Heat 2 teaspoons oil in a large nonstick skillet over medium-high heat. Add half of eggs; swirl to coat bottom of pan evenly. Sprinkle with 1/8 teaspoon pepper and dash of salt; cook 3 minutes or until egg is done. Remove egg from pan; thinly slice, and set aside.

Wipe pan clean with a paper towel. Heat remaining 4 teaspoons oil in pan over medium-high heat. Add 1 cup onions, ginger, and garlic; stir-fry 30 seconds. Add remaining eggs and rice; stir-fry 3 minutes. Stir in half of egg strips, remaining 3/4 cup onions, remaining 1/8 teaspoon pepper, soy sauce, 1/2 teaspoon salt, and peas; cook 30 seconds, stirring well to combine. Top with remaining egg strips and cilantro.

Recipe: Cauliflower Florets with Lemon Mustard Butte

Nutritionals

Calories 33.3	Sodium: 50.2	Protein: 1.09	Phos: 23.9
Fat: 2.053	Carbs: 2.053	Chol: 0	Pot: 162.3
Sat Fat: 0.416	Fiber: 1.384		
	Sugar: 1.414		

Ingredients

Amount	Ingredient
2 Tablespoon	Margarine Spread - reduced calorie, about 40% fat, tub, salted - Country Crock Light
1 Tablespoon	Dijon Mustard
4 Cup	Vegetable, Cauliflower, Raw
2 Teaspoon	Lemon, Rind

Serves: 8

Serving Size: 1/2 Cup

Instructions

In a small bowl, whisk together the margarine, Dijon mustard, lemon peel, and chopped onion. Steam cauliflower florets until tender crisp. In a large saucepan, add cauliflower and margarine mixture over low heat. Toss gently until cauliflower is coated.

Meal: *Tuna and White Bean Salad GDM*

Recipe		Ingredients	Instructions	Nutritionals				
Arugula, Tuna, and White Bean Salad	2 ounces	Lemon Juice, Bottled	1. Whisk together lemon juice, olive oil, garlic, salt, black pepper and Dijon mustard in a large bowl.	Calories 267.8	Sodium: 473.6	Protein: 21.6	Phos 332.7	
Serves: 4	4.5 Teaspoon	Oil, Olive		Fat: 9.334	Carbs: 25.2	Chol: 25.2	Pot: 512.2	
Serving Size: 2 1/4 Cups	0.25 Teaspoo	Herb, Garlic, Raw	2. Add tomatoes that have been cut in half, red onion, tuna, beans and arugula; toss. Top with cheese.	Sat Fat: 2.941	Fiber: 8.231			
	0.5 Tablespo	Mustard, Dijon			Sugar: 9.334			
	0.5 tsp	Spice, Black Pepper						
	0.5 teaspoon	Salt, Kosher						
	1 Cup	Vegetable, Tomato, Red, Cherry						
	16 Tablespoo	Vegetable, Onions, Red						
	2 Cup	Beans, Cannellini White, canned						
	4 cup	Vegetable, Lettuce, arugula, raw						
	4 Tablespoon	Cheese, Parmesan, dry grated, reduced fat						
	6 Ounce	Fish, Light Tuna, canned in H20 w/o salt, drained						

Recipe		Ingredients	Instructions	Nutritionals				
Orange	6 1	Fruit, Orange, All Varieties, peeled, raw	Piece of fruit.	Calories 86.5	Sodium: 0	Protein: 1.7	Phos 25.8	
Serves: 6				Fat: 0.2	Carbs: 21.6	Chol: 0	Pot: 333	
Serving Size: 1 Peeled Orange				Sat Fat: 0	Fiber: 4.4			
					Sugar: 17.2			

Recipe		Ingredients	Instructions	Nutritionals				
Rosemary Roasted Potatoes	5 each	Vegetable, Potato	Wash and dice potatoes into bite-sized pieces. Place into a large bowl or Ziplock bag; toss with olive oil. Sprinkle garlic, rosemary, paprika (optional), and pepper over potatoes and shake to coat. Layer potatoes in a single layer on a baking sheet coated with cooking spray. Bake at 400 F for 30 minutes or until slightly browned. Serves 5.	Calories 132.8	Sodium: 12.3	Protein: 3.094	Phos 85.4	
Serves: 6	1 Tablespoon	Oil, Vegetable or Olive		Fat: 2.581	Carbs: 25.5	Chol: 0	Pot: 642	
Serving Size: 3/4 cup Potatoes	0.75 Teaspoon	Herb, Garlic, Raw		Sat Fat: 0.407	Fiber: 3.056			
	3 teaspoon	Herb, Rosemary, Dried			Sugar: 1.443			
	2 teaspoon	Spice, Paprika						

Meal: *Chicken Milanese GDM*

Chicken Milanese
Serves: 4
Serving Size: 4 oz Breast

Amount	Ingredients
12 ounces	Chicken, Breast Boneless
0.25 tsp	Spice, Black Pepper
0.667 Cup	Breadcrumbs, Plain, Grated, Dry
2 Each	Egg White
0.25 Cup	Flour, Wheat, White, All Purpose, unbleached, enriched
4 Tablespoon	Cheese, Parmesan, dry grated, reduced fat
1 Tablespoon	Oil, Vegetable or Olive

Instructions: Place chicken between 2 sheets of heavy-duty plastic wrap; pound to 1/2-inch thickness using a meat mallet or small heavy skillet. Combine breadcrumbs and cheese in a shallow dish. Place flour in a shallow dish. Place egg white in a shallow dish. Sprinkle chicken with 1/8 teaspoon salt and 1/8 teaspoon pepper. Dredge chicken in flour; dip in egg white. Dredge in breadcrumb mixture. Place chicken on a wire rack; let stand 5 minutes. Heat 1 tablespoon oil in a large nonstick skillet over medium-high heat. Add chicken; cook 3 minutes. Turn chicken over; cook 2 minutes or until browned and done.

Nutritionals

Calories 298.2	Sodium: 330.5	Protein: 33.1	Phos 287.q
Fat: 8.838	Carbs: 19.2	Chol: 79.2	Pot: 301
Sat Fat: 2.529	Fiber: 1.056	Sugar: 1.256	

Couscous with Tomato and Dill
Serves: 4
Serving Size: 1/2 cup

Amount	Ingredients
3 Teaspoon	Oil, Olive
0.5 Cup	Grain, Couscous
0.5 cup	Soup, Chicken Broth Low Sodium
0.25 tsp	Salt
0.5 Cup	Vegetable, Tomato, Red, Cherry
5 Tablespoon	Vegetable, Onions, Red
3 Teaspoon	Herb, Dill Weed

Instructions: Heat a small saucepan over medium-high heat. Add olive oil to pan. Stir in couscous; sauté 1 minute. Add chicken broth and salt; bring to a boil. Cover, remove from heat, and let stand 5 minutes. Fluff with a fork. Stir in tomatoes, onion, and dill.

Nutritionals

Calories 125.3	Sodium: 159.5	Protein: 3.788	Phos 57.3
Fat: 3.774	Carbs: 19.2	Chol: 0	Pot: 146.1
Sat Fat: 0.556	Fiber: 1.58	Sugar: 0.953	

Corn On The Cob
Serves: 6
Serving Size: 1 ear of corn

Amount	Ingredients
6 Each	Vegetable, Corn on Cob, sm/med, ckd w/o fat or salt

Instructions: Shuck and clean corn. Boil until tender, about 4-6 minutes.

Nutritionals

Calories 82.7	Sodium: 1.5	Protein: 2.5	Phos 78.8
Fat: 0.9	Carbs: 19.2	Chol: 0	Pot: 190.6
Sat Fat: 0.1	Fiber: 2.8	Sugar: 0	

Broccoli Casserole
Serves: 8
Serving Size: 1/2 cup

Amount	Ingredients
4 Cup	Vegetable, Broccoli Florets, Raw
4 fluid ounces	Milk, Nonfat/Skim
0.125 tsp	Spice, Black Pepper
0.5 Cup	Cheese, Cheddar reduced fat
6 Ounces	Soup, Cream of Celery, Fat Free

Instructions: Preheat oven to 350°. In a large bowl, combine all ingredients. Pour into a medium casserole dish and bake for 30 min.

Nutritionals

Calories 53.3	Sodium: 300	Protein: 3.796	Phos 135.?
Fat: 2.291	Carbs: 5.245	Chol: 7.318	Pot: 231.2
Sat Fat: 1.228	Fiber: 0.179	Sugar: 1.884	

Meal: *Coconut Pork Stirfry GDM*

Coconut Curried Pork Sti Fry w Rice

Serves: 4

Serving Size: 1 1/4 c Pork Mixture + 1 c Rice

Nutritionals

Calories 444.4	Sodium: 1008	Protein: 29.1	Phos 385.2
Fat: 12.1	Carbs: 54.5	Chol: 73.7	Pot: 686.7
Sat Fat: 5.603	Fiber: 3.239		
	Sugar: 8.112		

Ingredients

Amount	Ingredient
2 Cup	Rice, white, cooked, instant
16 ounces	Pork, Tenderloin Lean
1 Tablespoon	Oil, Vegetable or Olive
1 tsp	Spice, Curry Powder
1 Cup	Vegetable, Peas, Snow/SugarSnap, ckd w/o fat or salt
0.333 Cup	Nuts, Coconut Milk, canned
1 Each	Fruit, Lime
1 Tablespoon	Sauce, Fish
1 Cup	Fruit, Mango, peeled, raw
0.5 Cup	Vegetable, Onions, Young Green, raw
2 Tablespoon	Nuts, Coconut, Sweetened, shredded, dried

Instructions

Prepare rice according to package directions, omitting salt and fat; drain.

Cut pork into 1-inch cubes. Heat oil in a large nonstick skillet over medium-high heat. Sprinkle pork evenly with curry powder. Add pork and snow peas to pan; stir-fry 3 minutes.

Combine coconut milk and fish sauce, stirring well. Add milk mixture to pan; bring to a simmer. Stir in chopped mango and 1/4 cup onions; cook 1 minute or until thoroughly heated. Remove from heat. Place 1 cup rice on each of 4 plates; top each serving with 1 1/4 cups pork mixture. Sprinkle each serving with 1 tablespoon of remaining 1/4 cup onions and 1 1/2 teaspoons shredded coconut. Serve with lime wedges, if desired.

Lemon Spinach

Serves: 4

Serving Size: 1/2 cup

Nutritionals

Calories 44.4	Sodium: 58.7	Protein: 2.2	Phos 43.6
Fat: 0.298	Carbs: 4.279	Chol: 0	Pot: 429.3
Sat Fat: 0.048	Fiber: 1.621		
	Sugar: 0.691		

Ingredients

Amount	Ingredient
4 Oz	Beverage, Alcoholic, Wine, Table, Dry White
2 ounces	Lemon Juice, Bottled
0.75 Teaspoo	Herb, Garlic, Raw
1.25 Ounces	Vegetable, Spinach, raw, torn

Instructions

In pan, stir in wine and lemon juice, cook 1 minute. Add garlic, and cook 1 minute. Add spinach, tossing 1 minute or until the spinach wilts.

Asparagus

Serves: 6

Serving Size: 1/2 Cup

Nutritionals

Calories 21.5	Sodium: 1.8	Protein: 2.3	Phos 48.3
Fat: 0.2	Carbs: 3.7	Chol: 0	Pot: 143.2
Sat Fat: 0	Fiber: 1.5		
	Sugar: 0		

Ingredients

Amount	Ingredient
54 Ounces	Vegetable, Asparagus Fresh

Instructions

Wash and clean asparagus by cutting off hard ends of stalk. Steam for 10 minutes in steamer or cook in 1 in water in microwaveable bowl for 5-7 minutes until desired tenderness.

152

Meal: *Prosciutto Stromboli GDM*

Recipe

Prosciutto and Gruyere Strombolis

Serves: 4

Serving Size: 1 biscuit

Ingredients

11 oz	Bread, Crusty French Loaf, refrigerated dough/Pillsbury	
2 Oz	Lunch Meat, Pork Ham, Prosciutto	
1 cup	Vegetable, Lettuce, arugula, raw	
0.5 cup	Cheese, Gruyere, shredded	
0.66 Tablesp	Herb, Parsley, dried	

Nutritionals

Calories 272.9	Sodium: 875	Protein: 14.1	Phos 129.9
Fat: 7.8	Carbs: 36.4	Chol: 24.7	Pot: 107.5
Sat Fat: 3.6	Fiber: 1.4		
	Sugar: 3.1		

Instructions

Preheat oven to 425°.

Unroll dough onto a baking sheet; pat into a 14 x 11-inch rectangle. Cut dough into quarters to form 4 (7 x 5 1/2-inch) rectangles. Top each rectangle with 1/2 ounce thinly sliced prosciutto, 1/4 cup chopped arugula, 2 tablespoons cheese, and .5 teaspoon parsley. Beginning at short side of each rectangle, roll up the dough, jelly-roll fashion; pinch seam to seal (do not seal ends of rolls). Arrange rolls 4 inches apart on baking sheet. Bake at 425° for 10 minutes or until rolls are lightly browned. Serve warm.

Recipe

Cucumber Salad

Serves: 4

Serving Size: 1/3 cup

Ingredients

1.5 Cup	Vegetable, Cucumber, peeled, raw	
8 Tablespoon	Vegetable, Onions, Red	
3 Teaspoon	Sweet, Sugar, granulated, white	
1 Tablespoon	Vinegar, Cider	
0.25 tsp	Salt	

Nutritionals

Calories 30	Sodium: 147.6	Protein: 0.647	Phos 22.5
Fat: 0.097	Carbs: 7.258	Chol: 0	Pot: 134.4
Sat Fat: 0.034	Fiber: 0.621		
	Sugar: 5.025		

Instructions

Combine 1 thinly sliced cucumber, red onion sliced, sugar, vinegar, and salt. Chill for 15 min.

Recipe

Oven Fries

Serves: 6

Serving Size: 1/2 potato

Ingredients

3 each	Vegetable, Potato	
1 Teaspoon	Spice, Mrs. Dash	
3 Each	Egg White	

Nutritionals

Calories 75	Sodium: 45	Protein: 3.3	Phos 55
Fat: 0.2	Carbs: 15	Chol: 0	Pot: 406
Sat Fat: 0	Fiber: 2		
	Sugar: 1		

Instructions

Cut potatoes into strips like fries. Beat egg whites and toss with fries. Sprinkle with Mrs. Dash type seasoning. Bake for 30 minutes at 400°F or until done.

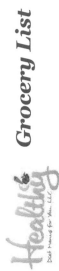

Healthy Grocery List

Diet Menus for You, LLC

Diet: **Gestational Diabetic - 2400**

Chicken and Bowtie Pasta GDM Meal

Chicken and Bowtie Pasta Salad

Quantity		Grocery Item
6	Teaspoon	Oil, Olive
1	Cup	Vegetable, Celery Raw
2	cup	Chicken, Lt & Dk meat, canned, meat only
24	oz	Pasta, Bow Tie
1.5	Teaspoon	Vinegar, rice
1.5	Cup	Fruit, Grapes, raw
1	Tablespoon	Herb, Parsley, dried
3	teaspoon	Mustard, Yellow
0.333	cup	Nuts, Walnut
5	Tablespoon	Vegetable, Onions, Red
2	ounces	Lemon Juice, Bottled
0.333	Cup	Fruit Juice, Orange, chilled
2	Teaspoon	Sweet, Sugar, granulated, white
1	tsp	Salt
1	Tablespoon	Herb, Chives, freeze-dried
0.5	tsp	Spice, Black Pepper

Cucumber and Tomato Salad

Quantity		Grocery Item
2	Cup	Vegetable, Tomato Red Raw
3	Teaspoon	Oil, Olive
2	Cup	Vegetable, Cucumber, peeled, raw
0.25	tsp	Spice, Black Pepper
6	Teaspoon	Vinegar, Red Wine
0.5	tsp	Salt

Oven Fries

Quantity		Grocery Item
3	Each	Egg White
3	each	Vegetable, Potato
1	Teaspoon	Spice, Mrs. Dash

London Broil GDM Meal

Marinated London Broil

Quantity		Grocery Item
1	teaspoon	Herb, Rosemary, Dried
16	Oz	Beef Steak, London Broil, lean only, broil or
0.25	tsp	Spice, Black Pepper
0.25	tsp	Salt
8	Tablespoon	Vinegar, balsamic
3	Teaspoon Pac	Sugar, Brown

Micro-Baked Potatoes

Quantity		Grocery Item
12	tablespoon	Butter, Light w/no added salt
6	Each	Vegetable, Potato, Flesh only,

Roasted Broccoli with Almonds

Quantity		Grocery Item
0.25	tsp	Spice, Black Pepper
1	Tablespoon	Oil, Vegetable or Olive
0.25	Cup	Nuts, Almond Sliced
5	Cup	Vegetable, Broccoli Florets, Raw
0.25	tsp	Salt

155

Fried Rice GDM Meal

Fried Rice

Quantity		Grocery Item
0.25	tsp	Salt
4	Tablespoon	Soy Sauce, Low Sodium
0.5	Teaspoon	Herb, Garlic, Raw
2	Cup	Vegetable, Peas, Green, Frozen
1.75	Cup	Vegetable, Onions, Young Green, raw
0.25	tsp	Spice, Black Pepper
2.5	Cup	Grain, Rice, Brown, Long grain
0.15	Cup	Herb, Cilantro Raw
4	Each	Egg, Whole
1	Teaspoon	Spice, Ginger
2	tablespoon	Oil, Canola

Cauliflower Florets with Lemon Mustard Butte

Quantity		Grocery Item
1	Tablespoon	Dijon Mustard
2	Tablespoon	Margarine Spread - reduced calorie, about
2	Teaspoon	Lemon, Rind
4	Cup	Vegetable, Cauliflower, Raw

Tuna and White Bean Salad GDM Meal

Arugula, Tuna, and White Bean Salad

Quantity		Grocery Item
1	Cup	Vegetable, Tomato, Red, Cherry
2	ounces	Lemon Juice, Bottled
6	Ounce	Fish, Light Tuna, canned in H2O w/o
0.25	Teaspoon	Herb, Garlic, Raw
4	cup	Vegetable, Lettuce, arugula, raw
0.5	tsp	Spice, Black Pepper
4	Tablespoon	Cheese, Parmesan, dry grated, reduced fat
4.5	Teaspoon	Oil, Olive
0.5	Tablespoon	Mustard, Dijon
0.5	teaspoon	Salt, Kosher
2	Cup	Beans, Cannellini White, canned
16	Tablespoon	Vegetable, Onions, Red

Orange

Quantity		Grocery Item
6	1	Fruit, Orange, All Varieties, peeled, raw

Rosemary Roasted Potatoes

Quantity		Grocery Item
2	teaspoon	Spice, Paprika
5	each	Vegetable, Potato
3	teaspoon	Herb, Rosemary, Dried
1	Tablespoon	Oil, Vegetable or Olive
0.75	Teaspoon	Herb, Garlic, Raw

Chicken Milanese GDM Meal

Chicken Milanese

Quantity		Grocery Item
12	ounces	Chicken, Breast Boneless
4	Tablespoon	Cheese, Parmesan, dry grated, reduced fat
2	Each	Egg White
1	Tablespoon	Oil, Vegetable or Olive
0.25	tsp	Spice, Black Pepper
0.25	Cup	Flour, Wheat, White, All Purpose,
0.667	Cup	Breadcrumbs, Plain, Grated, Dry

Couscous with Tomato and Dill

Quantity		Grocery Item
3	Teaspoon	Oil, Olive
0.25	tsp	Salt
0.5	Cup	Grain, Couscous
0.5	Cup	Vegetable, Tomato, Red, Cherry
5	Tablespoon	Vegetable, Onions, Red
0.5	cup	Soup, Chicken Broth Low Sodium
3	Teaspoon	Herb, Dill Weed

Corn On The Cob

Quantity		Grocery Item
6	Each	Vegetable, Corn on Cob, sm/med, ckd w/o

Oven Fries

Quantity		Grocery Item
3	each	Vegetable, Potato
1	Teaspoon	Spice, Mrs. Dash
3	Each	Egg White

Broccoli Casserole

Quantity		Grocery Item
4	fluid ounces	Milk, Nonfat/Skim
0.125	tsp	Spice, Black Pepper
4	Cup	Vegetable, Broccoli Florets, Raw
6	Ounces	Soup, Cream of Celery, Fat Free
0.5	Cup	Cheese, Cheddar reduced fat

Lemon Spinach

Quantity		Grocery Item
1.25	Ounces	Vegetable, Spinach, raw, torn
0.75	Teaspoon	Herb, Garlic, Raw
4	Oz	Beverage, Alcoholic, Wine, Table, Dry White
2	ounces	Lemon Juice, Bottled

Asparagus

Quantity		Grocery Item
54	Ounces	Vegetable, Asparagus Fresh

Coconut Pork Stirfry GDM Meal

Coconut Curried Pork Stir Fry w Rice

Quantity		Grocery Item
1	Cup	Vegetable, Peas, Snow/SugarSnap, ckd
1	Each	Fruit, Lime
1	Tablespoon	Oil, Vegetable or Olive
0.5	Cup	Vegetable, Onions, Young Green, raw
0.333	Cup	Nuts, Coconut Milk, canned
1	Tablespoon	Sauce, Fish
1	Cup	Fruit, Mango, peeled, raw
2	Tablespoon	Nuts, Coconut, Sweetened, shredded,
2	Cup	Rice, white, cooked, instant
16	ounces	Pork, Tenderloin Lean
1	tsp	Spice, Curry Powder

Prosciutto Stromboli GDM Meal

Prosciutto and Gruyere Strombolis

Quantity		Grocery Item
11	oz	Bread, Crusty French Loaf, refrigerated
0.5	cup	Cheese, Gruyere, shredded
1	cup	Vegetable, Lettuce, arugula, raw
0.66	Tablespoon	Herb, Parsley, dried
2	Oz	Lunch Meat, Pork Ham, Prosciutto

Cucumber Salad

Quantity		Grocery Item
3	Teaspoon	Sweet, Sugar, granulated, white
1	Tablespoons	Vinegar, Cider
1.5	Cup	Vegetable, Cucumber, peeled, raw
0.25	tsp	Salt
8	Tablespoon	Vegetable, Onions, Red

157

Week 10 Meals and Grocery Lists

Grilled Taco Chicken with Spanish Rice and Strawberries

Grilled Peaches and Pork with Down Home Baked Beans and Bananas

Beef Lettuce Wraps with Micro-Baked Potatoes and Creamy Lemon Coleslaw

Orzo Salad with Feta Vinaigrette with Asparagus, Corn on the Cob, and Steamed Carrots

Gnocchi with Shrimp, Asparagus and Pesto with Roasted Acorn Squash and Apples

Chicken and Cashews with Minute Rice, Tossed and Almond Salad and Roasted Broccoli with Almonds

Quick Chili with Roasted Parmesan Zucchini

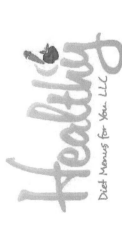

Healthy
Diet Menus for You, LLC

Meal Plan

www.healthydietmenusforyou.com

Diet: *Gestational Diabetic - 2400*

Meal: *Grilled Taco Chicken GDM*

Recipe | Ingredients | Instructions | Nutritionals

Grilled Taco Chicken

Serves: 6

Serving Size: 3 oz. chicken breast

	Ingredients
0.5 teaspoon	Spice, Chili Powder
0.25 tsp	Spice, Black Pepper
0.5 tsp	Spice, Cumin, Ground
1 Teaspoon	Herb, Oregano, Ground
0.25 Teaspoo	Spice, Onion Powder
1 Tablespoon	Oil, Vegetable or Olive
2 Tablespoon	Sauce, BBQ
24 ounces	Chicken, Breast Boneless

Instructions: Combine seasonings and oregano. Brush chicken with olive oil; sprinkle with seaoning mix. Grill chicken over medium heat; cook 10-15 minutes until done turning once. Combine BBQ and cumin. Heat in microwave and spread over chicken.

Nutritionals:

Calories	169.2	Sodium:	100.4	Protein:	26.8	Phos	199.1
Fat:	5.3	Carbs:	0.6	Chol:	73	Pot:	239.3
Sat Fat:	1.2	Fiber:	0.2				
		Sugar:	0				

Recipe | Ingredients | Instructions | Nutritionals

Spanish Rice

Serves: 6

Serving Size: 1/2 Cup

	Ingredients
2 Tablespoon	Oil, Vegetable or Olive
1 Cup	Vegetable, Onions
1 Teaspoon	Herb, Garlic, Raw
1.5 Cup	Grain, Rice, White, Medium grain, ckd
3 cup	Soup, Chicken Broth Low Sodium
1 Cup	Vegetable, Tomato Red Raw
0.25 Teaspoo	Herb, Oregano, Ground
0.5 tsp	Salt

Instructions: In a large skillet, brown rice in olive oil at a medium / high heat. Add onion and garlic. Cook onion / rice mixture, stirring frequently, about 4 minutes, or until onions are softened. In a separate pan, bring chicken broth to a simmer. Add tomato chopped, oregano and salt. Add rice to broth. Bring to a simmer. Cover. Lower heat and cook 15-25 minutes, depending on the type of rice and the instructions on the rice package. Turn off heat and let sit for 5 minutes.

Nutritionals:

Calories	248.2	Sodium:	232.7	Protein:	6.1	Phos	102
Fat:	5.5	Carbs:	43.2	Chol:	0	Pot:	246
Sat Fat:	0.9	Fiber:	1.3				
		Sugar:	1.7				

Recipe | Ingredients | Instructions | Nutritionals

Strawberries

Serves: 6

Serving Size: 1.5 Cups of Strawberries

	Ingredients
9 Cup	Fruit, Strawberries, halves/slices, raw

Instructions: Remove tops and wash prior to serving.

Nutritionals:

Calories	73	Sodium:	2.2	Protein:	1.5	Phos	54.7
Fat:	0.6	Carbs:	17.5	Chol:	0	Pot:	348.8
Sat Fat:	0	Fiber:	4.5				
		Sugar:	11.1				

161

Meal: Grilled Peaches and Pork GDM

Grilled Peaches and Pork

Serves: 4

Serving Size: 4 oz chop

Recipe / Ingredients	Instructions	Nutritionals			
		Calories 250.1	Sodium: 63.8	Protein: 26.3	Phos 271.1
		Fat: 7.828	Carbs: 18.4	Chol: 62.4	Pot: 797.9
		Sat Fat: 2.602	Fiber: 2.739		
			Sugar: 15.1		

Ingredients		Instructions
16 ounces	Pork, Center Rib Chop	Place each piece of pork between 2 sheets of heavy-duty plastic wrap, and pound each piece to 1/4-inch thickness using a meat mallet or a rolling pin.
4 Tablespoon	Vinegar, balsamic	
2 Tablespoon	Lime Juice	Combine 2 tablespoons vinegar, juice, thyme, salt, and pepper in a small bowl. Reserve 1 tablespoon juice mixture. Pour the remaining juice mixture in a large zip-top plastic bag. Add pork; seal and marinate in refrigerator for 1 hour, turning occasionally.
0.5 teaspoon	Salt, Kosher	
3 Teaspoon	Herb, Thyme Ground	
0.5 tsp	Spice, Black Pepper	
4 1	Fruit, Peach, peeled, raw	Preheat grill to medium heat.
		Place peaches, cut sides up, on a plate; drizzle with remaining 2 tablespoons vinegar. Place pork on grill rack coated with cooking spray; grill 3 minutes on each side or until pork is done. Set aside. Place peaches, cut sides down, on grill rack; grill 4 minutes or until soft and slightly browned. Turn and cook 2 minutes or until heated through. Cut each peach half into 4 slices. Slice pieces of pork into 1-inch-thick strips.

Down Home Baked Bean.

Serves: 4

Serving Size: 1/2 cup

Recipe / Ingredients	Instructions	Nutritionals			
		Calories 131	Sodium: 285	Protein: 6.03	Phos 114
		Fat: 1.5	Carbs: 23.7	Chol: 4.5	Pot: 276
		Sat Fat: 0.3	Fiber: 4.2		
			Sugar: 12.1		

Ingredients		Instructions
8 Tablespoon	Sauce, BBQ	In a small saucepan over high heat, combine the barbeque sauce with the dry mustard, onion, bacon bits, beans and kale. Bring to a boil, reduce the heat to low, and simmer the beans for 10 minutes, or until the kale is tender, stirring occasionally. The sauce should thicken slightly and the beans should be very tender.
0.25 Teaspoo	Spice, Dry Mustard	
0.33 Cup	Vegetable, Onions	
1 tablespoon	Bacon Bits	
1 Cup	Beans, Cannellini White, canned	
1 Cup	Vegetable, Kale, raw	

Banana

Serves: 6

Serving Size: 1 banana

Recipe / Ingredients	Instructions	Nutritionals			
		Calories 105	Sodium: 1.1	Protein: 1.2	Phos 26
		Fat: 0.3	Carbs: 27	Chol: 0	Pot: 422.4
		Sat Fat: 0.1	Fiber: 3		
			Sugar: 14.4		

Ingredients		Instructions
6 1	Fruit, Banana	Piece of fruit

Meal: *Beef, Lettuce Wraps GDM*

Beef Lettuce Wraps

Serves: 4

Serving Size: 2 wraps and 1 tsp sauce

Nutritionals

Calories	290.6	Sodium:	647.3	Protein:	35.9	Phos: 322.8
Fat:	11.1	Carbs:	11.2	Chol:	53.7	Pot: 678.1
Sat Fat:	3.6	Fiber:	1.9			
		Sugar:	6.6			

Ingredients

16 Ounces	Beef, Flank Lean Trimmed
0.25 teaspoo	Salt, Kosher
0.25 tsp	Spice, Black Pepper
3 Tablespoon	Lime Juice
1 Oz	Fish Sauce (Bagoong)
4 Teaspoon P	Sugar, Brown
1 Each	Vegetable, Pepper, Jalapeno, raw
8 Leaf	Vegetable, Lettuce, Butterhead (Boston/Bibb) leaves, raw
16 Tablespoo	Vegetable, Onions, Red
8 Tablespoon	Herb, Peppermint, fresh
0.5 Cup	Vegetable, Cucumber, peeled, raw
0.5 Cup	Herb, Cilantro Raw
1 oz	Peanuts, All Types, dry roasted w/o salt

Instructions

Heat a grill pan over medium-high heat. Coat pan with cooking spray. Sprinkle steak with salt and pepper. Place steak in pan; cook 5 minutes on each side or until desired degree of doneness. Remove from pan; let stand 10 minutes. Cut steak diagonally across the grain into thin slices. Mince jalapeno pepper and remove seeds. Cut cucumber into matchstick sized pieces. Chop peanuts.

Combine juice, fish sauce, sugar, and jalapeño in a medium bowl, stirring with a whisk. Reserve 4 teaspoons juice mixture in a small serving bowl. Pour remaining juice mixture in a large bowl; add steak, tossing to coat. Place 1 1/2 ounces beef in center of each lettuce leaf; top each with 2 tablespoons onion, 2 tablespoons mint, 1 tablespoon cucumber, and 1 tablespoon cilantro. Sprinkle evenly with peanuts; roll up. Serve with reserved juice mixture.

Micro-Baked Potatoes

Serves: 6

Serving Size: 1 potatoe + 2T Butter

Nutritionals

Calories	283.7	Sodium:	20.1	Protein:	4.1	Phos: 178.7
Fat:	14.3	Carbs:	36.3	Chol:	27.1	Pot: 659.3
Sat Fat:	8.8	Fiber:	2.4			
		Sugar:	0			

Ingredients

6 Each	Vegetable, Potato, Flesh only, microwaved w/skin, no salt
12 tablespoo	Butter, Light w/no added salt

Instructions

Pierce potatoes and coat with olive oil. Microwave on high 4 minutes. Turn each potato over, cook another 4 minutes. Turn all potatoes again. Cook another 3 minutes. They are done wehn a knife can slice through them easily. Remove from microwave. Cut open and serve with 2 T butter.

Creamy Lemon Coleslaw

Serves: 6

Serving Size: 1/6 of container

Nutritionals

Calories	81	Sodium:	158	Protein:	1.7	Phos: 34
Fat:	3	Carbs:	12	Chol:	4	Pot: 211
Sat Fat:	0.5	Fiber:	3			
		Sugar:	5.5			

Ingredients

1 Each	Vegetable, Cabbage Head
6 Each	Sugar Substitute Packet, Equal
0.125 Cup	Vegetable, Onions
0.5 teaspoon	Salt, Kosher
6 Tablespoon	Miracle Whip Light
2 Packet	True Lemon packet

Instructions

Shred cabbage and chop onions. Combine all ingredients in a bowl, and toss lightly. Refrigerate if not used immediately.

Meal: *Orzo Salad with Feta GDM*

Recipe		Ingredients	Instructions	Nutritionals					
Orzo Salad with Feta Vinaigrette	1 Cup	Pasta, Orzo Dry	Cook the orzo according to package directions, omitting salt and fat. Drain; rinse with cold water. Combine orzo, spinach, sun dried tomatoes, red onion, kalamata olives, pepper and salt in a large bowl. Drain artichokes, reserving marinade. Coarsely chop artichokes, and add artichokes, reserved marinade, and 1/2 cup feta cheese to orzo mixture, tossing gently to coat. Sprinkle each serving with remaining feta cheese.	Calories 312.5	Sodium: 936.9	Protein: 11.6	Phos 206
	2 Ounces	Vegetable, Spinach, raw, torn		Fat:	13.5	Carbs:	38	Chol:	25	Pot: 489.3
Serves: 4	0.5 Cup	Vegetable, Tomato, Sun–dried, oil packed, drained		Sat Fat:	5.268	Fiber:	6.407		
Serving Size: 1.25 cups salad + 1 T Cheese	4 Tablespoon	Vegetable, Onions, Red				Sugar:	2.523		
	0.5 tsp	Spice, Black Pepper							
	0.25 Cup	Vegetable, Olives							
	0.25 tsp	Salt							
	0.75 Cup	Cheese, Feta							
	0.75 Cup	Vegetable - Artichoke - canned artichoke hearts in oil							

Recipe		Ingredients	Instructions	Nutritionals					
Asparagus	54 Ounces	Vegetable, Asparagus Fresh	Wash and clean asparagus by cutting off hard ends of stalk. Steam for 10 minutes in steamer or cook in 1 in water in microwaveable bowl for 5-7 minutes until desired tenderness.	Calories 21.5	Sodium: 1.8	Protein: 2.3	Phos 48.3
Serves: 6				Fat:	0.2	Carbs:	3.7	Chol:	0	Pot: 143.2
Serving Size: 1/2 Cup				Sat Fat:	0	Fiber:	1.5		
						Sugar:	0		

Recipe		Ingredients	Instructions	Nutritionals					
Corn On The Cob	6 Each	Vegetable, Corn on Cob, sm/med, ckd w/o fat or salt	Shuck and clean corn. Boil until tender, about 4-6 minutes.	Calories 82.7	Sodium: 1.5	Protein: 2.5	Phos 78.8
Serves: 6				Fat:	0.9	Carbs:	19.2	Chol:	0	Pot: 190.6
Serving Size: 1 ear of cor,				Sat Fat:	0.1	Fiber:	2.8		
						Sugar:	0		

Recipe		Ingredients	Instructions	Nutritionals					
Steamed Carrots	3 Cup	Vegetable, Carrots	Steam carrots until tender, season with Mrs. Dash	Calories 33	Sodium: 2	Protein: 1	Phos 22
Serves: 6	1 Teaspoon	Spice, Mrs. Dash		Fat:	0	Carbs:	8	Chol:	0	Pot: 165
Serving Size: 1/2 cup				Sat Fat:	0	Fiber:	3		
						Sugar:	0		

Meal: *Gnocchi with Shrimp GDM*

Recipe: Gnocchi w Shrimp, Aspargus and Pesto
Serves: 4
Serving Size: 2 cups

Ingredients	
128 oz	Water
16 ounces	Pasta, Gnocchi, Potato, frozen
32 Ounces	Vegetable, Asparagus Fresh
16 Ounces	Shellfish, Shrimp, bkd, broil or saute, med/large sizes
16 Tablespoo	Herb, Basil, fresh
2 Tablespoon	Nuts, Pine nuts (Pignolias)
0.125 Cup	Cheese, Grated Parmesan, Reduced Fat
1 ounces	Lemon Juice, Bottled
2 Teaspoon	Herb, Garlic, Raw
1.3 Tablespo	Oil, Vegetable or Olive

Instructions

1. Bring 2 quarts water to a boil in a Dutch oven. Coarsely chop shrimp and asparagus. Add gnocchi to pan; cook 4 minutes or until done (gnocchi will rise to surface). Remove with a slotted spoon; place in a large bowl. Add asparagus and shrimp to pan; cook 5 minutes or until shrimp are done. Drain. Add shrimp mixture to gnocchi.

2. Combine remaining 1 tablespoon water, basil, and pine nuts, parmesan cheese, lemon juice and garlic in a food processor; process until smooth, scraping sides. Drizzle oil through food chute with food processor on; process until well blended. Add basil mixture to shrimp mixture; toss to coat. Serve immediately.

Nutritionals

Calories 450.4	Sodium: 720.9	Protein: 35.5	Phos 446.0
Fat: 22.3	Carbs: 28.2	Chol: 232.2	Pot: 739.9
Sat Fat: 7.4	Fiber: 4.2		
	Sugar: 2.9		

Recipe: Roasted Acorn Squash
Serves: 8
Serving Size: 1/8 recipe

Ingredients	
0.5 tsp	Salt
0.25 tsp	Spice, Black Pepper
2 Teaspoon	Oil, Olive
32 Ounces	Vegetable, Squash, Acorn, peeled, raw

Instructions

Preheat oven to 400°. Cut them off of each squash and cut in half lengthwise. Scoop out seeds; rinse and dry each squash, half. Spray all sides of squash halves with cooking spray. Season inside of each half with salt and pepper. Place cut side down on a nonstick cooking spray coated baking sheet. Bake for 45 min. Scoop squash meat out into a medium bowl; discard skins. Add olive oil and beat with a sturdy whisk until fluffy.

Nutritionals

Calories 100.8	Sodium: 72.5	Protein: 1.822	Phos 81.8
Fat: 1.354	Carbs: 23.7	Chol: 0	Pot: 787.9
Sat Fat: 0.204	Fiber: 3.419		
	Sugar: 0		

Recipe: Apple - Red
Serves: 6
Serving Size: 1 apple

Ingredients	
6 Each	Fruit, Apple, peeled, raw, medium

Instructions

Piece of fruit

Nutritionals

Calories 94.6	Sodium: 1.8	Protein: 0.4	Phos 20
Fat: 0.3	Carbs: 25.1	Chol: 0	Pot: 194.7
Sat Fat: 0	Fiber: 4.3		
	Sugar: 18.9		

Meal: *Cashew Chicken GDM*

Recipe | Ingredients | Instructions | Nutritionals

Chicken and Cashew
Serves: 4
Serving Size: 3/4 cup mixture

Amount	Ingredients
3 Tablespoon	Soy Sauce, Low Sodium
1 Ounces	Wine, table, red - dry sherry
4 Teaspoon	Cornstarch, hydrolyzed powder
0.5 cup	Soup, Chicken Broth Low Sodium
16 Ounce	Chicken, Breast, No Skin, Raw
0.5 ounces	Honey
2 Tablespoon	Sauce, Oyster
3 Teaspoon	Oil, Sesame Oil
0.75 Cup	Vegetable, Onions
0.5 Cup	Vegetable, Celery Raw
0.5 Cup	Vegetable, Onions, Young Green, raw
0.5 Cup	Vegetable, Pepper, Green
1 Teaspoon	Spice, Ginger
0.5 Teaspoon	Herb, Garlic, Raw
0.25 Cup	Nuts, Cashew, Dry Roasted, Chopped No Salt

Instructions:
1. Cook chicken well and chop into bite sized pieces. Combine 1 tablespoon soy sauce, sherry, 2 teaspoons cornstarch, and chicken in a large bowl; toss well to coat. Combine remaining 2 tablespoons soy sauce, remaining 2 teaspoons cornstarch, broth, oyster sauce, and honey in a small bowl.

2. Heat 1 teaspoon oil in a large nonstick skillet over medium-high heat. Add chicken mixture to pan; sauté 3 minutes. Remove from pan. Heat remaining 1 teaspoon oil in pan. Add onion, celery, and bell pepper to pan; sauté 2 minutes. Add ginger and garlic; sauté 1 minute. Return chicken mixture to pan; sauté 1 minute. Stir in broth mixture. Bring to a boil; cook 1 minute, stirring constantly. Remove from heat. Sprinkle with green onions and cashews.

Nutritionals:

Calories 280.7	Sodium: 802.8	Protein: 27.7	Phos 329.^
Fat: 10.7	Carbs: 17.5	Chol: 72.6	Pot: 687.7
Sat Fat: 2.012	Fiber: 1.851		
	Sugar: 7.299		

Minute Rice
Serves: 6
Serving Size: 1/2 Cup Ric

Amount	Ingredients
1.5 Cup	Rice, white, cooked, instant
12 oz	Water

Instructions:
Bring water to a boil. Stir in rice, cover and remove from heat. Let stand for 5 minutes or until water is absorbed. Fluff with fork.

Nutritionals:

Calories 96.3	Sodium: 294.8	Protein: 1.7	Phos 30.7
Fat: 0.4	Carbs: 20.6	Chol: 0	Pot: 8
Sat Fat: 0	Fiber: 0.4		
	Sugar: 0		

Tossed Pear and Almond Salad
Serves: 6
Serving Size: Salad

Amount	Ingredients
2 Fruit	Fruit, Pear Raw
6 Cup	Lettuce, Raw Iceberg
0.25 Cup	Nuts, Almond Sliced
6 Tablespoon	Salad Dressing, Vinaigrette

Instructions:
Toss Salad together and divide into 6 portions

Nutritionals:

Calories 127	Sodium: 222	Protein: 2	Phos 46
Fat: 7	Carbs: 16	Chol: 0	Pot: 191
Sat Fat: 1	Fiber: 3		
	Sugar: 7		

Recipe		Ingredients	Instructions	Nutritionals				
Roasted Broccoli with Almonds	5 Cup	Vegetable, Broccoli Florets, Raw	Cut broccoli off stem if necessary. Place broccoli in a sprayed baking dish. Drizzle broccoli with olive oil, garlic, salt and pepper. Bake 14 minutes at 450ºF. Sprinkle with almonds and divide into 6 servings.	Calories 123	Sodium: 164	Protein: 7	Phos 162	
	1 Tablespoon	Oil, Vegetable or Olive		Fat: 6	Carbs: 6	Chol: 0	Pot: 685	
	0.25 tsp	Salt		Sat Fat: 1	Fiber: 6			
Serves: 6	0.25 tsp	Spice, Black Pepper			Sugar: 4			
Serving Size: 3/4 Cup	0.25 Cup	Nuts, Almond Sliced						

Meal: *Turkey, Chili GDM*

Recipe		Ingredients	Instructions	Nutritionals				
Quick Chili	1 Cup	Rice, white, cooked, instant	Cook rice according to package directions, omitting salt and fat. Drain and rinse kidney beans.	Calories 526.2	Sodium: 905.4	Protein: 27.8	Phos 416.0	
	3 Teaspoon	Oil, Olive		Fat: 10.4	Carbs: 81.6	Chol: 46.3	Pot: 1114	
Serves: 4	1 Cup	Vegetable, Onions	While rice cooks, heat oil in a large nonstick skillet over medium-high heat. Add onion, bell pepper, and turkey, and cook 3 minutes or until done, stirring to crumble. Stir in chili powder, Worcestershire, cumin, oregano, black pepper, kidney beans, stewed tomatoes and tomato juice; bring to a boil. Cover, reduce heat, and simmer 10 minutes. Serve over rice, and sprinkle with cheese.	Sat Fat: 2.372	Fiber: 12.5			
Serving Size: 1 1/4 cup chili +1/2 cup Rice	0.75 Cup	Vegetable, Pepper, Green			Sugar: 8.064			
	0.5 Pound	Turkey, Ground Raw						
	3 teaspoon	Spice, Chili Powder						
	0.333 Tables	Worcestershire Sauce						
	0.5 tsp	Spice, Cumin, Ground						
	0.5 Teaspoon	Herb, Oregano, Ground						
	0.25 tsp	Spice, Black Pepper						
	0.25 Cup	Cheese, Cheddar reduced fat						
	14 Ounces	Vegetable, Tomatoes, canned, stewed						
	5 Ounce	Juice, Tomato, Low Sodium						
	1.8 Cup	Beans, Kidney, canned/Rinsed						

Recipe		Ingredients	Instructions	Nutritionals				
Roasted Parmesan Zucchini	2 Cup	Vegetable, Zucchini, slices	Preheat oven to 450°. Coat a roasting pan with cooking spray. Place zucchini, sliced in 2 inch wedges in pan. Drizzle olive oil over zucchini, and sprinkle evenly with garlic and Parmesan cheese. Roast for approximately 20 min.	Calories 33.1	Sodium: 50	Protein: 1.236	Phos 41.6	
	2 Teaspoon	Oil, Olive		Fat: 2.562	Carbs: 1.769	Chol: 2.64	Pot: 135.5	
Serves: 5	1 Teaspoon	Herb, Garlic, Raw		Sat Fat: 0.69	Fiber: 0.508			
Serving Size: 1/2 cup	3 Tablespoon	Cheese, Parmesan, dry grated, reduced fat			Sugar: 1.246			

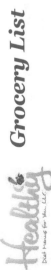

Grocery List

Grilled Taco Chicken GDM Meal

Grilled Taco Chicken

Quantity		Grocery Item
0.5	tsp	Spice, Cumin, Ground
1	Tablespoon	Oil, Vegetable or Olive
0.5	teaspoon	Spice, Chili Powder
24	ounces	Chicken, Breast Boneless
1	Teaspoon	Herb, Oregano, Ground
0.25	Teaspoon	Spice, Onion Powder
2	Tablespoon	Sauce, BBQ
0.25	tsp	Spice, Black Pepper

Spanish Rice

Quantity		Grocery Item
0.5	tsp	Salt
2	Tablespoon	Oil, Vegetable or Olive
1.5	Cup	Grain, Rice, White, Medium grain, ckd
0.25	Teaspoon	Herb, Oregano, Ground
1	Teaspoon	Herb, Garlic, Raw
3	cup	Soup, Chicken Broth Low Sodium
1	Cup	Vegetable, Onions
1	Cup	Vegetable, Tomato Red Raw

Strawberries

Quantity		Grocery Item
9	Cup	Fruit, Strawberries, halves/slices, raw

Grilled Peaches and Pork GDM Meal

Grilled Peaches and Pork

Quantity		Grocery Item
3	Teaspoon	Herb, Thyme Ground
0.5	tsp	Spice, Black Pepper
4	1	Fruit, Peach, peeled, raw
4	Tablespoon	Vinegar, balsamic
2	Tablespoon	Lime Juice
16	ounces	Pork, Center Rib Chop
0.5	teaspoon	Salt, Kosher

Down Home Baked Beans

Quantity		Grocery Item
1	tablespoon	Bacon Bits
1	Cup	Vegetable, Kale, raw
0.33	Cup	Vegetable, Onions
8	Tablespoon	Sauce, BBQ
0.25	Teaspoon	Spice, Dry Mustard
1	Cup	Beans, Cannellini White, canned

Banana

Quantity		Grocery Item
6	1	Fruit, Banana

Beef, Lettuce Wraps GDM Meal

Beef Lettuce Wraps

Quantity		Grocery Item
1	Oz	Fish Sauce (Bagoong)
8	Leaf	Vegetable, Lettuce, Butterhead
3	Tablespoon	Lime Juice
1	oz	Peanuts, All Types, dry roasted w/o salt
0.5	Cup	Vegetable, Cucumber, peeled, raw
8	Tablespoon	Herb, Peppermint, fresh
4	Teaspoon Pac	Sugar, Brown
0.5	Cup	Herb, Cilantro Raw
16	Ounces	Beef, Flank Lean Trimmed
16	Tablespoon	Vegetable, Onions, Red
0.25	teaspoon	Salt, Kosher
1	Each	Vegetable, Pepper, Jalapeno, raw
0.25	tsp	Spice, Black Pepper

Micro-Baked Potatoes

Quantity		Grocery Item
12	tablespoon	Butter, Light w/no added salt
6	Each	Vegetable, Potato, Flesh only,

Cashew Chicken GDM Meal

Chicken and Cashew

Quantity		Grocery Item
0.75	Cup	Vegetable, Onions
0.25	Cup	Nuts, Cashew, Dry Roasted, Chopped No
1	Teaspoon	Spice, Ginger
2	Tablespoon	Sauce, Oyster
0.5	Cup	Vegetable, Pepper, Green
0.5	ounces	Honey
3	Tablespoon	Soy Sauce, Low Sodium
4	Teaspoon	Cornstarch, hydrolyzed powder
3	Teaspoon	Oil, Sesame Oil
0.5	Cup	Vegetable, Celery Raw
0.5	Teaspoon	Herb, Garlic, Raw
0.5	Cup	Vegetable, Onions, Young Green, raw
16	Ounce	Chicken, Breast, No Skin, Raw
1	Ounces	Wine, table, red - dry sherry
0.5	cup	Soup, Chicken Broth Low Sodium

Minute Rice

Quantity		Grocery Item
12	oz	Water
1.5	Cup	Rice, white, cooked, instant

Steamed Carrots

Quantity		Grocery Item
1	Teaspoon	Spice, Mrs. Dash
3	Cup	Vegetable, Carrots

Gnocchi with Shrimp GDM Meal

Gnocchi w Shrimp, Aspargus and Pesto

Quantity		Grocery Item
128	oz	Water
1.3	Tablespoon	Oil, Vegetable or Olive
2	Teaspoon	Herb, Garlic, Raw
16	Tablespoon	Herb, Basil, fresh
16	ounces	Pasta, Gnocchi, Potato, frozen
2	Tablespoons	Nuts, Pine nuts (Pignolias)
1	ounces	Lemon Juice, Bottled
0.125	Cup	Cheese, Grated Parmesan, Reduced Fat
32	Ounces	Vegetable, Asparagus Fresh
16	Ounces	Shellfish, Shrimp, bkd, broil or saute,

Roasted Acorn Squash

Quantity		Grocery Item
32	Ounces	Vegetable, Squash, Acorn, peeled, raw
0.5	tsp	Salt
2	Teaspoon	Oil, Olive
0.25	tsp	Spice, Black Pepper

Apple - Red

Quantity		Grocery Item
6	Each	Fruit, Apple, peeled, raw, medium

Creamy Lemon Coleslaw

Quantity		Grocery Item
1	Each	Vegetable, Cabbage Head
6	Each	Sugar Substitute Packet, Equal
6	Tablespoon	Miracle Whip Light
0.125	Cup	Vegetable, Onions
2	Packet	True Lemon packet
0.5	teaspoon	Salt, Kosher

Orzo Salad with Feta GDM Meal

Orzo Salad with Feta Vinaigrette

Quantity		Grocery Item
4	Tablespoon	Vegetable, Onions, Red
0.25	Cup	Vegetable, Olives
0.5	Cup	Vegetable, Tomato, Sun-dried, oil packed,
0.75	Cup	Vegetable - Artichoke - canned artichoke
0.75	Cup	Cheese, Feta
1	Cup	Pasta, Orzo Dry
0.5	tsp	Spice, Black Pepper
0.25	tsp	Salt
2	Ounces	Vegetable, Spinach, raw, torn

Asparagus

Quantity		Grocery Item
54	Ounces	Vegetable, Asparagus Fresh

Corn On The Cob

Quantity		Grocery Item
6	Each	Vegetable, Corn on Cob, sm/med, ckd w/o

Turkey, Chili GDM Meal

Tossed Pear and Almond Salad

Quantity		Grocery Item
6	Cup	Lettuce, Raw Iceberg
2	Fruit	Fruit, Pear Raw
0.25	Cup	Nuts, Almond Sliced
6	Tablespoon	Salad Dressing, Vinaigrette

Roasted Broccoli with Almonds

Quantity		Grocery Item
0.25	tsp	Salt
1	Tablespoon	Oil, Vegetable or Olive
0.25	Cup	Nuts, Almond Sliced
0.25	tsp	Spice, Black Pepper
5	Cup	Vegetable, Broccoli Florets, Raw

Quick Chili

Quantity		Grocery Item
1	Cup	Rice, white, cooked, instant
0.333	Tablespoon	Worcestershire Sauce
0.5	tsp	Spice, Cumin, Ground
1	Cup	Vegetable, Onions
0.75	Cup	Vegetable, Pepper, Green
3	teaspoon	Spice, Chili Powder
1.8	Cup	Beans, Kidney, canned/Rinsed
0.5	Teaspoon	Herb, Oregano, Ground
3	Teaspoon	Oil, Olive
0.25	Cup	Cheese, Cheddar reduced fat
14	Ounces	Vegetable, Tomatoes, canned, stewed
0.25	tsp	Spice, Black Pepper
5	Ounce	Juice, Tomato, Low Sodium
0.5	Pound	Turkey, Ground Raw

Roasted Parmesan Zucchini

Quantity		Grocery Item
3	Tablespoon	Cheese, Parmesan, dry grated, reduced fat
2	Teaspoon	Oil, Olive
1	Teaspoon	Herb, Garlic, Raw
2	Cup	Vegetable, Zucchini, slices

Week 11 Meals and Grocery Lists

Chicken Kebabs with Creamy Pesto with Garlic Cheese Bread, Green Beans, and Tomato Ranch Salad

Pan Grilled Halibut with Rice and Noodle Pilaf and Strawberries with Broccoli Casserole

Beef Tips with Mushroom Gravy with Rice and Noodle Pilaf, Steamed Carrots and Bananas

Glazed Ham Steak with Broccoli Casserole, Creamy Herbed Mashed Potatoes and Garden Coleslaw with Almonds

Chinese Chicken Salad with Minute Rice and Italian Green Beans

Chipotle Bean Burrito with Tomato Ranch Salad

Baked Shrimp with Feta, Roasted Broccoli with Almonds and Corn Chowder Soup

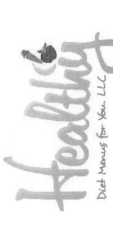

Diet Menus for You. LLC

Meal Plan

www.healthydietmenusforyou.com

Diet: *Gestational Diabetic - 2400*

Meal: *Chicken Kebabs with Pesto GDM*

Recipe		Ingredients	Instructions	Nutritionals					
Chicken Kebabs with Creamy Pesto	1 Each	Fruit, Lemon w/peel, raw	1. Preheat broiler. Cut yellow pepper into 2 inch pieces. Cut chicken breasts into 1 inch pieces. Grate lemon rind into bowl. Squeeze lemon juice into a separate bowl.	Calories 276.9	Sodium: 424.4	Protein: 37.5	Phos 312. 8	
	0.5 Teaspoon	Herb, Garlic, Raw		.				
	2 Teaspoon	Oil, Olive		Fat: 9.404	Carbs: 9.404	Chol: 101.2	Pot: 531.8	
Serves: 4	0.25 tsp	Spice, Black Pepper		Sat Fat: 2.543	Fiber: 1.78			
	16 ounces	Chicken, Breast Boneless	2. Combine rind, 1 tablespoon juice, garlic, oil, salt, and pepper. Toss with bell pepper, tomatoes, chicken, and onion. Thread vegetables and chicken onto 4 (12-inch) skewers. Place skewers on a broiler pan coated with cooking spray. Broil 12 minutes or until chicken is done, turning occasionally.		Sugar: 2.115			
Serving Size: 1 Kebab with 1 T Sauce	16 Tablespoo	Vegetable, Onions, Red						
	1 Oz	Yogurt, plain, lowfat milk						
	2 Tablespoon	Cream, Sour, Reduced Fat						
	8 Each	Vegetable, Tomato, Red, Cherry	3. Combine 1 teaspoon juice, yogurt, sour cream, and pesto. Serve sauce with kebabs.					
	1 Cup	Vegetable, Pepper, Yellow Raw						
	0.5 tsp	Salt						
	0.5 Ounces	Pesto						

175

Garlic Cheese Bread

Serves: 4
Serving Size: 2 oz baguett

Ingredients	
1 Loaf	Bread, French or Vienna - baguette
2 Teaspoon	Herb, Garlic, Raw
1.5 cup	Soup, Chicken Broth Low Sodium
1 teaspoon	Spice, Red Pepper
0.25 Cup	Cheese, Grated Parmesan, Reduced Fat
0.5 Cup	Cheese, Mozzarella Part Skim
10 Springs	Herb, Parsley, Raw, Fresh

Instructions: Preheat the oven to 450°F. Line a baking sheet with foil. Split the baguette in half crosswise, then lengthwise, to make 4 pieces. Rub the entire surface of each piece with garlic. Place the bread, cut side up, on the prepared baking sheet and bake until the bread begins to brown, about 8 minutes. Remove the bread from the oven. Turn the broiler on high. Pour the chicken broth into a small bowl, and dunk each piece of bread in the broth allowing it to absorb a good amount of liquid. Place the soaked pieces of baguette back on the baking sheet, cut side up. Season them with crushed red pepper to taste. Sprinkle with the Parmesan cheese and mozzarella. Broil the bread until the cheese is bubbly and beginning to brown about 3 minutes. Chop and sprinkle parsley over the bread, cut each piece in half and serve. Serves 4.

Nutritionals

Calories 252.6	Sodium: 567.7	Protein: 14.8	Phos 216.5
Fat: 6.3	Carbs: 34.8	Chol: 13.1	Pot: 202.1
Sat Fat: 3.08	Fiber: 1.6		
	Sugar: 1.7		

Green Beans

Serves: 6
Serving Size: 1/2 Cup

Ingredients	
3 Cup	Vegetable, Beans, String, Green, raw

Instructions: Rinse green beans, cook until just tender in steamer or microwave.

Nutritionals

Calories 17	Sodium: 3.3	Protein: 1	Phos 20.9
Fat: 0	Carbs: 3.9	Chol: 0	Pot: 115
Sat Fat: 0	Fiber: 0.9		
	Sugar: 0		

Tomato Ranch Salad

Serves: 6
Serving Size: 3/4 cup salad w/dressing

Ingredients	
2 Cup	Vegetable, Tomato Red Raw
4.5 Cup	Vegetable, Lettuce, Iceberg, head, raw
12 Tablespoo	Salad dressing, ranch dressing, reduced fat

Instructions: Toss lettuce and tomatoes and divide into 6 portions. Top each salad with 2T lite ranch dressing.

Nutritionals

Calories 75.6	Sodium: 280	Protein: 1.2	Phos 80.8
Fat: 3.9	Carbs: 10	Chol: 4.8	Pot: 242.1
Sat Fat: 0.3	Fiber: 1.5		
	Sugar: 3.5		

Meal: *Pan Grilled Halibut GDM*

Recipe: *Pan Grilled Halibut*

Serves: 4

Serving Size: 4 ounce file +2 teaspoons sauce

Ingredients		Instructions
2 Tablespoon	Herb, Basil, fresh	1. Combine cilantro, basil, onions, olive oil, fresh lemon juice in a medium bowl; stir in 1/4 teaspoon salt and 1/8 teaspoon pepper.
0.18 Cup	Vegetable, Onions, Young Green, raw	
1.5 Tablespo	Oil, Vegetable or Olive	2. Heat a grill pan over medium-high heat. Coat pan with cooking spray. Sprinkle remaining 1/4 teaspoon salt and 1/8 teaspoon pepper over fish. Add fish to pan; cook 4 minutes on each side or until desired degree of doneness. Serve with sauce.
0.667 ounces	Lemon Juice, Bottled	
0.5 tsp	Salt	
0.25 tsp	Spice, Black Pepper	
24 Ounces	Fish, Halibut, Atlantic & Pacific, raw	
0.18 Cup	Herb, Cilantro Raw	

Nutritionals

Calories 234.8	Sodium: 384.3	Protein: 35.5	Phos 380.1
Fat: 8.992	Carbs: 0.737	Chol: 54.4	Pot: 783.1
Sat Fat: 1.257	Fiber: 0.135		
	Sugar: 0.25		

Recipe: *Rice and Noodle Pilaf*

Serves: 6

Serving Size: 2/3 cup

Ingredients		Instructions
2 tablespoon	Butter, Light w/no added salt	Break spaghetti noodles into small sections about 1-2 inches long. Melt the butter in a large saucepan over medium heat, and add spaghetti.
0.3 Cup	Pasta, Spaghetti	
1 Cup	Rice, Medium Brown	Sauté spaghetti for 5 minutes or until lightly browned. Add the rice, stirring to coat. Stir in the boiling water, salt, and pepper, and bring to a boil. Cover; reduce heat, and simmer for 20 minutes or until the liquid is absorbed. Remove pilaf from heat, and let stand for 10 minutes. Fluff with a fork.
16 oz	Water	
0.25 tsp	Salt	
0.25 tsp	Spice, Black Pepper	

Nutritionals

Calories 188.2	Sodium: 103.8	Protein: 4.4	Phos 131.1
Fat: 3.4	Carbs: 34.5	Chol: 4.5	Pot: 105.3
Sat Fat: 1.6	Fiber: 1.5		
	Sugar: 0.6		

Recipe: *Strawberries*

Serves: 6

Serving Size: 1.5 Cups of Strawberries

Ingredients		Instructions
9 Cup	Fruit, Strawberries, halves/slices, raw	Remove tops and wash prior to serving.

Nutritionals

Calories 73	Sodium: 2.2	Protein: 1.5	Phos 54.7
Fat: 0.6	Carbs: 17.5	Chol: 0	Pot: 348.8
Sat Fat: 0	Fiber: 4.5		
	Sugar: 11.1		

Recipe: *Broccoli Casserole*

Serves: 8

Serving Size: 1/2 cup

Ingredients		Instructions
4 Cup	Vegetable, Broccoli Florets, Raw	Preheat oven to 350°. In a large bowl, combine all ingredients. Pour into a medium casserole dish and bake for 30 min.
4 fluid ounces	Milk, Nonfat/Skim	
0.125 tsp	Spice, Black Pepper	
0.5 Cup	Cheese, Cheddar reduced fat	
6 Ounces	Soup, Cream of Celery, Fat Free	

Nutritionals

Calories 53.3	Sodium: 300	Protein: 3.796	Phos 135.2
Fat: 2.291	Carbs: 5.245	Chol: 7.318	Pot: 231.2
Sat Fat: 1.228	Fiber: 0.179		
	Sugar: 1.884		

Meal: *Beef Tips GDM*

Recipe		Ingredients		Instructions	*Nutritionals*			
Beef Tips with Mushroom Gravy	16 Ounces	Beef, tenderloin, lean		Cut beef into small pieces of 1 to 2 ounces. Coat a large nonstick skillet with cooking spray over high heat. Add beef tips to skillet and sauté for 5 to 6 min. or until browned well. Remove beef from pan and set aside. Cover beef. Add mushrooms to pan and sauté for 4 to 5 min. In a small bowl, whisk together broth and cornstarch. Pour over mushrooms and bring to a boil, scraping browned bits of from the bottom of the pan. Reduce heat and simmer for 2 min. Stir in salt and pepper. Return beef tips and any juice and stir into gravy.	Calories 300.9	Sodium: 366	Protein: 23.5	Phos 232.4
	0.5 cup	Vegetable, Mushrooms, slices, raw			Fat: 21.3	Carbs: 2.688	Chol: 77.1	Pot: 421.4
Serves: 4	1 Cup	Soup, Beef broth, canned, low sodium			Sat Fat: 8.563	Fiber: 0.138		
Serving Size: 1/4 recipe	3 Teaspoon	Cornstarch, hydrolyzed powder				Sugar: 0.252		
	0.5 tsp	Salt						
	0.25 tsp	Spice, Black Pepper						

Recipe		Ingredients		Instructions	*Nutritionals*			
Rice and Noodle Pilaf	2 tablespoon	Butter, Light w/no added salt		Break spaghetti noodles into small sections about 1-2 inches long. Melt the butter in a large saucepan over medium heat, and add spaghetti. Sauté spaghetti for 5 minutes or until lightly browned. Add the rice, stirring to coat. Stir in the boiling water, salt, and pepper, and bring to a boil. Cover; reduce heat, and simmer for 20 minutes or until the liquid is absorbed. Remove pilaf from heat, and let stand for 10 minutes. Fluff with a fork.	Calories 188.2	Sodium: 103.8	Protein: 4.4	Phos 131.1
	0.3 Cup	Pasta, Spaghetti			Fat: 3.4	Carbs: 34.5	Chol: 4.5	Pot: 105.3
Serves: 6	1 Cup	Rice, Medium Brown			Sat Fat: 1.6	Fiber: 1.5		
Serving Size: 2/3 cup	16 oz	Water				Sugar: 0.6		
	0.25 tsp	Salt						
	0.25 tsp	Spice, Black Pepper						

Recipe		Ingredients	Instructions	*Nutritionals*			
Banana	6 1	Fruit, Banana	Piece of fruit	Calories 105	Sodium: 1.1	Protein: 1.2	Phos 26
Serves: 6				Fat: 0.3	Carbs: 27	Chol: 0	Pot: 422.4
Serving Size: 1 banana				Sat Fat: 0.1	Fiber: 3		
					Sugar: 14.4		

Recipe		Ingredients	Instructions	*Nutritionals*			
Steamed Carrots	3 Cup	Vegetable, Carrots	Steam carrots until tender, season with Mrs. Dash	Calories 33	Sodium: 2	Protein: 1	Phos 22
Serves: 6	1 Teaspoon	Spice, Mrs. Dash		Fat: 0	Carbs: 8	Chol: 0	Pot: 165
Serving Size: 1/2 cup				Sat Fat: 0	Fiber: 3		
					Sugar: 0		

Meal: Glazed Ham Steaks GDM

Glazed Ham Steaks
Serves: 4
Serving Size: 4 ounce ham steak

Ingredients	Instructions	Nutritionals
1 Tablespoon Soy Sauce, Low Sodium 0.125 Cup Condiment, Tomato catsup - ketchup 12 Teaspoon Sweet, Jams & Preserves, apricot 16 Ounce Pork Ham Steak, Cured, extra lean, boneless	Preheat oven to 375°. In a small saucepan, bring the preserves, soy sauce, and catchup to a boil. Reduce heat and simmer for 45 min. Coat a shallow baking pan with cooking spray. Arrange ham steaks in the bottom of the dish. Brush glaze on top and sides of ham steaks. Bake for 15 to 20 min.	Calories 192.5 Sodium: 1622 Protein: 22.6 Phos 301.1 Fat: 4.874 Chol: 51 Pot: 405.5 Sat Fat: 1.637 Fiber: 0.103 Sugar: 9.602

Broccoli Casserole
Serves: 8
Serving Size: 1/2 cup

Ingredients	Instructions	Nutritionals
4 Cup Vegetable, Broccoli Florets, Raw 4 fluid ounces Milk, Nonfat/Skim 0.125 tsp Spice, Black Pepper 0.5 Cup Cheese, Cheddar reduced fat 6 Ounces Soup, Cream of Celery, Fat Free	Preheat oven to 350°. In a large bowl, combine all ingredients. Pour into a medium casserole dish and bake for 30 min.	Calories 53.3 Sodium: 300 Protein: 3.796 Phos 135.2 Fat: 2.291 Chol: 5.245 Pot: 231.2 Sat Fat: 1.228 Fiber: 0.179 Sugar: 1.884

Creamy Herbed Mashed Potatoes
Serves: 6
Serving Size: 3/4 Cup

Ingredients	Instructions	Nutritionals
4 Cup Vegetable, Potato, Flesh only, diced, raw 4 fluid ounces Milk, Nonfat/Skim 1 Tablespoon Cream, Sour, Reduced Fat 3 tablespoon Butter, Light w/no added salt 3 Tablespoon Herb, Chives, raw 4 Springs Herb, Parsley, Raw, Fresh 0.5 tsp Salt 0.5 tsp Spice, Black Pepper	Peel and cube potatoes. Place potato in a saucepan; cover with water. Bring to a boil; cover, reduce heat, and simmer 10 minutes or until tender. Drain. Return potato to pan. Add milk and remaining ingredients; mash with a potato masher to desired consistency.	Calories 147.1 Sodium: 215.1 Protein: 3.1 Phos 73 Fat: 4.6 Chol: 23.8 Pot: 422.7 Sat Fat: 2.8 Fiber: 2.1 Sugar: 2.3

Recipe	Ingredients		Instructions	Nutritionals			
Garden Coleslaw With Almonds	0.25 Cup	Nuts, Almond Sliced	Start by toasting the almonds; put them in a small skillet, without oil, over medium heat and shake until almonds start to get golden brown. Remove and set aside.	Calories 162.8	Sodium: 69.3	Protein: 5.15	Phos 103.5
	1 Each	Vegetable, Cabbage Head		Fat: 7.843	Carbs: 21.2	Chol: 0	Pot: 479.2
Serves: 6	1 Cup	Vegetable, Carrots	Make slaw by shredding cabbage and dicing. Put in bowl.	Sat Fat: 0.936	Fiber: 6.47		
Serving Size: 3/4 Cup	6 Teaspoon	Oil, Olive	Shredded carrots, add to bowl.		Sugar: 13.9		
	9 Teaspoon	Vinegar, rice	Make dressing by whisking together the remaining ingredients until smooth; then pour the dressing over the slaw.				
	1 ounces	Honey	Add the toasted almonds, tossing to combine. Let stand for 30 minutes, tossing several times.				
	2 ounces	Yogurt, Greek Non Fat	To serve, spoon portions onto individual salad plates. You will have enough salad for 4 to 6 people.				
	0.4 Tablespo	Dijon Mustard					
	0.25 tsp	Spice, Black Pepper					

Meal: *Chinese Chicken Salad GDM*

Recipe		Ingredients	Instructions	Nutritionals

Chinese Chicken Salad
Serves: 4
Serving Size: 1/4 Mixture

Calories 258.5	Sodium: 1097	Protein: 25	Phos 268.5
Fat: 8.577	Carbs: 22	Chol: 52.9	Pot: 669.4
Sat Fat: 1.575	Fiber: 4.288		
	Sugar: 8.411		

Amount	Ingredient
3 Teaspoon	Oil, Sesame Oil
15 teaspoons	Herb, Ginger Root, peeled, sliced, raw
1.5 Teaspoon	Herb, Garlic, Raw
0.5 Cup	Vegetable, Onions, Young Green, raw
3 Teaspoon	Cornstarch, hydrolyzed powder
6 Tablespoon	Soy Sauce, Low Sodium
0.5 cup	Soup, Chicken Broth Low Sodium
9 Teaspoon	Vinegar, rice
3 tsp	Spice, Black Pepper
5 Tablespoon	Lime Juice
3 teaspoon	Spice, Chili Powder
0.25 Cup	Condiment, Tomato catsup - ketchup
12 ounces	Chicken, Breast Boneless
0.5 Cup	Vegetable, Peas, Snow/SugarSnap, ckd w/o fat or salt
0.5 Cup	Herb, Cilantro Raw
4 Cup	Vegetable, Cabbage Heads, Red, raw
6 Teaspoon	Spice, Sesame Seed

Instructions: Heat a large nonstick sauté pan over high heat. When the pan is hot, add the sesame oil. Add the ginger, garlic, and onions, and sauté, stirring often, about 2 min. Meanwhile, place the cornstarch in a medium bowl. Add the soy sauce, chicken broth, vinegar, and catchup and whisk to blend. Whisk the cornstarch mixture into the sauté pan and bring sauce to a simmer. Reduce the heat to medium and simmer, whisking constantly, until the sauce has thickened, about 2 min. Cook chicken, then shred into small pieces.

In a large bowl, whisk together the sauce you just made, lime juice and chili powder. Add the shredded chicken, red cabbage, snow peas, cilantro, and sesame seeds. Toss the salad to combine. Chill in the refrigerator until serving time, up to 6 hours.

Recipe		Ingredients	Instructions	Nutritionals

Minute Rice
Serves: 6
Serving Size: 1/2 Cup Ric

Calories 96.3	Sodium: 294.8	Protein: 1.7	Phos 30.7
Fat: 0.4	Carbs: 20.6	Chol: 0	Pot: 8
Sat Fat: 0	Fiber: 0.4		
	Sugar: 0		

Amount	Ingredient
1.5 Cup	Rice, white, cooked, instant
12 oz	Water

Instructions: Bring water to a boil. Stir in rice, cover and remove from heat. Let stand for 5 minutes or until water is absorbed. Fluff with fork.

Recipe: Italian Green Beans

Serves: 6

Serving Size: 1/2 cup

Ingredients

3 Teaspoon	Oil, Olive
1 Cup	Vegetable, Onions
2 Teaspoon	Herb, Garlic, Raw
1 Can	Vegetable, Tomato Diced Canned
0.25 Teaspoo	Herb, Oregano, Ground
0.25 Teaspoo	Herb, Basil, Ground
16 Ounces	Vegetable, Beans, Italian, Frozen

Instructions

Steam green beans until tender crisp. Set aside. Heat olive oil in a medium nonstick skillet over medium-high heat. Sauté onions until clear. Add garlic; sauté 30 seconds. Add tomatoes, basil, and oregano, and simmer for 15 to 20 min. for tomato mixture over steamed green beans and mix well.

Nutritionals

Calories 67.1	Sodium: 217.2	Protein: 2.111	Phos 46.7
Fat: 2.519	Carbs: 10.9	Chol: 0	Pot: 315.5
Sat Fat: 0.37	Fiber: 3.596		
	Sugar: 3.97		

Meal: *Bean Burrito GDM*

Recipe: Chipotle Bean Burrito

Serves: 6

Serving Size: 1 Burrito

Ingredients

1 Tablespoon	Oil, Vegetable or Olive
0.25 Teaspoon	Herb, Garlic, Raw
0.5 Teaspoon	Spice, Chipotle Chili Powder
3 oz	Water
1.75 Cup	Beans, Black, Canned
1.75 Cup	Beans, Kidney, canned/Rinsed
3 Tablespoon	Condiment, Salsa
6 Each	Tortilla, Flour (Wheat)
0.5 Cup	Cheese, Mexican blend, reduced fat - Kraft Mexican Four Cheese made with 2% Milk
0.5 Cup	Vegetable, Onions, Young Green, raw
1.5 Cup	Vegetable, Tomato, Plum/Italian
1.5 Cup	Vegetable, Lettuce, Cos/Romaine, raw
6 Tablespoon	Cream, Sour, Reduced Fat

Instructions

1. Heat oil in a large nonstick skillet over medium heat. Add garlic to pan; cook 1 minute., stirring frequently. Stir in chile powder and salt; cook 30 seconds, stirring constantly. Stir in 1/3 cup water and beans; bring to a boil. Reduce heat, and simmer 10 minutes. Remove from heat; stir in salsa. Partially mash bean mixture with a fork.
2. Warm tortillas according to package directions. Spoon about 1/3 cup bean mixture into center of each tortilla. Top each serving with about 2 1/2 tablespoons cheese, 1/4 cup tomato, 1/4 cup lettuce, 1 tablespoon onions, and 1 tablespoon sour cream; roll up.

Nutritionals

Calories 399.5	Sodium: 758.7	Protein: 18.7	Phos 343
Fat: 12.2	Carbs: 57.7	Chol: 17.3	Pot: 668.7
Sat Fat: 4.085	Fiber: 10.3		
	Sugar: 2.273		

Recipe: Tomato Ranch Salad

Serves: 6

Serving Size: 3/4 cup salad w/dressing

Ingredients

2 Cup	Vegetable, Tomato Red Raw
4.5 Cup	Vegetable, Lettuce, Iceberg, head, raw
12 Tablespoo	Salad dressing, ranch dressing, reduced fat

Instructions

Toss lettuce and tomatoes and divide into 6 portions. Top each salad with 2T lite ranch dressing.

Nutritionals

Calories 75.6	Sodium: 280	Protein: 1.2	Phos 80.8
Fat: 3.9	Carbs: 10	Chol: 1.5	Pot: 242.1
Sat Fat: 0.3	Fiber: 0.3		
	Sugar: 3.5		

Meal: Baked Shrimp GDM

Recipe		Ingredients	Instructions	Nutritionals				
Baked Shrimp with Feta	0.5 ounces	Lemon Juice, Bottled	1. Preheat oven to 450°.			Phos	441.0	
Serves: 4	0.333 Tables	Oil, Vegetable or Olive				Pot:	594.3	
Serving Size: 1 Cup	24 Ounces	Shrimp, peeled and deveined	2. Combine lemon juice and peeled and deveined shrimp in a large bowl; toss well. Heat a large nonstick skillet over medium-high heat. Coat pan with cooking spray. Add oil to pan, swirling to coat. Add onion to pan; sauté 1 minute. Add garlic; sauté 1 minute. Add clam juice, wine, oregano, pepper, and tomatoes; bring to a boil. Reduce heat, and simmer 5 minutes. Stir in shrimp mixture. Place mixture in an 11 x 7-inch baking dish coated with cooking spray. Sprinkle cheese evenly over mixture. Bake at 450° for 12 minutes or until shrimp are done and cheese melts. Sprinkle with parsley; serve immediately.	Calories	274.9	Sodium:	503.4	Protein: 38.5
	0.5 Cup	Vegetable, Onions		Fat:	8.278	Carbs:	9.337	Chol: 275.2
	0.25 Teaspoo	Herb, Garlic, Raw		Sat Fat:	3.548	Fiber:	1.641	
	1 Ounce	Juice, Clam & Tomato, canned				Sugar:	4.032	
	0.5 Teaspoon	Herb, Oregano, Ground						
	0.5 Oz	Beverage, Alcoholic, Wine, Table, Dry White						
	0.25 tsp	Spice, Black Pepper						
	2 Tablespoon	Herb, Parsley, Raw, Chopped						
	0.5 Cup	Cheese, Feta						
	15 Oz	Vegetable, Tomatoes, canned, low sodium crushed						

Recipe		Ingredients	Instructions	Nutritionals				
Roasted Broccoli with Almonds	5 Cup	Vegetable, Broccoli Florets, Raw	Cut broccoli off stem if necessary. Place broccoli in a sprayed baking dish. Drizzle broccoli with olive oil, garlic, salt and pepper. Bake 14 minutes at 450F. Sprinkle with almonds and divide into 6 servings.			Phos	162	
Serves: 6	1 Tablespoon	Oil, Vegetable or Olive				Pot:	685	
Serving Size: 3/4 Cup	0.25 tsp	Salt		Calories	123	Sodium:	164	Protein: 7
	0.25 tsp	Spice, Black Pepper		Fat:	6	Carbs:	15	Chol: 0
	0.25 Cup	Nuts, Almond Sliced		Sat Fat:	1	Fiber:	6	
						Sugar:	4	

Recipe	Ingredients		Instructions	Nutritionals			
Corn Chowder Soup	1 Cup	Vegetable, Onions	Heat a large 5 quart Dutch oven over medium heat. When the pot is hot, spray it with cooking spray. Add the onion and corn. Season with salt and pepper to taste. Saute, stirring occasionally, for 6 minutes or until the vegetables have started to soften. Add the cauliflower and milk, cover, and bring the soup to a boil. Reduce the heat to medium-low. Simmer the soup until the corn and cauliflower are tender, about 20 minutes. Strain 1 cup of the soup through a colander, saving the solids and returning the liquid to the pot. Using a stick blender or food processor, puree the liquid and rest of the pot (except the solids you just strained out) until smooth. Return the soup to the pot, add the strained solids and bring to a boil. Remove the soup from the heat; stir in the yogurt and scallions. Season with salt and pepper and serve.	Calories 209.5	Sodium: 99	Protein: 13	Phos 331.4
Serves: 6	4 Cup	Vegetable, Corn Frozen		Fat: 1.57	Carbs: 40.3	Chol: 2.45	Pot: 701.9
Serving Size: 1 cup of sou	1 teaspoon	Salt, Kosher		Sat Fat: 0.3	Fiber: 5.5		
	0.5 tsp	Spice, Black Pepper			Sugar: 10.2		
	2 Cup	Vegetable, Cauliflower, Raw					
	24 fluid ounce	Milk, Nonfat/Skim					
	10 ounces	Yogurt, Greek Non Fat					
	0.5 Cup	Vegetable, Onions, Young Green, raw					

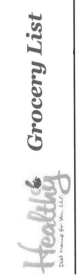

Grocery List

Chicken Kebabs with Pesto GDM Meal

Chicken Kebabs with Creamy Pesto

Quantity		Grocery Item
0.25	tsp	Spice, Black Pepper
0.5	Ounces	Pesto
1	Cup	Vegetable, Pepper, Yellow Raw
2	Teaspoon	Oil, Olive
2	Tablespoons	Cream, Sour, Reduced Fat
1	Oz	Yogurt, plain, lowfat milk
1	Each	Fruit, Lemon w/peel, raw
0.5	Teaspoon	Herb, Garlic, Raw
16	Tablespoon	Vegetable, Onions, Red
0.5	tsp	Salt
8	Each	Vegetable, Tomato, Red, Cherry
16	ounces	Chicken, Breast Boneless

Pan Grilled Halibut GDM Meal

Pan Grilled Halibut

Quantity		Grocery Item
24	Ounces	Fish, Halibut, Atlantic & Pacific, raw
1.5	Tablespoon	Oil, Vegetable or Olive
0.18	Cup	Herb, Cilantro Raw
2	Tablespoon	Herb, Basil, fresh
0.25	tsp	Spice, Black Pepper
0.5	tsp	Salt
0.18	Cup	Vegetable, Onions, Young Green, raw
0.667	ounces	Lemon Juice, Bottled

Garlic Cheese Bread

Quantity		Grocery Item
1	teaspoon	Spice, Red Pepper
1	Loaf	Bread, French or Vienna - baguette
0.25	Cup	Cheese, Grated Parmesan, Reduced Fat
1.5	cup	Soup, Chicken Broth Low Sodium
2	Teaspoon	Herb, Garlic, Raw
10	Springs	Herb, Parsley, Raw, Fresh
0.5	Cup	Cheese, Mozzarella Part Skim

Rice and Noodle Pilaf

Quantity		Grocery Item
1	Cup	Rice, Medium Brown
0.3	Cup	Pasta, Spaghetti
0.25	tsp	Spice, Black Pepper
16	oz	Water
2	tablespoon	Butter, Light w/no added salt
0.25	tsp	Salt

Green Beans

Quantity		Grocery Item
3	Cup	Vegetable, Beans, String, Green, raw

Tomato Ranch Salad

Quantity		Grocery Item
4.5	Cup	Vegetable, Lettuce, Iceberg, head, raw
2	Cup	Vegetable, Tomato Red Raw
12	Tablespoon	Salad dressing, ranch dressing, reduced fat

Strawberries

Quantity		Grocery Item
9	Cup	Fruit, Strawberries, halves/slices, raw

185

Broccoli Casserole

Quantity		Grocery Item
4	Cup	Vegetable, Broccoli Florets, Raw
0.5	Cup	Cheese, Cheddar reduced fat
0.125	tsp	Spice, Black Pepper
4	fluid ounces	Milk, Nonfat/Skim
6	Ounces	Soup, Cream of Celery, Fat Free

Beef Tips GDM Meal

Beef Tips with Mushroom Gravy

Quantity		Grocery Item
0.5	tsp	Salt
0.25	tsp	Spice, Black Pepper
1	Cup	Soup, Beef broth, canned, low sodium
3	Teaspoon	Cornstarch, hydrolyzed powder
0.5	cup	Vegetable, Mushrooms, slices, raw
16	Ounces	Beef, tenderloin, lean

Rice and Noodle Pilaf

Quantity		Grocery Item
1	Cup	Rice, Medium Brown
0.3	Cup	Pasta, Spaghetti
2	tablespoon	Butter, Light w/no added salt
0.25	tsp	Spice, Black Pepper
16	oz	Water
0.25	tsp	Salt

Banana

Quantity		Grocery Item
6	1	Fruit, Banana

Steamed Carrots

Quantity		Grocery Item
1	Teaspoon	Spice, Mrs. Dash
3	Cup	Vegetable, Carrots

Glazed Ham Steaks GDM Meal

Glazed Ham Steaks

Quantity		Grocery Item
1	Tablespoon	Soy Sauce, Low Sodium
0.125	Cup	Condiment, Tomato catsup - ketchup
16	Ounce	Pork Ham Steak, Cured, extra lean,
12	Teaspoon	Sweet, Jams & Preserves, apricot

Broccoli Casserole

Quantity		Grocery Item
4	fluid ounces	Milk, Nonfat/Skim
0.125	tsp	Spice, Black Pepper
4	Cup	Vegetable, Broccoli Florets, Raw
0.5	Cup	Cheese, Cheddar reduced fat
6	Ounces	Soup, Cream of Celery, Fat Free

Creamy Herbed Mashed Potatoes

Quantity		Grocery Item
3	tablespoon	Butter, Light w/no added salt
4	fluid ounces	Milk, Nonfat/Skim
0.5	tsp	Spice, Black Pepper
4	Cup	Vegetable, Potato, Flesh only, diced, raw
4	Springs	Herb, Parsley, Raw, Fresh
3	Tablespoon	Herb, Chives, raw
0.5	tsp	Salt
1	Tablespoons	Cream, Sour, Reduced Fat

Garden Coleslaw With Almonds

Quantity		Grocery Item
1	ounces	Honey
0.25	tsp	Spice, Black Pepper
9	Teaspoon	Vinegar, rice
2	ounces	Yogurt, Greek Non Fat
0.4	Tablespoon	Dijon Mustard
1	Each	Vegetable, Cabbage Head
1	Cup	Vegetable, Carrots
0.25	Cup	Nuts, Almond Sliced
6	Teaspoon	Oil, Olive

Chinese Chicken Salad GDM Meal

Chinese Chicken Salad

Quantity		Grocery Item
0.5	Cup	Herb, Cilantro Raw
0.5	Cup	Vegetable, Onions, Young Green, raw
4	Cup	Vegetable, Cabbage Heads, Red, raw
3	Teaspoon	Oil, Sesame Oil
9	Teaspoon	Vinegar, rice
6	Teaspoon	Spice, Sesame Seed
0.5	Cup	Vegetable, Peas, Snow/SugarSnap, ckd
3	Teaspoon	Cornstarch, hydrolyzed powder
15	teaspoons	Herb, Ginger Root, peeled, sliced, raw
12	ounces	Chicken, Breast Boneless
3	teaspoon	Spice, Chili Powder
5	Tablespoon	Lime Juice
0.5	cup	Soup, Chicken Broth Low Sodium
6	Tablespoon	Soy Sauce, Low Sodium
3	tsp	Spice, Black Pepper
0.25	Cup	Condiment, Tomato catsup - ketchup
1.5	Teaspoon	Herb, Garlic, Raw

Minute Rice

Quantity		Grocery Item
12	oz	Water
1.5	Cup	Rice, white, cooked, instant

Italian Green Beans

Quantity		Grocery Item
0.25	Teaspoon	Herb, Oregano, Ground
2	Teaspoon	Herb, Garlic, Raw
0.25	Teaspoon	Herb, Basil, Ground
1	Can	Vegetable, Tomato Diced Canned
1	Cup	Vegetable, Onions
3	Teaspoon	Oil, Olive
16	Ounces	Vegetable, Beans, Italian, Frozen

Bean Burrito GDM Meal

Chipotle Bean Burrito

Quantity		Grocery Item
0.5	Teaspoon	Spice, Chipotle Chili Powder
0.25	Teaspoon	Herb, Garlic, Raw
1	Tablespoon	Oil, Vegetable or Olive
1.75	Cup	Beans, Kidney, canned/Rinsed
3	Tablespoon	Condiment, Salsa
1.5	Cup	Vegetable, Tomato, Plum/Italian
3	oz	Water
0.5	Cup	Vegetable, Onions, Young Green, raw
1.75	Cup	Beans, Black, Canned
6	Each	Tortilla, Flour (Wheat)
0.5	Cup	Cheese, Mexican blend, reduced fat -
1.5	Cup	Vegetable, Lettuce, Cos/Romaine, raw
6	Tablespoons	Cream, Sour, Reduced Fat

Tomato Ranch Salad

Quantity		Grocery Item
4.5	Cup	Vegetable, Lettuce, Iceberg, head, raw
12	Tablespoon	Salad dressing, ranch dressing, reduced fat
2	Cup	Vegetable, Tomato Red Raw

Baked Shrimp GDM Meal

Baked Shrimp with Feta

Quantity		Grocery Item
0.5	Cup	Vegetable, Onions
0.5	Oz	Beverage, Alcoholic, Wine, Table, Dry White
0.5	Cup	Cheese, Feta
0.5	ounces	Lemon Juice, Bottled
0.333	Tablespoon	Oil, Vegetable or Olive
0.25	Teaspoon	Herb, Garlic, Raw
15	Oz	Vegetable, Tomatoes, canned, low sodium
1	Ounce	Juice, Clam & Tomato, canned
2	Tablespoon	Herb, Parsley, Raw, Chopped
0.25	tsp	Spice, Black Pepper
24	Ounces	Shrimp, peeled and deveined
0.5	Teaspoon	Herb, Oregano, Ground

187

Roasted Broccoli with Almonds

Quantity		Grocery Item
0.25	tsp	Spice, Black Pepper
0.25	tsp	Salt
5	Cup	Vegetable, Broccoli Florets, Raw
1	Tablespoon	Oil, Vegetable or Olive
0.25	Cup	Nuts, Almond Sliced

Corn Chowder Soup

Quantity		Grocery Item
0.5	tsp	Spice, Black Pepper
24	fluid ounces	Milk, Nonfat/Skim
2	Cup	Vegetable, Cauliflower, Raw
1	Cup	Vegetable, Onions
4	Cup	Vegetable, Corn Frozen
10	ounces	Yogurt, Greek Non Fat
1	teaspoon	Salt, Kosher
0.5	Cup	Vegetable, Onions, Young Green, raw

Week 12 Meals and Grocery Lists

Chicken Couscous Salad with Italian Tomatoes

Quesadilla with Cranberry Salsa with Creamy Lemon Coleslaw and Oven Fries

Grilled Salmon with Corn Relish with Cucumber and Tomato Salad, Brussels Sprouts and Bacon and Strawberries

Chipotle Rubbed Flank Steak with Steamed Carrots, Fried Rice, and Grapes

Spinach Linguine with Asparagus, Savory Grits and Cauliflower Florets with Lemon Mustard Butter

Chicken Butternut Tagine with Minute Rice, Broccoli Casserole, and Italian Green Beans

Pork Chops Oregano with Bacon Potato Salad, Braised Red Cabbage and Apples

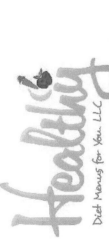

Meal Plan

www.healthydietmenusforyou.com

Diet: *Gestational Diabetic - 2400*

Meal: *Chicken Couscous Salad GDM*

Recipe		Ingredients	Instructions	Nutritionals	
Chicken Couscous Salad	2 ounces	Lemon Juice, Bottled	In a medium bowl, whisk together lemon juice, honey, olive oil, salt and ground pepper. This becomes dressing for meal. Fully cook couscous, omitting salt and fat. Allow to cool. In another medium bowl, toss couscous chicken raisins and walnuts. Drizzle dressing over couscous and toss to coat. Arrange greens on a plate and mount 1 cup of couscous salad in center. Repeat for remaining 5 plates.	Calories 486	Sodium: 201.6	Protein: 26.3	Phos 245.5
Serves: 6	6 Teaspoon	Oil, Olive		Fat: 13.9	Carbs: 64.4	Chol: 34.2	Pot: 417.7
Serving Size: 1/6 recipe	1 ounces	Honey		Sat Fat: 2.564	Fiber: 4.484		
	0.25 tsp	Salt			Sugar: 14.6		
	0.25 tsp	Spice, Black Pepper					
	2 Cup	Grain, Couscous					
	2 cup	Chicken, Lt & Dk meat, canned, meat only					
	0.25 Cup	Fruit, Rasins, Golden, Seedless					
	0.25 cup	Nuts, Walnut					
	0.25 Cup	Fruit, Raisins, seedless					
	4 Cup	Vegetable, Lettuce, Cos/Romaine, raw					

Recipe		Ingredients	Instructions	Nutritionals	
Italian Tomatoes	4 Cup	Vegetable, Tomato Red Raw	Slice tomatoes into 1/4 in thick slices. Whisk olive oil, hot sauce and pepper together. Drizzle onto tomatoes, and sprinkle with cheese and basil. Refrigerate for 30 or more minutes.	Calories 69	Sodium: 45	Protein: 2	Phos 48
Serves: 6	2 Tablespoon	Oil, Vegetable or Olive		Fat: 5	Carbs: 5	Chol: 5	Pot: 300
Serving Size: 3/4 Tomato	0.33 Tablesp	Sauce, Hot Pepper		Sat Fat: 1	Fiber: 1.5		
	0.5 tsp	Spice, Black Pepper			Sugar: 3		
	0.25 Cup	Cheese, Grated Parmesan, Reduced Fat					
	2 Teaspoon	Herb, Basil, Ground					

Meal: *Turkey Quesadilla GDM*

Recipe		Ingredients	Instructions	Nutritionals			
Quesadilla with Cranberry Salsa	0.75 Cup	Fruit, Cranberry Sauce, canned, sweetened	To prepare salsa, combine cranberry sauce, cilantro, green onion, lime juice, cumin, pear and pepper ingredients. Cover and chill.	Calories 353.8	Sodium: 515.4	Protein: 16.5	Phos 224.6
	0.25 Cup	Herb, Cilantro Raw		Fat: 10.5	Carbs: 48.7	Chol: 34	Pot: 265.3
Serves: 6	0.25 Cup	Vegetable, Onions, Young Green, raw	To prepare quesadillas, heat a large nonstick skillet over medium-high heat. Coat pan with cooking spray. Add 1/4 cup sliced onions to pan; sauté 3 minutes or until tender. Remove onions from pan; reduce heat to medium. Sprinkle 2 tablespoons cheese over each of 4 tortillas. Top each cheese-covered tortilla with one-fourth of onions, 1/2 cup turkey, 2 tablespoons cheese, and 1 tortilla.	Sat Fat: 4.799	Fiber: 3.16		
Serving Size: 1 tortilla folded in half	3 Tablespoon	Lime Juice			Sugar: 17.6		
	1 Fruit	Fruit, Pear Raw					
	0.5 tsp	Spice, Cumin, Ground					
	0.25 Cup	Vegetable, Green Onion					
	1 Each	Vegetable, Pepper, Jalapeno, raw	Recoat pan with cooking spray. Add 1 quesadilla to pan; cook 2 minutes on each side or until lightly browned and cheese melts. Repeat with remaining quesadillas. Cut each quesadilla into 6 wedges. Serve with cranberry salsa and sour cream.				
	6 Each	Tortilla, Flour (Wheat)					
	12 Tablespoo	Cream, Sour, Reduced Fat					
	1 Cup	Cheese, Monterey - Monterey Jack cheese					
	8 Ounces	Turkey, light meat, cooked					

Recipe		Ingredients	Instructions	Nutritionals			
Creamy Lemon Coleslaw	1 Each	Vegetable, Cabbage Head	Shred cabbage and chop onions. Combine all ingredients in a bowl, and toss lightly. Refrigerate if not used immediately.	Calories 81	Sodium: 158	Protein: 1.7	Phos 34
Serves: 6	6 Each	Sugar Substitute Packet, Equal		Fat: 3	Carbs: 12	Chol: 4	Pot: 211
	0.125 Cup	Vegetable, Onions		Sat Fat: 0.5	Fiber: 3		
Serving Size: 1/6 of container	0.5 teaspoon	Salt, Kosher			Sugar: 5.5		
	6 Tablespoon	Miracle Whip Light					
	2 Packet	True Lemon packet					

Recipe		Ingredients	Instructions	Nutritionals			
Oven Fries	3 each	Vegetable, Potato	Cut potatoes into strips like fries. Beat egg whites and toss with fries. Sprinkle with Mrs. Dash type seasoning. Bake 30 minutes at 400°F or until done.	Calories 75	Sodium: 45	Protein: 3.3	Phos 55
Serves: 6	1 Teaspoon	Spice, Mrs. Dash		Fat: 0.2	Carbs: 15	Chol: 0	Pot: 406
	3 Each	Egg White		Sat Fat: 0	Fiber: 2		
Serving Size: 1/2 potato					Sugar: 1		

192

Meal: *Grilled Salmon with Corn Relish GDM*

Recipe		Ingredients	Instructions	Nutritionals					

Grilled Salmon with Corn Relish

Serves: 4

Serving Size: 6 ounce fillet +3/4 cup relish

	Ingredients	Instructions
2 Tablespoon	Vegetable, Peppers, hot, chili, adobo, chili sauce	Chop chilies and set aside. Place corn on grill rack coated with cooking spray; grill 10 minutes or until lightly browned, turning occasionally. Cool slightly. Cut kernels from cobs.
2 Each	Vegetable, Corn on Cob, sm/med, ckd w/o fat or salt	
1 Cup	Vegetable, Tomato Red Raw	Combine chiles, corn, tomato, cilantro, and juice; toss gently. Add 1/2 teaspoon salt and 1/4 teaspoon black pepper.
0.25 Cup	Herb, Cilantro Raw	
4 Tablespoon	Lime Juice	Combine remaining 1/2 teaspoon salt, remaining 1/4 teaspoon black pepper, and cumin, stirring well. Rub spice mixture evenly over both sides of salmon. Place salmon on grill rack coated with cooking spray; grill 4 minutes on each side or until fish flakes easily when tested with a fork or until desired degree of doneness. Serve with relish.
0.5 tsp	Salt	
0.5 tsp	Spice, Black Pepper	
1 tsp	Spice, Cumin, Ground	
24 Oz	Fish, Salmon, baked or broiled	

Nutritionals

Calories 413.4	Sodium: 406.7	Protein: 37	Phos 470.7
Fat: 23.8	Carbs: 13.1	Chol: 93.6	Pot: 933.6
Sat Fat: 5.387	Fiber: 1.827		
	Sugar: 4.801		

Cucumber and Tomato Salad

Serves: 5

Serving Size: 1/5 recipe

	Ingredients	Instructions
2 Cup	Vegetable, Cucumber, peeled, raw	Peel and dice cucumbers. Chop or dice tomatoes. In a medium bowl, toss cucumbers and tomatoes. Drizzle oil and vinegar over vegetables and toss to coat. Season with salt and pepper.
3 Teaspoon	Oil, Olive	
2 Cup	Vegetable, Tomato Red Raw	
6 Teaspoon	Vinegar, Red Wine	
0.5 tsp	Salt	
0.25 tsp	Spice, Black Pepper	

Nutritionals

Calories 44.6	Sodium: 237.8	Protein: 0.961	Phos 29.1
Fat: 2.933	Carbs: 4.056	Chol: 0	Pot: 246.7
Sat Fat: 0.401	Fiber: 1.264		
	Sugar: 2.628		

Brussel Sprouts and Bacon

Serves: 4

Serving Size: 4 ounces

	Ingredients	Instructions
0.5 tsp	Salt	Cut the brussels sprouts in half and trim bottoms. Heat a large skillet or saute pan over medium heat. Add the bacon and cook until crispy, about 5 minutes. Remove to a plate lined with paper towels. Discard all but 1 tablespoon of the rendered bacon fat. Add the garlic, pepper flakes, brussels sprouts and salt to the skillet. Saute until the sprouts are lightly browned on the outside and tender - but still firm - throughout. Approx 10-12 minutes. Add the almonds and bacon (crumbled) and saute for another minute or two. Season with salt and pepper.
1 tsp	Spice, Black Pepper	
4 Slices	Pork Bacon, Cured or Smoked, lower sodium, slices	
2 Teaspoon	Herb, Garlic, Raw	
1 teaspoon	Spice, Red Pepper	
0.06 Cup	Nuts, Almond Sliced	
1 Pounds	Vegetable, Brussels Sprouts, raw	

Nutritionals

Calories 121	Sodium: 402.1	Protein: 7.2	Phos 127
Fat: 6.2	Carbs: 12	Chol: 5	Pot: 528.2
Sat Fat: 1.6	Fiber: 5		
	Sugar: 2.7		

Recipe: Strawberries

Serves: 6

Serving Size: 1.5 Cups of Strawberries

Ingredients	Instructions
9 Cup — Fruit, Strawberries, halves/slices, raw	Remove tops and wash prior to serving.

Nutritionals

Calories 73	Sodium: 2.2	Protein: 1.5	Phos 54.7
Fat: 0.6	Carbs: 17.5	Chol: 0	Pot: 348.8
Sat Fat: 0	Fiber: 4.5		
	Sugar: 11.1		

Meal: Chipotle Flank Steak GDM

Recipe: Chipotle Rubbed Flank Steak

Serves: 4

Serving Size: 3 oz steak + 3 T sauce

Ingredients	Instructions
1 Teaspoon — Spice, Ancho Chile Powder	1. Preheat broiler to high.
1 teaspoon — Spice, Paprika	2. Combine chipotle pepper, paprika, and salt ingredients. Sprinkle steak with chipotle mixture. Place on a broiler pan; broil 5 minutes on each side. Let stand 5 minutes. Cut thinly across grain.
0.25 tsp — Salt	
16 Ounces — Beef, Flank Lean Trimmed	
1 Teaspoon — Oil, Olive	3. Heat oil in a saucepan over medium heat. Add shallots and garlic; cook 1 minute. Add flour; cook 30 seconds, stirring. Add milk; boil. Cook until reduced by half. Remove from heat; stir in cheese and remaining ingredients.
2 tablespoons — Vegetable, Shallots, peeled, raw	
0.25 Teaspoo — Herb, Garlic, Raw	
1 teaspoon — Flour, Wheat or White, All Purpose	
1 Tablespoon — Herb, Parsley, Raw, Chopped	
0.333 tablesp — Butter, Light w/no added salt	
0.667 Cup — Milk, Lowfat, 1% fat w/added vitamin A	
0.25 Cup — Cheese, Gorgonzola	

Nutritionals

Calories 284.3	Sodium: 349.6	Protein: 35.6	Phos 338.5
Fat: 12	Carbs: 6.633	Chol: 58.9	Pot: 538.3
Sat Fat: 5.442	Fiber: 0.348		
	Sugar: 2.238		

Recipe: Steamed Carrots

Serves: 6

Serving Size: 1/2 cup

Ingredients	Instructions
3 Cup — Vegetable, Carrots	Steam carrots until tender, season with Mrs. Dash
1 Teaspoon — Spice, Mrs. Dash	

Nutritionals

Calories 33	Sodium: 2	Protein: 1	Phos 22
Fat: 0	Carbs: 8	Chol: 0	Pot: 165
Sat Fat: 0	Fiber: 3		
	Sugar: 0		

Recipe: Fried Rice

Nutritionals

Calories 194.2	Sodium: 291.4	Protein: 7.416	Phos 84.7
Fat: 3.609	Carbs: 32	Chol: 0.314	Pot: 200.8
Sat Fat: 0.534	Fiber: 2.083		
	Sugar: 1.384		

Ingredients

Amount	Ingredient
1.5 Cup	Rice, white, cooked, instant
0.125 cup	Soup, Chicken Broth Low Sodium
2 Teaspoon	Vinegar, Red Wine
1 Tablespoon	Soy Sauce, Low Sodium
0.5 tsp	Salt
1 Teaspoon	Oil, Sesame Oil
0.25 tsp	Spice, Black Pepper
1 tablespoon	Oil, Canola
1 Cup	Egg Substitute
1 Cup	Vegetable, Onions, Young Green, raw
1 Cup	Vegetable, Peas, Green, Frozen

Instructions

Cook Rice according to directions on package, omitting salt and fat. Spread Rice in a shallow baking pan and separate grains with a fork. In a small bowl, whisk together broth, vinegar, soy sauce, salt, sesame oil, and black pepper. Set aside. Coat a large nonstick skillet or wok with cooking spray and heat canola oil over moderately high heat until hot. Stirfry, egg substitute until scrambled about 30 seconds. Add scallions and stirfry 1 min. Add peas and stirfry until heated through. Add Rice and stirfry, stirring frequently 2 to 3 min. or until heated throughout. Stir liquid and add to fried rice, tossing to coat evenly.

Serves: 8

Serving Size: 1/2 cup

Recipe: Grapes

Nutritionals

Calories 92.5	Sodium: 2.7	Protein: 0.8	Phos 13.8
Fat: 0.4	Carbs: 23.7	Chol: 0	Pot: 263.6
Sat Fat: 0.1	Fiber: 1.2		
	Sugar: 22.4		

Ingredients

Amount	Ingredient
9 Cup	Fruit, Grapes, raw

Instructions

Wash and remove stems from grapes prior to eating.

Serves: 6

Serving Size: 1.5 cups of grapes

Meal: Spinach Linguine GDM

Recipe: Spinach Linguine

Nutritionals

Calories 300.5	Sodium: 637.6	Protein: 21.1	Phos 378.
Fat: 13.5	Carbs: 24.7	Chol: 35.6	Pot: 392.9
Sat Fat: 7.2	Fiber: 3.4		
	Sugar: 3		

Ingredients

Amount	Ingredient
1.25 Cup	Cheese, Ricotta, Part Skim Milk
1.5 Cup	Cheese, Mozzarella Part Skim
0.25 Cup	Cheese, Grated Parmesan, Reduced Fat
8 fluid ounces	Milk, Nonfat/Skim
2 Tablespoon	Margarine Spread - reduced calorie, about 40% fat, tub, salted - Country Crock Light
2 Teaspoon	Herb, Garlic, Raw
2 Cup	Vegetable, Spinach Frozen
1.5 Cup	Pasta, Spaghetti

Instructions

In a blender or with a whisk (blender preferred) combine and puree ricotta, milk, mozzarella and parmesan. In a sprayed skillet, saute garlic in margarine. Add cheese mixture and spinach in skillet and cook until heated. Add linguine and toss gently. Divide into 6 portions of 1/2 cup linguine with sauce.

Serves: 6

Serving Size: 1/2 cup linguine with sauce

Asparagus

Serves: 6
Serving Size: 1/2 Cup

Ingredients

Amount	Ingredient
54 Ounces	Vegetable, Asparagus Fresh

Instructions

Wash and clean asparagus by cutting off hard ends of stalk. Steam for 10 minutes in steamer or cook in 1 in water in microwaveable bowl for 5-7 minutes until desired tenderness.

Nutritionals

Calories 21.5	Sodium: 1.8	Protein: 2.3	Phos 48.3
Fat: 0.2	Carbs: 3.7	Chol: 0	Pot: 143.2
Sat Fat: 0	Fiber: 1.5		
	Sugar: 0		

Savory Grits

Serves: 7
Serving Size: 1/2 cup

Ingredients

Amount	Ingredient
28 oz	Water
0.75 Cup	Cereal, Grits, White, Regular, dry
0.5 tsp	Salt
0.25 Cup	Vegetable, Onions
0.25 Cup	Cheese, Cheddar reduced fat

Instructions

In a medium saucepan, bring water to a boil. Stir in grits and salt, stirring vigorously. Reduce heat and simmer, covered, for 15 to 20 min., stirring occasionally. Stir in cheese and onions until cheese melts.

Nutritionals

Calories 74.6	Sodium: 199.5	Protein: 2.659	Phos 54.4
Fat: 0.983	Carbs: 14.5	Chol: 2.26	Pot: 39
Sat Fat: 0.516	Fiber: 0.941		
	Sugar: 0.441		

Cauliflower Florets with Lemon Mustard Butte

Serves: 8
Serving Size: 1/2 Cup

Ingredients

Amount	Ingredient
2 Tablespoon	Margarine Spread - reduced calorie, about 40% fat, tub, salted - Country Crock Light
1 Tablespoon	Dijon Mustard
4 Cup	Vegetable, Cauliflower, Raw
2 Teaspoon	Lemon, Rind

Instructions

In a small bowl, whisk together the margarine, Dijon mustard, lemon peel, and chopped onion. Steam cauliflower florets until tender crisp. In a large saucepan, add cauliflower and margarine mixture over low heat. Toss gently until cauliflower is coated.

Nutritionals

Calories 33.3	Sodium: 50.2	Protein: 1.09	Phos 23.9
Fat: 2.053	Carbs: 3.431	Chol: 0	Pot: 162.3
Sat Fat: 0.416	Fiber: 1.384		
	Sugar: 1.414		

Recipe: Chicken Butternut Tagine

Serves: 4

Serving Size: 1 1/4 cup

Nutritionals

Calories	349.6	Sodium:	982.6	Protein:	39.8	Phos	358.6	Pot:	850.8
Fat:	11.9	Carbs:	22.9	Chol:	96.3				
Sat Fat:	2.2	Fiber:	4.3						
		Sugar:	4.9						

Ingredients

1	Tablespoon	Oil, Vegetable or Olive
2	Cup	Vegetable, Onions
2	tsp	Spice, Cumin, Ground
1	teaspoon	Spice, Paprika
1	Teaspoon	Spice, Turmeric, ground
0.25	tsp	Salt
0.25	Teaspoo	Spice, Cinnamon, ground
0.25	Teaspoo	Spice, Ginger
2	Teaspoon	Herb, Garlic, Raw
16	ounces	Chicken, Breast Boneless
2	cup	Soup, Chicken Broth Low Sodium
8	Oz	Vegetable, Squash, Butternut, peeled, raw
3	Oz	Fruit, Olives, Green, Halved
8	Each	Fruit, Plum, Japanese, dried, Chopped
10	Springs	Herb, Parsley, Raw, Fresh

Instructions

Heat oil in a Dutch oven over medium heat. Add onion; cook 8 minutes or until golden, stirring occasionally. Stir in cumin and paprika, turmeric, salt, cinnamon, ginger, garlic and chicken that was cut into bite sized pieces; cook 1 minute, stirring constantly. Stir in broth, squash, olives, and dried plums; bring to a boil. Cover, reduce heat to medium-low, and simmer 10 minutes or until squash is tender. Garnish with parsley, if desired.

Recipe: Minute Rice

Serves: 6

Serving Size: 1/2 Cup Ric

Nutritionals

Calories	96.3	Sodium:	294.8	Protein:	1.7	Phos	30.7	Pot:	8
Fat:	0.4	Carbs:	20.6	Chol:	0				
Sat Fat:	0	Fiber:	0.4						
		Sugar:	0						

Ingredients

1.5	Cup	Rice, white, cooked, instant
12	oz	Water

Instructions

Bring water to a boil. Stir in rice, cover and remove from heat. Let stand for 5 minutes or until water is absorbed. Fluff with fork.

Recipe: Broccoli Casserole

Serves: 8

Serving Size: 1/2 cup

Nutritionals

Calories	53.3	Sodium:	300	Protein:	3.796	Phos	135.3	Pot:	231.2
Fat:	2.291	Carbs:	5.245	Chol:	0.179				
Sat Fat:	1.228	Fiber:	7.318						
		Sugar:	1.884						

Ingredients

4	Cup	Vegetable, Broccoli Florets, Raw
4	fluid ounces	Milk, Nonfat/Skim
0.125	tsp	Spice, Black Pepper
0.5	Cup	Cheese, Cheddar reduced fat
6	Ounces	Soup, Cream of Celery, Fat Free

Instructions

Preheat oven to 350°. In a large bowl, combine all ingredients. Pour into a medium casserole dish and bake for 30 min.

Recipe: Italian Green Beans

Serves: 6
Serving Size: 1/2 cup

Ingredients
Amount	Ingredient
3 Teaspoon	Oil, Olive
1 Cup	Vegetable, Onions
2 Teaspoon	Herb, Garlic, Raw
1 Can	Vegetable, Tomato Diced Canned
0.25 Teaspoon	Herb, Oregano, Ground
0.25 Teaspoo	Herb, Basil, Ground
16 Ounces	Vegetable, Beans, Italian, Frozen

Instructions
Steam green beans until tender crisp. Set aside. Heat olive oil in a medium nonstick skillet over medium-high heat. Sauté onions until clear. Add garlic; sauté 30 seconds. Add tomatoes, basil, and oregano, and simmer for 15 to 20 min. for tomato mixture over steamed green beans and mix well.

Nutritionals
Calories 67.1	Sodium: 217.2	Protein: 2.111	Phos 46.7
Fat: 2.519	Carbs: 10.9	Chol: 0	Pot: 315.5
Sat Fat: 0.37	Fiber: 3.596		
	Sugar: 3.97		

Meal: Pork Chops Oregano GDM

Recipe: Pork Chops Oregano

Serves: 4
Serving Size: 1 4oz pork chop

Ingredients
Amount	Ingredient
1 Tablespoon	Oil, Vegetable or Olive
2 Teaspoon	Lemon, Rind
2 ounces	Lemon Juice, Bottled
0.75 Teaspoo	Herb, Garlic, Raw
1 Teaspoon	Herb, Oregano, Ground
16 ounces	Pork, Center Rib Chop
1 tsp	Spice, Black Pepper

Instructions
1. Grate lemon rind and squeeze lemon for juice. Combine olive oil, lemon juice, lemon juice, oregano and garlic in an 11 x 7 inch baking dish. Add pork, turning to coat. Let stand 30 minutes, turning pork occasionally.

2. Preheat broiler.

3. Remove pork from baking dish; discard marinade. Place pork on a broiler pan coated with cooking spray. Broil 4 minutes on each side or until done.

Nutritionals
Calories 183.1	Sodium: 58.7	Protein: 24.1	Phos 252.4
Fat: 8.199	Carbs: 2.221	Chol: 71.4	Pot: 452.4
Sat Fat: 2.133	Fiber: 0.336		
	Sugar: 0.317		

Recipe: Bacon Potato Salad

Serves: 6
Serving Size: 1/2 cup

Ingredients
Amount	Ingredient
2 Slices	Beef, Bacon, lean, ckd
4 each	Vegetable, Potato
0.25 Cup	Mayonnaise, reduced kcal, cholest free/Hellmann
0.33 Tablesp	Dijon Mustard

Instructions
Fry bacon, drain and pat grease off. Crumble. Peel potatoes, cook until tender - about 40 minutes at a low boil, and cube/slice them. Toss the warm potatoes with mayo, mustard, salt and pepper. Add bacon and serve.

Nutritionals
Calories 131.3	Sodium: 124.9	Protein: 2.5	Phos 47.9
Fat: 3.3	Carbs: 23	Chol: 0.82	Pot: 280.2
Sat Fat: 0.5	Fiber: 2		
	Sugar: 0.9		

Recipe		Ingredients	Instructions	Nutritionals					
Braised Red Cabbage			In a large saucepan, bring broth, vinegar, honey, and allspice to a boil. Add cabbage and cubed apples. Reduce heat and simmer, uncovered, for 30 min.	Calories 96.9	Sodium: 57.4	Protein: 3.612		Phos 67.7
	2 cup	Soup, Chicken Broth Low Sodium		.				.
Serves: 4				Fat: 0.938	Carbs: 2.39	Chol: 0		Pot: 362.6
	8 Tablespoon	Vinegar, Cider						
Serving Size: 1/2 cup	6 Teaspoon	Vinegar, Red Wine		Sat Fat: 0.249	Fiber: 2.39			
	0.5 ounces	Honey						
					Sugar: 13.9			
	0.5 Teaspoon	Spice, Allspice, ground						
	4 Cup	Vegetable, Cabbage Heads, Red, raw						
	2 Each	Fruit, Apple, peeled, Granny Smith, medium						

Recipe		Ingredients	Instructions	Nutritionals					
Apple - Red			Piece of fruit	Calories 94.6	Sodium: 1.8	Protein: 0.4		Phos 20
	6 Each	Fruit, Apple, peeled, raw, medium		.				
Serves: 6				Fat: 0.3	Carbs: 25.1	Chol: 0		Pot: 194.7
Serving Size: 1 apple				Sat Fat: 0	Fiber: 4.3			
					Sugar: 18.9			

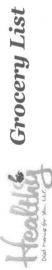

Grocery List

Oven Fries

Quantity		Grocery Item
1	Teaspoon	Spice, Mrs. Dash
3	each	Vegetable, Potato
3	Each	Egg White

Grilled Salmon with Corn Relish GDM Meal

Grilled Salmon with Corn Relish

Quantity		Grocery Item
2	Tablespoon	Vegetable, Peppers, hot, chili, adobo, chili
0.5	tsp	Spice, Black Pepper
1	Cup	Vegetable, Tomato Red Raw
24	Oz	Fish, Salmon, baked or broiled
0.5	tsp	Salt
2	Each	Vegetable, Corn on Cob, sm/med, ckd w/o
		Herb, Cilantro Raw
0.25	Cup	Spice, Cumin, Ground
1	tsp	Lime Juice
4	Tablespoon	

Turkey Quesadilla GDM Meal

Quesadilla with Cranberry Salsa

Quantity		Grocery Item
0.25	Cup	Herb, Cilantro Raw
8	Ounces	Turkey, light meat, cooked
0.5	tsp	Spice, Cumin, Ground
0.75	Cup	Fruit, Cranberry Sauce, canned, sweetened
3	Tablespoon	Lime Juice
1	Fruit	Fruit, Pear Raw
6	Each	Tortilla, Flour (Wheat)
0.25	Cup	Vegetable, Onions, Young Green, raw
1	Each	Vegetable, Pepper, Jalapeno, raw
12	Tablespoons	Cream, Sour, Reduced Fat
1	Cup	Cheese, Monterey - Monterey Jack cheese
0.25	Cup	Vegetable, Green Onion

Creamy Lemon Coleslaw

Quantity		Grocery Item
6	Each	Sugar Substitute Packet, Equal
0.125	Cup	Vegetable, Onions
2	Packet	True Lemon packet
0.5	teaspoon	Salt, Kosher
6	Tablespoon	Miracle Whip Light
1	Each	Vegetable, Cabbage Head

Chicken Couscous Salad GDM Meal

Chicken Couscous Salad

Quantity		Grocery Item
2	cup	Chicken, Lt & Dk meat, canned, meat only
0.25	tsp	Salt
0.25	cup	Nuts, Walnut
2	ounces	Lemon Juice, Bottled
4	Cup	Vegetable, Lettuce, Cos/Romaine, raw
6	Teaspoon	Oil, Olive
2	Cup	Grain, Couscous
0.25	Cup	Fruit, Rasins, Golden, Seedless
0.25	Cup	Fruit, Raisins, seedless
0.25	tsp	Spice, Black Pepper
1	ounces	Honey

Italian Tomatoes

Quantity		Grocery Item
2	Teaspoon	Herb, Basil, Ground
0.25	Cup	Cheese, Grated Parmesan, Reduced Fat
2	Tablespoon	Oil, Vegetable or Olive
0.33	Tablespoon	Sauce, Hot Pepper
4	Cup	Vegetable, Tomato Red Raw
0.5	tsp	Spice, Black Pepper

Chipotle Flank Steak GDM Meal

Cucumber and Tomato Salad

Quantity		Grocery Item
0.25	tsp	Spice, Black Pepper
2	Cup	Vegetable, Tomato Red Raw
6	Teaspoon	Vinegar, Red Wine
2	Cup	Vegetable, Cucumber, peeled, raw
3	Teaspoon	Oil, Olive
0.5	tsp	Salt

Brussel Sprouts and Bacon

Quantity		Grocery Item
0.5	tsp	Salt
4	Slices	Pork Bacon, Cured or Smoked, lower
2	Teaspoon	Herb, Garlic, Raw
0.06	Cup	Nuts, Almond Sliced
1	tsp	Spice, Black Pepper
1	Pounds	Vegetable, Brussels Sprouts, raw
1	teaspoon	Spice, Red Pepper

Strawberries

Quantity		Grocery Item
9	Cup	Fruit, Strawberries, halves/slices, raw

Chipotle Rubbed Flank Steak

Quantity		Grocery Item
1	teaspoon	Spice, Paprika
1	Tablespoon	Herb, Parsley, Raw, Chopped
0.25	tsp	Salt
0.333	tablespoon	Butter, Light w/no added salt
16	Ounces	Beef, Flank Lean Trimmed
2	tablespoons	Vegetable, Shallots, peeled, raw
1	Teaspoon	Spice, Ancho Chile Powder
0.667	Cup	Milk, Lowfat, 1% fat w/added vitamin A
1	Teaspoon	Oil, Olive
0.25	Cup	Cheese, Gorgonzola
0.25	Teaspoon	Herb, Garlic, Raw
1	teaspoon	Flour, Wheat or White, All Purpose

Steamed Carrots

Quantity		Grocery Item
3	Cup	Vegetable, Carrots
1	Teaspoon	Spice, Mrs. Dash

Fried Rice

Quantity		Grocery Item
1	Cup	Egg Substitute
1	tablespoon	Oil, Canola
1	Teaspoon	Oil, Sesame Oil
1.5	Cup	Rice, white, cooked, instant
1	Cup	Vegetable, Onions, Young Green, raw
1	Cup	Vegetable, Peas, Green, Frozen
0.125	cup	Soup, Chicken Broth Low Sodium
1	Tablespoon	Soy Sauce, Low Sodium
0.5	tsp	Salt
0.25	tsp	Spice, Black Pepper
2	Teaspoon	Vinegar, Red Wine

Grapes

Quantity		Grocery Item
9	Cup	Fruit, Grapes, raw

Spinach Linguine GDM Meal

Spinach Linguine

Quantity		Grocery Item
1.5	Cup	Cheese, Mozzarella Part Skim
1.25	Cup	Cheese, Ricotta, Part Skim Milk
1.5	Cup	Pasta, Spaghetti
2	Cup	Vegetable, Spinach Frozen
0.25	Cup	Cheese, Grated Parmesan, Reduced Fat
8	fluid ounces	Milk, Nonfat/Skim
2	Teaspoon	Herb, Garlic, Raw
2	Tablespoon	Margarine Spread - reduced calorie, about

Asparagus

Quantity		Grocery Item
54	Ounces	Vegetable, Asparagus Fresh

Savory Grits

Quantity		Grocery Item
0.75	Cup	Cereal, Grits, White, Regular, dry
0.5	tsp	Salt
0.25	Cup	Vegetable, Onions
28	oz	Water
0.25	Cup	Cheese, Cheddar reduced fat

Cauliflower Florets with Lemon Mustard Butte

Quantity		Grocery Item
4	Cup	Vegetable, Cauliflower, Raw
2	Teaspoon	Lemon, Rind
1	Tablespoon	Dijon Mustard
2	Tablespoon	Margarine Spread - reduced calorie, about

Chicken Butternut Tagine Meal

Chicken Butternut Tagine

Quantity		Grocery Item
1	teaspoon	Spice, Paprika
2	Cup	Vegetable, Onions
2	cup	Soup, Chicken Broth Low Sodium
1	Tablespoon	Oil, Vegetable or Olive
0.25	tsp	Salt
16	ounces	Chicken, Breast Boneless
2	tsp	Spice, Cumin, Ground
1	Teaspoon	Spice, Turmeric, ground
0.25	Teaspoon	Spice, Ginger
2	Teaspoon	Herb, Garlic, Raw
10	Springs	Herb, Parsley, Raw, Fresh
0.25	Teaspoon	Spice, Cinnamon, ground
3	Oz	Fruit, Olives, Green, Halved
8	Each	Fruit, Plum, Japanese, dried, Chopped
8	Oz	Vegetable, Squash, Butternut, peeled, raw

Minute Rice

Quantity		Grocery Item
12	oz	Water
1.5	Cup	Rice, white, cooked, instant

Broccoli Casserole

Quantity		Grocery Item
4	fluid ounces	Milk, Nonfat/Skim
4	Cup	Vegetable, Broccoli Florets, Raw
0.5	Cup	Cheese, Cheddar reduced fat
6	Ounces	Soup, Cream of Celery, Fat Free
0.125	tsp	Spice, Black Pepper

Italian Green Beans

Quantity		Grocery Item
1	Cup	Vegetable, Onions
1	Can	Vegetable, Tomato Diced Canned
3	Teaspoon	Oil, Olive
2	Teaspoon	Herb, Garlic, Raw
16	Ounces	Vegetable, Beans, Italian, Frozen
0.25	Teaspoon	Herb, Basil, Ground
0.25	Teaspoon	Herb, Oregano, Ground

Pork Chops Oregano GDM Meal

Pork Chops Oregano

Quantity		Grocery Item
16	ounces	Pork, Center Rib Chop
2	Teaspoon	Lemon, Rind
1	tsp	Spice, Black Pepper
1	Teaspoon	Herb, Oregano, Ground
0.75	Teaspoon	Herb, Garlic, Raw
1	Tablespoon	Oil, Vegetable or Olive
2	ounces	Lemon Juice, Bottled

Bacon Potato Salad

Quantity		Grocery Item
0.33	Tablespoon	Dijon Mustard
0.25	Cup	Mayonnaise, reduced kcal, cholest
2	Slices	Beef, Bacon, lean, ckd
4	each	Vegetable, Potato

Braised Red Cabbage

Quantity		Grocery Item
2	Each	Fruit, Apple, peeled, Granny Smith, medium
8	Tablespoons	Vinegar, Cider
0.5	ounces	Honey
6	Teaspoon	Vinegar, Red Wine
2	cup	Soup, Chicken Broth Low Sodium
4	Cup	Vegetable, Cabbage Heads, Red, raw
0.5	Teaspoons	Spice, Allspice, ground

Apple - Red

Quantity		Grocery Item
6	Each	Fruit, Apple, peeled, raw, medium

Week 13 Meals and Grocery Lists

Chicken Penne with Tomato Sauce Light with Cucumber and Tomato Salad

Egg Noodles with Bacon and Vegetables Light with Cauliflower with Lemon Mustard Butter, Creamy Lemon Coleslaw and Brussels Sprouts and Bacon

Sirloin Tip Roast with Rosemary Roasted Potatoes and Ratatouille and Black-Eyed Peas

Chicken with Red Wine Vinegar Sauce with Coconut Rice, Broccoli Casserole and Strawberries

Grilled Mushroom Burgers with Oven Fries, Roasted Parmesan Zucchini and Red Apple Coleslaw

Blackened Cumin-Cayenne Tilapia with Couscous with Tomato and Dill, Down Home Baked Beans and Bananas

Ham and Pear Sandwich with Creamy Lemon Coleslaw, Steamed Carrots, and Corn on the Cob

Week 13 Meals and Grocery Lists

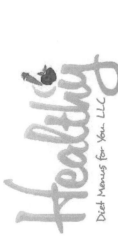

Meal: *Chicken Penne GDM*

Recipe | Ingredients | Instructions | Nutritionals

Chicken Penne with Tomato Sauce Light

Serves: 4

Serving Size: 1 1/4 cups

	Ingredients	
1 Teaspoon	Spice, Fennel Seed, Crushed	
2 Tablespoon	Herb, Basil, fresh	
1 Teaspoon	Herb, Basil, Ground	
0.5 Teaspoon	Spice, Coriander Seed	
0.25 tsp	Spice, Black Pepper	
12 Ounces	Chicken, Breast Tenders Boneless	
3 Teaspoon	Oil, Olive	
1 Teaspoon	Herb, Garlic, Raw	
8 Oz	Beverage, Alcoholic, Wine, Table, Dry White	
8 Ounce	Pasta, Penne, dry noodles	
1 Ounces	Cheese, Parmesan, shredded	
1.5 Can	Vegetable, Tomato Diced Canned	

Instructions:

Combine ground fennel, dried basil, ground coriander and black pepper in a small bowl; rub over chicken. Cut chicken into 1 inch pieces.

Heat oil in a large nonstick skillet over medium-high heat. Add chicken; cook 4 minutes, turning once. Remove from heat; set aside.

Reduce heat to medium. Add garlic; sauté 30 seconds or until garlic is soft. Add tomatoes and wine, scraping pan to loosen browned bits. Bring to a boil. Reduce heat, and simmer 15 minutes. Add chicken, and simmer 5 minutes.

Cook pasta according to package directions, omitting salt and fat. Drain. Toss pasta with sauce in a large bowl. Sprinkle with cheese and basil.

Nutritionals:

Calories 565.4	Sodium: 469.2	Protein: 23.1	Phos 367.7
Fat: 19	Carbs: 65.6	Chol: 37.4	Pot: 732.1
Sat Fat: 4.052	Fiber: 5.099		
	Sugar: 6.748		

Recipe | Ingredients | Instructions | Nutritionals

Cucumber and Tomato Salad

Serves: 5

Serving Size: 1/5 recipe

	Ingredients	
2 Cup	Vegetable, Cucumber, peeled, raw	
3 Teaspoon	Oil, Olive	
2 Cup	Vegetable, Tomato Red Raw	
6 Teaspoon	Vinegar, Red Wine	
0.5 tsp	Salt	
0.25 tsp	Spice, Black Pepper	

Instructions:

Peel and dice cucumbers. Chop or dice tomatoes. In a medium bowl, toss cucumbers and tomatoes. Drizzle oil and vinegar over vegetables and toss to coat. Season with salt and pepper.

Nutritionals:

Calories 44.6	Sodium: 237.8	Protein: 0.961	Phos 29.1
Fat: 2.933	Carbs: 4.056	Chol: 0	Pot: 246.7
Sat Fat: 0.401	Fiber: 1.264		
	Sugar: 2.628		

Meal: *Egg Noodles, with Bacon GDM*

Recipe	Ingredients	Instructions	Nutritionals

Egg Noodles with Bacon and Vegetables Light

Serves: 4

Serving Size: 2 cups pasta + 1 T Cheese

5 Cup	Noodles, Egg, enriched, dry
4 Slices	Pork Bacon, Cured or Smoked, lower sodium, slices
3 Teaspoon	Oil, Olive
0.5 Cup	Vegetable, Onions
1 Cup	Vegetable, Tomato, Red, Cherry
0.5 Teaspoon	Herb, Garlic, Raw
1.5 Cup	Vegetable, Zucchini, slices
0.75 Cup	Vegetable, Corn Frozen
8 Tablespoon	Cheese, Parmesan, dry grated, reduced fat
2 Tablespoon	Herb, Basil, fresh
0.25 tsp	Spice, Black Pepper

Instructions:

1. Cook pasta according to package directions, omitting salt and fat; drain.

2. While pasta cooks, cook bacon in a large nonstick skillet over medium-high heat 5 minutes or until crisp. Remove bacon from pan with a slotted spoon, reserving drippings in pan; add oil to drippings. Add onion and garlic to pan; sauté 2 minutes, stirring occasionally. Add zucchini; cook 3 minutes, stirring occasionally. Stir in corn and tomatoes; cook 5 minutes or until tomatoes burst, stirring occasionally. Add pasta to tomato mixture; toss. Cook 1 minute or until thoroughly heated, stirring frequently. Remove from heat. Add 1/4 cup cheese, basil, and pepper; toss to combine. Sprinkle with remaining cheese.

Nutritionals:

Calories 298.4	Sodium: 266.3	Protein: 11.6	Phos 266.1
Fat: 10.5	Carbs: 41.5	Chol: 45	Pot: 525
Sat Fat: 3.514	Fiber: 3.573		
	Sugar: 6.536		

Recipe	Ingredients	Instructions	Nutritionals

Cauliflower Florets with Lemon Mustard Butte

Serves: 8

Serving Size: 1/2 Cup

Qty	Ingredient
2 Tablespoon	Margarine Spread - reduced calorie, about 40% fat, tub, salted - Country Crock Light
1 Tablespoon	Dijon Mustard
4 Cup	Vegetable, Cauliflower, Raw
2 Teaspoon	Lemon, Rind

Instructions:

In a small bowl, whisk together the margarine, Dijon mustard, lemon peel, and chopped onion. Steam cauliflower florets until tender crisp. In a large saucepan, add cauliflower and margarine mixture over low heat. Toss gently until cauliflower is coated.

Nutritionals:

Calories 33.3	Sodium: 50.2	Protein: 1.09	Phos 23.9
Fat: 2.053	Carbs: 3.431	Chol: 0	Pot: 162.3
Sat Fat: 0.416	Fiber: 1.384		
	Sugar: 1.414		

Recipe	Ingredients	Instructions	Nutritionals

Creamy Lemon Coleslaw

Serves: 6

Serving Size: 1/6 of container

Qty	Ingredient
1 Each	Vegetable, Cabbage Head
6 Each	Sugar Substitute Packet, Equal
0.125 Cup	Vegetable, Onions
0.5 teaspoon	Salt, Kosher
6 Tablespoon	Miracle Whip Light
2 Packet	True Lemon packet

Instructions:

Shred cabbage and chop onions. Combine all ingredients in a bowl, and toss lightly. Refrigerate if not used immediately.

Nutritionals:

Calories 81	Sodium: 158	Protein: 1.7	Phos 34
Fat: 3	Carbs: 12	Chol: 4	Pot: 211
Sat Fat: 0.5	Fiber: 3		
	Sugar: 5.5		

Recipe: Brussel Sprouts and Baco

Serves: 4
Serving Size: 4 ounces

Ingredients

Amount	Ingredient
0.5 tsp	Salt
1 tsp	Spice, Black Pepper
4 Slices	Pork Bacon, Cured or Smoked, lower sodium, slices
2 Teaspoon	Herb, Garlic, Raw
1 teaspoon	Spice, Red Pepper
0.06 Cup	Nuts, Almond Sliced
1 Pounds	Vegetable, Brussels Sprouts, raw

Instructions

Cut the brussels sprouts in half and trim bottoms. Heat a large skillet or saute pan over medium heat. Add the bacon and cook until crispy, about 5 minutes. Remove to a plate lined with paper towels. Discard all but 1 tablespoon of the rendered bacon fat. Add the garlic, pepper flakes, brussels sprouts and salt to the skillet. Saute until the sprouts are lightly browned on the outside and tender - but still firm - throughout. Approx 10-12 minutes. Add the almonds and bacon (crumbled) and saute for another minute or two. Season with salt and pepper.

Nutritionals

Calories 121	Sodium: 402.1	Protein: 7.2	Phos 127
Fat: 6.2	Carbs: 12	Chol: 6.8	Pot: 528.2
Sat Fat: 1.6	Fiber: 5		
	Sugar: 2.7		

Meal: Sirloin Tip Roast GDM

Recipe: Sirloin Tip Roast

Serves: 6
Serving Size: 4-5 oz portion

Ingredients

Amount	Ingredient
2 Pound	Beef, bottom sirloin, tri-tip roast, raw
0.5 teaspoon	Spice, Garlic Powder
0.5 tsp	Spice, Black Pepper
0.5 teaspoon	Salt, Kosher
0.5 Cup	Vegetable, Onions
2 Ounces	Vegetable, Mushrooms Canned
1.2 Cup	Soup, Beef broth, canned, low sodium

Instructions

Place meat in roast pan with broth, wine and sprinkle with spices. Bake covered at 300' for 45 min. Remove cover and baste, sprinkle again with spices, add mushrooms and onions and bake for 15 more minutes. Cut into 6 portions.

Nutritionals

Calories 280.4	Sodium: 120.1	Protein: 32.6	Phos 305.4
Fat: 14.7	Carbs: 2.2	Chol: 108.9	Pot: 575.3
Sat Fat: 5.3	Fiber: 0.5		
	Sugar: 0.5		

Recipe: Rosemary Roasted Potatoes

Serves: 6
Serving Size: 3/4 cup Potatoes

Ingredients

Amount	Ingredient
5 each	Vegetable, Potato
1 Tablespoon	Oil, Vegetable or Olive
0.75 Teaspoo	Herb, Garlic, Raw
3 teaspoon	Herb, Rosemary, Dried
2 teaspoon	Spice, Paprika

Instructions

Wash and dice potatoes into bite-sized pieces. Place into a large bowl or Ziplock bag; toss with olive oil. Sprinkle garlic, rosemary, paprika (optional), and pepper over potatoes and shake to coat. Layer potatoes in a single layer on a baking sheet coated with cooking spray. Bake at 400 F for 30 minutes or until slightly browned. Serves 5.

Nutritionals

Calories 132.8	Sodium: 12.3	Protein: 3.094	Phos 85.4
Fat: 2.581	Carbs: 25.5	Chol: 0	Pot: 642
Sat Fat: 0.407	Fiber: 3.056		
	Sugar: 1.443		

Recipe: Ratatouille

Serves: 6

Serving Size: 1 Cup

Ingredients

Amount	Ingredient
3 Teaspoon	Oil, Olive
2 Teaspoon	Herb, Garlic, Raw
1 Each	Vegetable, Eggplant
1.5 Cup	Vegetable, Zucchini, slices
1 Cup	Vegetable, Pepper, Green
0.5 tsp	Salt
0.25 tsp	Spice, Black Pepper
8 ounces	Vegetable, Tomato, Red Canned, No Added Salt

Instructions

Add oil to a large nonstick skillet over medium to high heat. Add garlic and sauté for 30 seconds. Add remaining ingredients and cook 10 to 15 min., stirring occasionally, until vegetables are tender.

Nutritionals

Calories 41.4	Sodium: 201.3	Protein: 1.074	Phos 28.3
Fat: 2.468	Carbs: 4.775	Chol: 0	Pot: 228.7
Sat Fat: 0.362	Fiber: 1.612		
	Sugar: 2.585		

Recipe: Black-Eyed Peas

Serves: 7

Serving Size: 1/2 cup

Ingredients

Amount	Ingredient
6 Teaspoon	Oil, Olive
1 Cup	Vegetable, Pepper, Green
2 Teaspoon	Herb, Garlic, Raw
30 Ounces	Vegetable, Peas, Black Eyed, Canned
0.5 Teaspoon	Spice, Pepper, Cayenne

Instructions

Add oil to a large nonstick skillet over medium-high heat. Add green pepper and sauté for approximately 10 min. Add garlic and sauté for 30 seconds. Rinse and drain black-eyed peas prior to use. Add black eyed peas, and red pepper flakes and sauté 5 to 10 more minutes

Nutritionals

Calories 131.9	Sodium: 163.9	Protein: 5.938	Phos 89.3
Fat: 4.574	Carbs: 17.5	Chol: 0	Pot: 237.8
Sat Fat: 0.72	Fiber: 4.285		
	Sugar: 0.337		

Meal: Chicken with Red Wine Vinegar GDM

Recipe: Chicken with Red Wine Vinegar Sauce

Serves: 4

Serving Size: 4 oz breast - sauce

Ingredients

Amount	Ingredient
16 ounces	Chicken, Breast Boneless
0.5 tsp	Salt
0.5 tsp	Spice, Black Pepper
0.33 tablespo	Butter, Light w/no added salt
0.33 Tablesp	Oil, Vegetable or Olive
0.5 Cup	Vegetable, Onions, Young Green, raw
0.75 cup	Soup, Chicken Broth Low Sodium
9 Teaspoon	Vinegar, Red Wine
2 Tablespoon	Cream, Light Whipping
5 Springs	Herb, Parsley, Raw, Fresh

Instructions

Sprinkle chicken with salt and pepper. Heat the butter and oil in a large nonstick skillet over medium-high heat. Add chicken; cook 4 minutes on each side. Remove from pan; keep warm. Add onions to pan; sauté 1 minute. Stir in chicken broth and vinegar, and cook 2 minutes. Add whipping cream; cook 1 minute. Serve sauce with the chicken. Sprinkle with parsley.

Nutritionals

Calories 193.5	Sodium: 374.7	Protein: 28.1	Phos 221
Fat: 7.3	Carbs: 1.9	Chol: 82.5	Pot: 314.2
Sat Fat: 2.9	Fiber: 0.4		
	Sugar: 0		

Recipe

Coconut Rice
Serves: 4
Serving Size: 1/2 cup

Ingredients

Amount	Ingredient
10 oz	Water
0.25 tsp	Salt
4 Ounces	Milk, Coconut, canned
8 Ounces	Grain, Rice, Basmati, raw

Instructions

Combine basmati rice, water, coconut milk and salt in a small saucepan. Bring to a boil. Cover, reduce heat and simmer 16 min. or until liquid is absorbed.

Nutritionals

Calories 224.5	Sodium: 153.5	Protein: 3.868	Phos 80.3
Fat: 6.331	Carbs: 37.8	Chol: 0	Pot: 116.1
Sat Fat: 5.427	Fiber: 0.601		
	Sugar: 0.056		

Recipe

Broccoli Casserole
Serves: 8
Serving Size: 1/2 cup

Ingredients

Amount	Ingredient
4 Cup	Vegetable, Broccoli Florets, Raw
4 fluid ounces	Milk, Nonfat/Skim
0.125 tsp	Spice, Black Pepper
0.5 Cup	Cheese, Cheddar reduced fat
6 Ounces	Soup, Cream of Celery, Fat Free

Instructions

Preheat oven to 350°. In a large bowl, combine all ingredients. Pour into a medium casserole dish and bake for 30 min.

Nutritionals

Calories 53.3	Sodium: 300	Protein: 3.796	Phos 135.3
Fat: 2.291	Carbs: 5.245	Chol: 7.318	Pot: 231.2
Sat Fat: 0.179	Fiber:		
	Sugar: 1.884		

Recipe

Strawberries
Serves: 6
Serving Size: 1.5 Cups of Strawberries

Ingredients

Amount	Ingredient
9 Cup	Fruit, Strawberries, halves/slices, raw

Instructions

Remove tops and wash prior to serving.

Nutritionals

Calories 73	Sodium: 2.2	Protein: 1.5	Phos 54.7
Fat: 0.6	Carbs: 17.5	Chol: 0	Pot: 348.8
Sat Fat: 0	Fiber: 4.5		
	Sugar: 11.1		

Meal: Grilled Mushroom Burger GDM

Recipe

Grilled Mushroom Burgers
Serves: 6
Serving Size: 4 oz plus bu

Ingredients

Amount	Ingredient
1 tsp	Garlic, Minced
1 tsp	Spice, Black Pepper
24 ounces	Beef, Ground Sirloin (85-89% lean)
1 Tablespoon	Worcestershire Sauce
6 Each	Bread, Hamburger Bun

Instructions

Combine all ingredients and form into 6 patties. Place patties on a broiler pan and place under broiler. Broil for 3-5 minutes on each side or until done. Serve each burger on a hamburger bun.

Nutritionals

Calories 312	Sodium: 533	Protein: 24	Phos 178
Fat: 13.5	Carbs: 22	Chol: 68	Pot: 309
Sat Fat: 4.9	Fiber: 1		
	Sugar: 3		

Recipe

Oven Fries
Serves: 6
Serving Size: 1/2 potato

Ingredients

Amount	Ingredient
3 each	Vegetable, Potato
1 Teaspoon	Spice, Mrs. Dash
3 Each	Egg White

Instructions

Cut potatoes into strips like fries. Beat egg whites and toss with fries. Sprinkle with Mrs. Dash type seasoning. Bake for 30 minutes at 400'F or until done.

Nutritionals

Calories 75	Sodium: 45	Protein: 3.3	Phos 55
Fat: 0.2	Carbs: 15	Chol: 0	Pot: 406
Sat Fat: 0	Fiber: 2		
	Sugar: 1		

Recipe: Roasted Parmesan Zucchini

Serves: 5

Serving Size: 1/2 cup

Nutritionals

Calories 33.1	Sodium: 50	Protein: 1.236	Phos 41.6
Fat: 2.562	Carbs: 1.769	Chol: 2.64	Pot: 135.5
Sat Fat: 0.69	Fiber: 0.508		
	Sugar: 1.246		

Ingredients

2 Cup	Vegetable, Zucchini, slices
2 Teaspoon	Oil, Olive
1 Teaspoon	Herb, Garlic, Raw
3 Tablespoon	Cheese, Parmesan, dry grated, reduced fat

Instructions

Preheat oven to 450°. Coat a roasting pan with cooking spray. Place zucchini, sliced in 2 inch wedges in pan. Drizzle olive oil over zucchini, and sprinkle evenly with garlic and Parmesan cheese. Roast for approximately 20 min.

Recipe: Red Apple Coleslaw

Serves: 4

Serving Size: 3/4 cup

Nutritionals

Calories 149.2	Sodium: 217.1	Protein: 1.4	Phos 39.9
Fat: 10.3	Carbs: 15.2	Chol: 10.5	Pot: 237.5
Sat Fat: 1.6	Fiber: 2.8		
	Sugar: 8.6		

Ingredients

0.5 Cup	Mayonnaise, reduced kcal, cholest free/Hellmann
3 Teaspoon	Vinegar, Red Wine
1 Each	Sugar Substitute Packet, Equal
1 Teaspoon	Spice, Celery Seed
2 Cup	Vegetable, Cabbage Heads, Red, raw
1 Cup	Vegetable, Onions, Young Green, raw
1 Each	Fruit, Apple w/skin, raw
0.5 tsp	Spice, Black Pepper

Instructions

In a large bowl, whisk the mayo, vinegar, sweetener, and celery seeds together. Add the shredded cabbage, scallions, and grated apple. Season with pepper. Toss to thoroughly combine ingredients. Chill, covered, until cold about 2 hours. Serves 4.

Meal: Blackened Tilapia GDM

Recipe: Blackened Cumin-Cayenne Tilapia

Serves: 4

Serving Size: 6 ounce file

Nutritionals

Calories 199.3	Sodium: 381.3	Protein: 34.4	Phos 296.8
Fat: 6.545	Carbs: 0.959	Chol: 85	Pot: 543.2
Sat Fat: 1.794	Fiber: 0.241		
	Sugar: 0.057		

Ingredients

3 Teaspoon	Oil, Olive
24 Oz	Fish, Tilapia, baked or broiled
2 tsp	Spice, Cumin, Ground
0.5 tsp	Salt
0.5 teaspoon	Spice, Garlic Powder
0.5 teaspoon	Spice, Red Pepper
0.25 tsp	Spice, Black Pepper

Instructions

1. Preheat broiler.

2. Rub oil evenly over fish. Combine cumin, salt, garlic powder, and peppers; sprinkle over fish. Arrange fish on a broiler pan coated with cooking spray; broil 5 minutes or until fish flakes easily when tested with a fork or desired degree of doneness.

Couscous with Tomato and Dill

Recipe

Couscous with Tomato and Dill

Serves: 4

Serving Size: 1/2 cup

	Ingredients
3 Teaspoon	Oil, Olive
0.5 Cup	Grain, Couscous
0.5 cup	Soup, Chicken Broth Low Sodium
0.25 tsp	Salt
0.5 Cup	Vegetable, Tomato, Red, Cherry
5 Tablespoon	Vegetable, Onions, Red
3 Teaspoon	Herb, Dill Weed

Instructions

Heat a small saucepan over medium-high heat. Add olive oil to pan. Stir in couscous; sauté 1 minute. Add chicken broth and salt; bring to a boil. Cover, remove from heat, and let stand 5 minutes. Fluff with a fork. Stir in tomatoes, onion, and dill.

Nutritionals

Calories 125.3	Sodium: 159.5	Protein: 3.788	Phos 57.3
Fat: 3.774	Carbs: 19.2	Chol: 0	Pot: 146.1
Sat Fat: 0.556	Fiber: 1.58		
	Sugar: 0.953		

Recipe

Down Home Baked Bean.

Serves: 4

Serving Size: 1/2 cup

	Ingredients
8 Tablespoon	Sauce, BBQ
0.25 Teaspoo	Spice, Dry Mustard
0.33 Cup	Vegetable, Onions
1 tablespoon	Bacon Bits
1 Cup	Beans, Cannellini White, canned
1 Cup	Vegetable, Kale, raw

Instructions

In a small saucepan over high heat, combine the barbeque sauce with the dry mustard, onion, bacon bits, beans and kale. Bring to a boil, reduce the heat to low, and simmer the beans for 10 minutes, or until the kale is tender, stirring occasionally. The sauce should thicken slightly and the beans should be very tender.

Nutritionals

Calories 131	Sodium: 285	Protein: 6.03	Phos 114
Fat: 1.5	Carbs: 23.7	Chol: 4.5	Pot: 276
Sat Fat: 0.3	Fiber: 4.2		
	Sugar: 12.1		

Recipe

Banana

Serves: 6

Serving Size: 1 banana

		Ingredients
6	1	Fruit, Banana

Instructions

Piece of fruit

Nutritionals

Calories 105	Sodium: 1.1	Protein: 1.2	Phos 26
Fat: 0.3	Carbs: 27	Chol: 0	Pot: 422.4
Sat Fat: 0.1	Fiber: 3		
	Sugar: 14.4		

Meal: *Ham and Pear Sandwiches GDM*

Recipe	Ingredients	Instructions	Nutritionals

Ham and Pear Sandwich

Serves: 4

Serving Size: 1 Sandwich

Ingredients:

8 Each	Bread, Sandwich Thin, Multigrain
1 tablespoon	Butter, Light w/no added salt
3 cup	Vegetable, Lettuce, arugula, raw
0.5 Cup	Vegetable, Onions, Young Green, raw
1 Tablespoon	Oil, Vegetable or Olive
2 Teaspoon	Vinegar, Red Wine
0.25 tsp	Spice, Black Pepper
1 Fruit	Fruit, Pear Raw
2 Ounce	Cheese, Blue or Roquefort
2 Oz	Lunch Meat, Pork Ham, Prosciutto

Instructions: Preheat broiler. Arrange bread in a single layer on a baking sheet; broil 3 minutes or until toasted. Turn bread slices over; spread butter evenly over bread slices. Broil an additional 2 minutes or until toasted. Slice pears and green onions in thin slices. Combine arugula and shallot in a medium bowl. Drizzle arugula mixture with oil and vinegar; sprinkle with pepper. Toss well to coat. Divide arugula mixture evenly among 4 bread slices, buttered side up; top evenly with ham. Divide pear slices and cheese evenly among sandwiches; top each sandwich with 1 bread slice, buttered side down.

Nutritionals:

Calories 295.3	Sodium: 799.5	Protein: 14.8
Fat: 12.8	Carbs: 31.1	Chol: 23.8
Sat Fat: 5.076	Fiber: 6.66	
	Sugar: 8.548	

Phos 236
Pot: 379.8

Creamy Lemon Coleslaw

Serves: 6

Serving Size: 1/6 of container

Ingredients:

1 Each	Vegetable, Cabbage Head
6 Each	Sugar Substitute Packet, Equal
0.125 Cup	Vegetable, Onions
0.5 teaspoon	Salt, Kosher
6 Tablespoon	Miracle Whip Light
2 Packet	True Lemon packet

Instructions: Shred cabbage and chop onions. Combine all ingredients in a bowl, and toss lightly. Refrigerate if not used immediately.

Nutritionals:

Calories 81	Sodium: 158	Protein: 1.7
Fat: 3	Carbs: 12	Chol: 4
Sat Fat: 0.5	Fiber: 3	
	Sugar: 5.5	

Phos 34
Pot: 211

Steamed Carrots

Serves: 6

Serving Size: 1/2 cup

Ingredients:

3 Cup	Vegetable, Carrots
1 Teaspoon	Spice, Mrs. Dash

Instructions: Steam carrots until tender, season with Mrs. Dash

Nutritionals:

Calories 33	Sodium: 2	Protein: 1
Fat: 0	Carbs: 8	Chol: 0
Sat Fat: 0	Fiber: 3	
	Sugar: 0	

Phos 22
Pot: 165

Corn On The Cob

Serves: 6

Serving Size: 1 ear of corn

Ingredients:

6 Each	Vegetable, Corn on Cob, sm/med, ckd w/o fat or salt

Instructions: Shuck and clean corn. Boil until tender, about 4-6 minutes.

Nutritionals:

Calories 82.7	Sodium: 1.5	Protein: 2.5
Fat: 0.9	Carbs: 19.2	Chol: 0
Sat Fat: 0.1	Fiber: 2.8	
	Sugar: 0	

Phos 78.8
Pot: 190.6

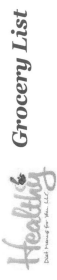
Grocery List

Chicken Penne GDM Meal

Chicken Penne with Tomato Sauce Light

Quantity		Grocery Item
8	Ounce	Pasta, Penne, dry noodles
3	Teaspoon	Oil, Olive
1	Ounces	Cheese, Parmesan, shredded
8	Oz	Beverage, Alcoholic, Wine, Table, Dry White
2	Tablespoon	Herb, Basil, fresh
1	Teaspoon	Herb, Basil, Ground
12	Ounces	Chicken, Breast Tenders Boneless
1.5	Can	Vegetable, Tomato Diced Canned
0.5	Teaspoon	Spice, Coriander Seed
0.25	tsp	Spice, Black Pepper
1	Teaspoon	Herb, Garlic, Raw
1	Teaspoon	Spice, Fennel Seed, Crushed

Cucumber and Tomato Salad

Quantity		Grocery Item
3	Teaspoon	Oil, Olive
6	Teaspoon	Vinegar, Red Wine
2	Cup	Vegetable, Tomato Red Raw
0.25	tsp	Spice, Black Pepper
2	Cup	Vegetable, Cucumber, peeled, raw
0.5	tsp	Salt

Egg Noodles, with Bacon GDM Meal

Egg Noodles with Bacon and Vegetables Light

Quantity		Grocery Item
1	Cup	Vegetable, Tomato, Red, Cherry
0.5	Cup	Vegetable, Onions
0.25	tsp	Spice, Black Pepper
2	Tablespoon	Herb, Basil, fresh
0.5	Teaspoon	Herb, Garlic, Raw
5	Cup	Noodles, Egg, enriched, dry
1.5	Cup	Vegetable, Zucchini, slices
4	Slices	Pork Bacon, Cured or Smoked, lower
8	Tablespoon	Cheese, Parmesan, dry grated, reduced fat
3	Teaspoon	Oil, Olive
0.75	Cup	Vegetable, Corn Frozen

Cauliflower Florets with Lemon Mustard Butte

Quantity		Grocery Item
4	Cup	Vegetable, Cauliflower, Raw
1	Tablespoon	Dijon Mustard
2	Tablespoon	Margarine Spread - reduced calorie, about
2	Teaspoon	Lemon, Rind

Creamy Lemon Coleslaw

Quantity		Grocery Item
6	Tablespoon	Miracle Whip Light
6	Each	Sugar Substitute Packet, Equal
0.125	Cup	Vegetable, Onions
1	Each	Vegetable, Cabbage Head
2	Packet	True Lemon packet
0.5	teaspoon	Salt, Kosher

Brussel Sprouts and Bacon

Quantity		Grocery Item
4	Slices	Pork Bacon, Cured or Smoked, lower
1	Pounds	Vegetable, Brussels Sprouts, raw
2	Teaspoon	Herb, Garlic, Raw
0.06	Cup	Nuts, Almond Sliced
1	teaspoon	Spice, Red Pepper
1	tsp	Spice, Black Pepper
0.5	tsp	Salt

Sirloin Tip Roast GDM Meal

Sirloin Tip Roast

Quantity		Grocery Item
0.5	tsp	Spice, Black Pepper
0.5	teaspoon	Salt, Kosher
2	Ounces	Vegetable, Mushrooms Canned
0.5	Cup	Vegetable, Onions
2	Pound	Beef, bottom sirloin, tri-tip roast, raw
1.2	Cup	Soup, Beef broth, canned, low sodium
0.5	teaspoon	Spice, Garlic Powder

Rosemary Roasted Potatoes

Quantity		Grocery Item
2	teaspoon	Spice, Paprika
3	teaspoon	Herb, Rosemary, Dried
5	each	Vegetable, Potato
1	Tablespoon	Oil, Vegetable or Olive
0.75	Teaspoon	Herb, Garlic, Raw

Ratatouille

Quantity		Grocery Item
0.25	tsp	Spice, Black Pepper
0.5	tsp	Salt
1	Cup	Vegetable, Pepper, Green
1	Each	Vegetable, Eggplant
1.5	Cup	Vegetable, Zucchini, slices
8	ounces	Vegetable, Tomato, Red Canned, No Added
3	Teaspoon	Oil, Olive
2	Teaspoon	Herb, Garlic, Raw

Black-Eyed Peas

Quantity		Grocery Item
2	Teaspoon	Herb, Garlic, Raw
6	Teaspoon	Oil, Olive
0.5	Teaspoon	Spice, Pepper, Cayenne
30	Ounces	Vegetable, Peas, Black Eyed, Canned
1	Cup	Vegetable, Pepper, Green

Chicken with Red Wine Vinegar GDM Meal

Chicken with Red Wine Vinegar Sauce

Quantity		Grocery Item
9	Teaspoon	Vinegar, Red Wine
2	Tablespoon	Cream, Light Whipping
0.5	Cup	Vegetable, Onions, Young Green, raw
16	ounces	Chicken, Breast Boneless
0.5	tsp	Salt
0.5	tsp	Spice, Black Pepper
0.75	cup	Soup, Chicken Broth Low Sodium
0.33	Tablespoon	Oil, Vegetable or Olive
0.33	tablespoon	Butter, Light w/no added salt
5	Springs	Herb, Parsley, Raw, Fresh

Coconut Rice

Quantity		Grocery Item
4	Ounces	Milk, Coconut, canned
8	Ounces	Grain, Rice, Basmati, raw
10	oz	Water
0.25	tsp	Salt

Broccoli Casserole

Quantity		Grocery Item
0.5	Cup	Cheese, Cheddar reduced fat
4	fluid ounces	Milk, Nonfat/Skim
6	Ounces	Soup, Cream of Celery, Fat Free
4	Cup	Vegetable, Broccoli Florets, Raw
0.125	tsp	Spice, Black Pepper

Strawberries

Quantity		Grocery Item
9	Cup	Fruit, Strawberries, halves/slices, raw

Grilled Mushroom Burger GDM Meal

Grilled Mushroom Burgers

Quantity		Grocery Item
1	tsp	Spice, Black Pepper
6	Each	Bread, Hamburger Bun
24	ounces	Beef, Ground Sirloin (85-89% lean)
1	Tablespoon	Worcestershire Sauce
1	tsp	Garlic, Minced

Oven Fries

Quantity		Grocery Item
1	Teaspoon	Spice, Mrs. Dash
3	Each	Egg White
3	each	Vegetable, Potato

Ham and Pear Sandwiches GDM Meal

Ham and Pear Sandwiches

Quantity		Grocery Item
3	cup	Vegetable, Lettuce, arugula, raw
0.5	Cup	Vegetable, Onions, Young Green, raw
2	Ounce	Cheese, Blue or Roquefort
2	Teaspoon	Vinegar, Red Wine
8	Each	Bread, Sandwich Thin, Multigrain
2	Oz	Lunch Meat, Pork Ham, Prosciutto
0.25	tsp	Spice, Black Pepper
1	tablespoon	Butter, Light w/no added salt
1	Fruit	Fruit, Pear Raw
1	Tablespoon	Oil, Vegetable or Olive

Creamy Lemon Coleslaw

Quantity		Grocery Item
2	Packet	True Lemon packet
0.125	Cup	Vegetable, Onions
0.5	teaspoon	Salt, Kosher
1	Each	Vegetable, Cabbage Head
6	Each	Sugar Substitute Packet, Equal
6	Tablespoon	Miracle Whip Light

Steamed Carrots

Quantity		Grocery Item
3	Cup	Vegetable, Carrots
1	Teaspoon	Spice, Mrs. Dash

Couscous with Tomato and Dill

Quantity		Grocery Item
0.5	cup	Soup, Chicken Broth Low Sodium
3	Teaspoon	Herb, Dill Weed
0.5	Cup	Grain, Couscous
3	Teaspoon	Oil, Olive
5	Tablespoon	Vegetable, Onions, Red
0.25	tsp	Salt
0.5	Cup	Vegetable, Tomato, Red, Cherry

Down Home Baked Beans

Quantity		Grocery Item
1	Cup	Vegetable, Kale, raw
0.25	Teaspoon	Spice, Dry Mustard
1	Cup	Beans, Cannellini White, canned
8	Tablespoon	Sauce, BBQ
1	tablespoon	Bacon Bits
0.33	Cup	Vegetable, Onions

Banana

Quantity		Grocery Item
6	1	Fruit, Banana

Roasted Parmesan Zucchini

Quantity		Grocery Item
2	Teaspoon	Oil, Olive
1	Teaspoon	Herb, Garlic, Raw
3	Tablespoon	Cheese, Parmesan, dry grated, reduced fat
2	Cup	Vegetable, Zucchini, slices

Red Apple Coleslaw

Quantity		Grocery Item
3	Teaspoon	Vinegar, Red Wine
0.5	Cup	Mayonnaise, reduced kcal, cholest
1	Each	Fruit, Apple w/skin, raw
2	Cup	Vegetable, Cabbage Heads, Red, raw
1	Teaspoon	Spice, Celery Seed
1	Cup	Vegetable, Onions, Young Green, raw
0.5	tsp	Spice, Black Pepper
1	Each	Sugar Substitute Packet, Equal

Blackened Tilapia GDM Meal

Blackened Cumin-Cayenne Tilapia

Quantity		Grocery Item
2	tsp	Spice, Cumin, Ground
24	Oz	Fish, Tilapia, baked or broiled
3	Teaspoon	Oil, Olive
0.5	teaspoon	Spice, Garlic Powder
0.25	tsp	Spice, Black Pepper
0.5	tsp	Salt
0.5	teaspoon	Spice, Red Pepper

Corn On The Cob

Quantity	Grocery Item
6 Each	Vegetable, Corn on Cob, sm/med, ckd w/o

Week 14 Meals and Grocery Lists

Stir Fried Chicken Salad with Creamy Lemon Coleslaw, Oven Fries and Grapes

Chicken with Sherry Soy Sauce with Warm Bulgur Salad and Garden Coleslaw with Almonds

Beef Ribs with Cilantro Relish with Black-Eyed Peas, Brussels Sprouts and Bacon and Broccoli Casserole

Easy Baked Fish Fillet with Creamy Herbed Mashed Potatoes, Roasted Acorn Squash and Tomato Ranch Salad

Moroccan Pork with Caramelized Radicchio with Rosemary Roasted Potatoes, Down Home Baked Beans and Ratatouille

Greek Sandwich on Sourdough with Cucumber and Tomato Salad and Oven Fries

Turkey and White Bean Chili with Spring Salad with Craisins, Steamed Carrots and Warm Bulgur Salad

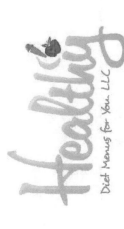

Diet Menus for You, LLC

Meal Plan

www.healthydietmenusforyou.com

Diet: *Gestational Diabetic - 2400*

Meal: *Chicken with Sherry Soy Sauce GDM*

Recipe	Ingredients		Instructions	Nutritionals			
Chicken with Sherry Soy Sauce	24 ounces	Chicken, Breast Boneless	Heat a large nonstick skillet over medium-high heat. Coat pan with cooking spray. Sprinkle chicken with salt and black pepper. Add chicken to pan; cook 4 minutes on each side or until lightly browned. Remove from pan; keep warm.	Calories 243.1	Sodium: 611.9	Protein: 36.7	Phos 374.5
Serves: 4	0.25 tsp	Salt		Fat: 5.573	Carbs: 5.033	Chol: 108.9	Pot: 695.9
	0.25 tsp	Spice, Black Pepper		Sat Fat: 1.132	Fiber: 0.292		
Serving Size: 6 ounce breast	3 Ounces	Wine, table, red - dry sherry	Add sherry, sugar, soy sauce, vinegar, and red pepper to pan; scrape pan to loosen browned bits. Bring to a boil; cook 1 minute. Stir in oil. Drizzle over chicken and serve.		Sugar: 3.575		
	3 Teaspoon	Sweet, Sugar, granulated, white					
	2 Tablespoon	Soy Sauce, Low Sodium					
	6 Teaspoon	Vinegar, Red Wine					
	0.25 teaspoo	Spice, Red Pepper					
	1 Teaspoon	Oil, Sesame Oil					
	0.25 Cup	Vegetable, Onions, Young Green, raw					

Recipe	Ingredients		Instructions	Nutritionals			
Warm Bulgur Salad	3 Cup	Bulgar	Combine 3 cups hot cooked bulgur and 5 ounces baby spinach; cover and let stand 15 minutes or until spinach wilts. Stir in 1 cup halved cherry tomatoes, 3 tablespoons fresh lemon juice, 2 tablespoons extra-virgin olive oil, 1/2 teaspoon salt, and 1/4 teaspoon black pepper. Sprinkle with 1/4 cup (1 ounce) crumbled feta cheese.	Calories 169.9	Sodium: 292.9	Protein: 4.988	Phos 79.7
Serves: 4	0.75 Ounces	Vegetable, Spinach, raw, torn		Fat: 7.986	Carbs: 22.2	Chol: 3.154	Pot: 366.6
Serving Size: 1 cup	1 Cup	Vegetable, Tomato, Red, Cherry		Sat Fat: 1.541	Fiber: 5.848		
	1 ounces	Lemon Juice, Bottled			Sugar: 1.559		
	2 Tablespoon	Oil, Vegetable or Olive					
	0.25 tsp	Spice, Black Pepper					
	0.15 Cup	Cheese, Feta					

221

Garden Coleslaw With Almonds

Serves: 6

Serving Size: 3/4 Cup

Ingredients

Amount	Ingredient
0.25 Cup	Nuts, Almond Sliced
1 Each	Vegetable, Cabbage Head
1 Cup	Vegetable, Carrots
6 Teaspoon	Oil, Olive
9 Teaspoon	Vinegar, rice
1 ounces	Honey
2 ounces	Yogurt, Greek Non Fat
0.4 Tablespo	Dijon Mustard
0.25 tsp	Spice, Black Pepper

Instructions

Start by toasting the almonds; put them in a small skillet, without oil, over medium heat and shake until almonds start to get golden brown. Remove and set aside.

Make slaw by shredding cabbage and dicing. Put in bowl.

Shredded carrots, add to bowl.

Make dressing by whisking together the remaining ingredients until smooth; then pour the dressing over the slaw.

Add the toasted almonds, tossing to combine. Let stand for 30 minutes, tossing several times.

To serve, spoon portions onto individual salad plates. You will have enough salad for 4 to 6 people.

Nutritionals

Calories 162.8	Sodium: 69.3	Protein: 5.15	Phos 103.5
Fat: 7.843	Carbs: 21.2	Chol: 0	Pot: 479.2
Sat Fat: 0.936	Fiber: 6.47		
	Sugar: 13.9		

Meal: Stirfried Chicken Salad GDM

Stirfried Chicken Salad

Serves: 4

Serving Size: 1 1/4 cup mix

Ingredients

Amount	Ingredient
0.25 cup	Soup, Chicken Broth Low Sodium
6 Teaspoon	Vinegar, Red Wine
1 Tablespoo	Soy Sauce, Low Sodium
0.75 Teaspoo	Herb, Garlic, Raw
2 Teaspoon	Sweet, Sugar, granulated, white
16 Ounces	Chicken, Breast Tenders Boneless
1 Tablespoon	Oil, Peanut oil
4 Cup	Vegetable, Lettuce, Mixed Salad Greens
2 Tablespoon	Herb, Basil, fresh
4 Tablespoon	Vegetable, Onions, Red
0.15 Cups	Nuts, Peanuts, All Types, dry roasted w/o salt

Instructions

Combine chicken broth, wine vinegar, soy sauce, garlic, and sugar in a medium bowl. Add chicken to broth mixture, stirring to coat. Let stand 3 minutes.

Heat oil in a large nonstick skillet over medium-high heat. Drain chicken, reserving marinade. Add chicken to the pan; cook 4 minutes or until done, stirring frequently. Stir in the reserved marinade. Reduce heat; cook 1 minute or until slightly thickened. Remove pan from heat.

Combine greens and basil in a large bowl. Add chicken mixture, tossing to coat. Place 1 1/4 cups salad mixture on each of 4 plates. Top each serving with 2 tablespoons onion and 1 1/2 teaspoons peanuts. Add pan sauce as dressing for salad. Serve immediately. Serve with lime wedges, if desired.

Nutritionals

Calories 207.1	Sodium: 521.8	Protein: 25.2	Phos 345.8
Fat: 8.995	Carbs: 66.9	Chol: 66.9	Pot: 566.6
Sat Fat: 1.675	Fiber: 1.809		
	Sugar: 3.515		

Grapes

Serves: 6

Serving Size: 1.5 cups of grapes

Ingredients

Amount	Ingredient
9 Cup	Fruit, Grapes, raw

Instructions

Wash and remove stems from grapes prior to eating.

Nutritionals

Calories 92.5	Sodium: 2.7	Protein: 0.8	Phos 13.8
Fat: 0.4	Carbs: 23.7	Chol: 0	Pot: 263.6
Sat Fat: 0.1	Fiber: 1.2		
	Sugar: 22.4		

Recipe: Creamy Lemon Coleslaw

Serves: 6

Serving Size: 1/6 of container

Ingredients

Amount	Ingredient
1 Each	Vegetable, Cabbage Head
6 Each	Sugar Substitute Packet, Equal
0.125 Cup	Vegetable, Onions
0.5 teaspoon	Salt, Kosher
6 Tablespoon	Miracle Whip Light
2 Packet	True Lemon packet

Instructions

Shred cabbage and chop onions. Combine all ingredients in a bowl, and toss lightly. Refrigerate if not used immediately.

Nutritionals

Calories 81	Sodium: 158	Protein: 1.7	Phos 34
Fat: 3	Carbs: 12	Chol: 4	Pot: 211
Sat Fat: 0.5	Fiber: 3		
	Sugar: 5.5		

Recipe: Oven Fries

Serves: 6

Serving Size: 1/2 potato

Ingredients

Amount	Ingredient
3 each	Vegetable, Potato
1 Teaspoon	Spice, Mrs. Dash
3 Each	Egg White

Instructions

Cut potatoes into strips like fries. Beat egg whites and toss with fries. Sprinkle with Mrs. Dash type seasoning. Bake for 30 minutes at 400'F or until done.

Nutritionals

Calories 75	Sodium: 45	Protein: 3.3	Phos 55
Fat: 0.2	Carbs: 15	Chol: 0	Pot: 406
Sat Fat: 0	Fiber: 2		
	Sugar: 1		

Meal: Beef Ribs with Cilantro Relish GDM

Recipe: Beef Ribs with Cilantro Relish

Serves: 4

Serving Size: 2 chops +3 tablespoons rel

Ingredients

Amount	Ingredient
3 Teaspoon	Oil, Olive
0.75 Cup	Herb, Cilantro Raw
0.5 ounces	Lemon Juice, Bottled
1 Each	Vegetable, Pepper, Jalapeno, raw
1 Cup	Vegetable, Onions
0.25 tsp	Spice, Black Pepper
0.5 teaspoon	Salt, Kosher
16 Ounce	Beef, Ribs lean
0.5 teaspoon	Fruit, Lemon Peel, Raw
0.25 tsp	Spice, Cumin, Ground

Instructions

1. Preheat oven to 400°.

2. Combine 1 teaspoon olive oil, lemon rind and cumin ingredients.

3. Heat a large ovenproof skillet over medium-high heat. Coat pan with cooking spray. Sprinkle beef with 1/4 teaspoon salt and black pepper. Add beef to pan; cook 2 minutes on each side. Spread oil mixture over beef; place pan in oven. Bake at 400° for 15 minutes or until a thermometer registers 138°. Remove beef from pan; let stand 8 minutes. Cut into chops.

4. Heat a skillet over medium-high heat. Coat pan with cooking spray. Add onion and jalapeño; sauté 5 minutes. Combine onion mixture, cilantro, lemon juice, 2 teaspoons olive oil, and kosher salt. Serve on side with beef.

Nutritionals

Calories 236.4	Sodium: 304	Protein: 22.9	Phos 228.6
Fat: 13.7	Carbs: 4.479	Chol: 66.9	Pot: 476.5
Sat Fat: 4.652	Fiber: 0.952		
	Sugar: 1.947		

Black-Eyed Peas

Serves: 7

Serving Size: 1/2 cup

Ingredients	
6 Teaspoon	Oil, Olive
1 Cup	Vegetable, Pepper, Green
2 Teaspoon	Herb, Garlic, Raw
30 Ounces	Vegetable, Peas, Black Eyed, Canned
0.5 Teaspoon	Spice, Pepper, Cayenne

Instructions

Add oil to a large nonstick skillet over medium-high heat. Add green pepper and sauté for approximately 10 min. Add garlic and sauté for 30 seconds. Rinse and drain black-eyed peas prior to use. Add black eyed peas, and red pepper flakes and sauté 5 to 10 more minutes

Nutritionals

Calories 131.9	Sodium: 163.9	Protein: 5.938	Phos 89.3	
Fat: 4.574	Carbs: 17.5	Chol: 0	Pot: 237.8	
Sat Fat: 0.72	Fiber: 4.285			
	Sugar: 0.337			

Brussel Sprouts and Bacon

Serves: 4

Serving Size: 4 ounces

Ingredients	
0.5 tsp	Salt
1 tsp	Spice, Black Pepper
4 Slices	Pork Bacon, Cured or Smoked, lower sodium, slices
2 Teaspoon	Herb, Garlic, Raw
1 teaspoon	Spice, Red Pepper
0.06 Cup	Nuts, Almond Sliced
1 Pounds	Vegetable, Brussels Sprouts, raw

Instructions

Cut the brussels sprouts in half and trim bottoms. Heat a large skillet or saute pan over medium heat. Add the bacon and cook until crispy, about 5 minutes. Remove to a plate lined with paper towels. Discard all but 1 tablespoon of the rendered bacon fat. Add the garlic, pepper flakes, brussels sprouts and salt to the skillet. Saute until the sprouts are lightly browned on the outside and tender - but still firm - throughout. Approx 10-12 minutes. Add the almonds and bacon (crumbled) and saute for another minute or two. Season with salt and pepper.

Nutritionals

Calories 121	Sodium: 402.1	Protein: 7.2	Phos 127
Fat: 6.2	Carbs: 12	Chol: 6.8	Pot: 528.2
Sat Fat: 1.6	Fiber: 5		
	Sugar: 2.7		

Broccoli Casserole

Serves: 8

Serving Size: 1/2 cup

Ingredients	
4 Cup	Vegetable, Broccoli Florets, Raw
4 fluid ounces	Milk, Nonfat/Skim
0.125 tsp	Spice, Black Pepper
0.5 Cup	Cheese, Cheddar reduced fat
6 Ounces	Soup, Cream of Celery, Fat Free

Instructions

Preheat oven to 350°. In a large bowl, combine all ingredients. Pour into a medium casserole dish and bake for 30 min.

Nutritionals

Calories 53.3	Sodium: 300	Protein: 3.796	Phos 135.3
Fat: 2.291	Carbs: 5.245	Chol: 7.318	Pot: 231.2
Sat Fat: 1.228	Fiber: 0.179		
	Sugar: 1.884		

Meal: *Baked Fish Filet GDM*

Recipe

Easy Baked Fish Fillet

Serves: 4

Serving Size: 5 oz Fish

Ingredients

4 Tablespoon	Lime Juice
24 oz	Fish, Cod, Pacific, Raw
0.5 Teaspoon	Spice, Onion Powder
1 tablespoon	Salad Dressing, Mayo, LT/Kraft
0.15 tsp	Spice, Black Pepper
0.5 Cup	Breadcrumbs, Plain, Grated, Dry
1.5 tablespoo	Butter, Light w/no added salt
2 Tablespoon	Herb, Parsley, Raw, Chopped

Instructions

Preheat oven to 425°.
Place fish in an 11 x 7-inch baking dish coated with cooking spray. Combine lime juice, mayonnaise, onion powder, and pepper in a small bowl, and spread over fish. Sprinkle with breadcrumbs; drizzle with butter. Bake at 425° for 20 minutes or until fish flakes easily when tested with a fork. Sprinkle with parsley.

Nutritionals

Calories	232.7	Sodium:	253.8	Protein:	32.5	Phos	324.0
Fat:	5.699	Carbs:	10.9	Chol:	69.3	Pot:	736.9
Sat Fat:	2.141	Fiber:	0.762			
		Sugar:	1.137			

Recipe

Creamy Herbed Mashed Potatoes

Serves: 6

Serving Size: 3/4 Cup

Ingredients

4 Cup	Vegetable, Potato, Flesh only, diced, raw
4 fluid ounces	Milk, Nonfat/Skim
1 Tablespoon	Cream, Sour, Reduced Fat
3 tablespoon	Butter, Light w/no added salt
3 Tablespoon	Herb, Chives, raw
4 Springs	Herb, Parsley, Raw, Fresh
0.5 tsp	Salt
0.5 tsp	Spice, Black Pepper

Instructions

Peel and cube potatoes. Place potato in a saucepan; cover with water. Bring to a boil; cover, reduce heat, and simmer 10 minutes or until tender. Drain. Return potato to pan. Add milk and remaining ingredients; mash with a potato masher to desired consistency.

Nutritionals

Calories	147.1	Sodium:	215.1	Protein:	3.1	Phos	73
Fat:	4.6	Carbs:	23.8	Chol:	11	Pot:	422.7
Sat Fat:	2.8	Fiber:	2.1			
		Sugar:	2.3			

Recipe

Roasted Acorn Squash

Serves: 8

Serving Size: 1/8 recipe

Ingredients

0.5 tsp	Salt
0.25 tsp	Spice, Black Pepper
2 Teaspoon	Oil, Olive
32 Ounces	Vegetable, Squash, Acorn, peeled, raw

Instructions

Preheat oven to 400°. Cut them off of each squash and cut in half lengthwise. Scoop out seeds; rinse and dry each squash, half. Spray all sides of squash halves with cooking spray. Season inside of each half with salt and pepper. Place cut side down on a nonstick cooking spray coated baking sheet. Bake for 45 min.. Scoop squash meat out into a medium bowl; discard skins. Add olive oil and beat with a sturdy whisk until fluffy.

Nutritionals

Calories	100.8	Sodium:	72.5	Protein:	1.822	Phos	81.8
Fat:	1.354	Carbs:	23.7	Chol:	0	Pot:	787.9
Sat Fat:	0.204	Fiber:	3.419			
		Sugar:	0			

Tomato Ranch Salad

Serves: 6

Serving Size: 3/4 cup salad w/dressing

Ingredients		Instructions
2 Cup	Vegetable, Tomato Red Raw	Toss lettuce and tomatoes and divide into 6 portions. Top each salad with 2T lite ranch dressing.
4.5 Cup	Vegetable, Lettuce, Iceberg, head, raw	
12 Tablespoo	Salad dressing, ranch dressing, reduced fat	

Nutritionals

Calories 75.6	Sodium: 280	Protein: 1.2	Phos 80.8
Fat: 3.9	Carbs: 10	Chol: 4.8	Pot: 242.1
Sat Fat: 0.3	Fiber: 1.5		
	Sugar: 3.5		

Meal: Moroccan Pork GDM

Moroccan Pork with Carmelized Radicchio

Serves: 4

Serving Size: 4 oz pork chop

Ingredients		Instructions
1 tsp	Spice, Cumin, Ground	In a small bowl, combine the cumin, paprika, cayenne pepper, ground cinnamon and dry mustard. Dredge one-side of each pork chop in spice mixture. Add oil and a generous amount of cooking spray to a large nonstick skillet over high heat. Place chop spice side down in the skillet. Cook for 6 min. on each side. Remove from pan and set aside. Spray skillet generously again and add radicchio to the pan. Sauté radicchio for 2 min. Add sugar, salt and pepper. Sauté 5 to 6 more minutes or until radicchio begins to caramelize. Serve radicchio on top of each pork chop.
1 teaspoon	Spice, Paprika	
0.25 Teaspoo	Spice, Pepper, Cayenne	
0.25 Teaspoo	Spice, Cinnamon, ground	
0.25 teaspoo	Spice, Mustard Powder	
16 ounces	Pork, Center Rib Chop	
2 Teaspoon	Oil, Olive	
2 Cup	Vegetable, Radicchio, raw	
1 Teaspoon	Sweet, Sugar, granulated, white	
0.5 tsp	Salt	
0.25 tsp	Spice, Black Pepper	

Nutritionals

Calories 206.1	Sodium: 347.4	Protein: 25.2	Phos 248.0
Fat: 9.904	Carbs: 2.786	Chol: 62.4	Pot: 565.2
Sat Fat: 2.89	Fiber: 0.598		
	Sugar: 1.258		

Rosemary Roasted Potatoes

Serves: 6

Serving Size: 3/4 cup Potatoes

Ingredients		Instructions
5 each	Vegetable, Potato	Wash and dice potatoes into bite-sized pieces. Place into a large bowl or Ziplock bag; toss with olive oil. Sprinkle garlic, rosemary, paprika (optional), and pepper over potatoes and shake to coat. Layer potatoes in a single layer on a baking sheet coated with cooking spray. Bake at 400 F for 30 minutes or until slightly browned. Serves 5.
1 Tablespoo	Oil, Vegetable or Olive	
0.75 Teaspoo	Herb, Garlic, Raw	
3 teaspoon	Herb, Rosemary, Dried	
2 teaspoon	Spice, Paprika	

Nutritionals

Calories 132.8	Sodium: 12.3	Protein: 3.094	Phos 85.4
Fat: 2.581	Carbs: 25.5	Chol: 0	Pot: 642
Sat Fat: 0.407	Fiber: 3.056		
	Sugar: 1.443		

Down Home Baked Bean

Serves: 4

Serving Size: 1/2 cup

Ingredients	Instructions	Nutritionals
8 Tablespoon Sauce, BBQ 0.25 Teaspoo Spice, Dry Mustard 0.33 Cup Vegetable, Onions 1 tablespoon Bacon Bits 1 Cup Beans, Cannellini White, canned 1 Cup Vegetable, Kale, raw	In a small saucepan over high heat, combine the barbeque sauce with the dry mustard, onion, bacon bits, beans and kale. Bring to a boil, reduce the heat to low, and simmer the beans for 10 minutes, or until the kale is tender, stirring occasionally. The sauce should thicken slightly and the beans should be very tender.	Calories 131 · Sodium: 285 · Protein: 6.03 · Phos 114 Fat: 1.5 · Carbs: 23.7 · Chol: 4.5 · Pot: 276 Sat Fat: 0.3 · Fiber: 4.2 Sugar: 12.1

Ratatouille

Serves: 6

Serving Size: 1 Cup

Ingredients	Instructions	Nutritionals
3 Teaspoon Oil, Olive 2 Teaspoon Herb, Garlic, Raw 1 Each Vegetable, Eggplant 1.5 Cup Vegetable, Zucchini, slices 1 Cup Vegetable, Pepper, Green 0.5 tsp Salt 0.25 tsp Spice, Black Pepper 8 ounces Vegetable, Tomato, Red Canned, No Added Salt	Add oil to a large nonstick skillet over medium to high heat. Add garlic and sauté for 30 seconds. Add remaining ingredients and cook 10 to 15 min., stirring occasionally, until vegetables are tender.	Calories 41.4 · Sodium: 201.3 · Protein: 1.074 · Phos 28.3 Fat: 2.468 · Carbs: 4.775 · Chol: 0 · Pot: 228.7 Sat Fat: 0.362 · Fiber: 1.612 Sugar: 2.585

Meal: Greek Sandwich GDM

Greek Sandwich On Sourdough

Serves: 4

Serving Size: 1 sandwich

Ingredients	Instructions	Nutritionals
0.15 Cup Cheese, Feta 1 ounces Lemon Juice, Bottled 3 Teaspoon Oil, Olive 0.5 Teaspoon Sweet, Sugar, granulated, white 0.5 Teaspoon Herb, Oregano, Ground 0.25 Teaspoon Herb, Garlic, Raw 0.25 tsp Spice, Black Pepper 1 Cup Vegetable, Tomato Red Raw 8 Tablespoon Vegetable, Onions, Red 0.5 Cup Vegetable, Cucumber, peeled, raw 8 Each Bread, Sourdough 3 cup Vegetable, Lettuce, arugula, raw 2 Tablespoon Vegetable, Olives, Kalamata	To prepare the vinaigrette, combine the feta cheese, lemon juice, olive oil, sugar, oregano, and garlic in a medium bowl, stirring with a whisk. To prepare the sandwich, put pepper in a medium bowl. Place 2 tomato slices on each of 4 bread slices, and sprinkle evenly with half of the pepper. Arrange the cucumber slices over the tomato slices; sprinkle evenly with remaining pepper. Add arugula, onion, and chopped olives to the vinaigrette; toss to coat. Arrange the arugula mixture evenly over the cucumber slices. Top with the remaining bread slices.	Calories 256.7 · Sodium: 514.5 · Protein: 9.358 · Phos 117.1 Fat: 6.203 · Carbs: 42.2 · Chol: 4.172 · Pot: 302.2 Sat Fat: 1.583 · Fiber: 2.927 Sugar: 4.869

Recipe: Cucumber and Tomato Salad

Serves: 5
Serving Size: 1/5 recipe

Amount	Ingredients
2 Cup	Vegetable, Cucumber, peeled, raw
3 Teaspoon	Oil, Olive
2 Cup	Vegetable, Tomato Red Raw
6 Teaspoon	Vinegar, Red Wine
0.5 tsp	Salt
0.25 tsp	Spice, Black Pepper

Instructions: Peel and dice cucumbers. Chop or dice tomatoes. In a medium bowl, toss cucumbers and tomatoes. Drizzle oil and vinegar over vegetables and toss to coat. Season with salt and pepper.

Nutritionals:

Calories 44.6	Sodium: 237.8	Protein: 0.961	Phos 29.1
Fat: 2.933	Carbs: 4.056	Chol: 0	Pot: 246.7
Sat Fat: 0.401	Fiber: 1.264		
	Sugar: 2.628		

Recipe: Oven Fries

Serves: 6
Serving Size: 1/2 potato

Amount	Ingredients
3 each	Vegetable, Potato
1 Teaspoon	Spice, Mrs. Dash
3 Each	Egg White

Instructions: Cut potatoes into strips like fries. Beat egg whites and toss with fries. Sprinkle with Mrs. Dash type seasoning. Bake for 30 minutes at 400°F or until done.

Nutritionals:

Calories 75	Sodium: 45	Protein: 3.3	Phos 55
Fat: 0.2	Carbs: 15	Chol: 15	Pot: 406
Sat Fat: 0	Fiber: 2		
	Sugar: 1		

Meal: Turkey and White Bean Chili GDM

Recipe: Turkey and White Bean Chili

Serves: 4
Serving Size: 1 1/4 cup

Amount	Ingredients
1 Pound	Turkey, Ground Raw
8 Tablespoon	Vegetable, Onions, chopped, raw
2 Teaspoon	Herb, Garlic, Raw
3 Teaspoon	Oil, Olive
3 teaspoon	Spice, Chili Powder
1 tsp	Spice, Cumin, Ground
2 Cup	Beans, Cannellini White, canned
12 Ounces	Vegetable, Tomatoes, canned, stewed
1 cup	Soup, Chicken Broth Low Sodium

Instructions: Heat oil in a large saucepan over medium-high heat. Add onion and cook, stirring occasionally, until softened, about 5 min. Add garlic and cook 1 min. more. Add Turkey, chili powder, and cumin; cook, stirring often, until Turkey is no longer pink inside, about 5 min. Rinse and drain beans. Add beans, tomatoes with juice, and broth; bring to a boil. Reduce heat to medium to low, cover, and simmer until flavors blend about 15 min.

Nutritionals:

Calories 358.7	Sodium: 487.1	Protein: 29.2	Phos 346.α
Fat: 14.2	Carbs: 30.1	Chol: 89.6	Pot: 921.6
Sat Fat: 3.332	Fiber: 8.934		
	Sugar: 6.833		

Recipe: Spring Salad with Craisin

Serves: 6
Serving Size: 3/4 cup salad + 2T drsing

Amount	Ingredients
4.5 Cups	Vegetables, Mixed salad greens, raw
0.5 Cups	Fruit, Cranberries, dried - Craisins
12 Tablespoo	Salad Dressing, Dijon Vinaigrette, light/Wishbone

Instructions: Toss salad items together. Divide into 6 portions of 3/4 cup each. Add 2 T dressing to each salad.

Nutritionals:

Calories 66.9	Sodium: 248.3	Protein: 0.6	Phos 15
Fat: 3.1	Carbs: 10.3	Chol: 1.3	Pot: 128.2
Sat Fat: 0.4	Fiber: 1.3		
	Sugar: 6.3		

Recipe	Ingredients		Instructions	Nutritionals			
Steamed Carrots	3 Cup	Vegetable, Carrots	Steam carrots until tender, season with Mrs. Dash	Calories 33	Sodium: 2	Protein: 1	Phos 22 .
	1 Teaspoon	Spice, Mrs. Dash		Fat: 0	Carbs: 8	Chol: 0	Pot: 165
Serves: 6				Sat Fat: 0	Fiber: 3		
Serving Size: 1/2 cup					Sugar: 0		

Recipe	Ingredients		Instructions	Nutritionals			
Warm Bulgur Salad	3 Cup	Bulgar	Combine 3 cups hot cooked bulgur and 5 ounces baby spinach; cover and let stand 15 minutes or until spinach wilts. Stir in 1 cup halved cherry tomatoes, 3 tablespoons fresh lemon juice, 2 tablespoons extra-virgin olive oil, 1/2 teaspoon salt, and 1/4 teaspoon black pepper. Sprinkle with 1/4 cup (1 ounce) crumbled feta cheese.	Calories 169.9 .	Sodium: 292.9	Protein: 4.988	Phos 79.7 .
	0.75 Ounces	Vegetable, Spinach, raw, torn		Fat: 7.986	Carbs: 22.2	Chol: 3.154	Pot: 366.6
Serves: 4	1 Cup	Vegetable, Tomato, Red, Cherry		Sat Fat: 1.541	Fiber: 5.848		
	1 ounces	Lemon Juice, Bottled			Sugar: 1.559		
Serving Size: 1 cup	2 Tablespoon	Oil, Vegetable or Olive					
	0.25 tsp	Spice, Black Pepper					
	0.15 Cup	Cheese, Feta					

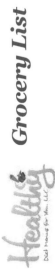

Grocery List

Diet: *Gestational Diabetic - 2400*

Stirfried Chicken Salad GDM Meal

Stirfried Chicken Salad

Quantity		Grocery Item
4	Cup	Vegetable, Lettuce, Mixed Salad Greens
2	Teaspoon	Sweet, Sugar, granulated, white
0.15	Cups	Nuts, Peanuts, All Types, dry roasted w/o
1	Tablespoon	Oil, Peanut oil
0.75	Teaspoon	Herb, Garlic, Raw
16	Ounces	Chicken, Breast Tenders Boneless
4	Tablespoon	Vegetable, Onions, Red
0.25	cup	Soup, Chicken Broth Low Sodium
1	Tablespoon	Soy Sauce, Low Sodium
2	Tablespoon	Herb, Basil, fresh
6	Teaspoon	Vinegar, Red Wine

Grapes

Quantity		Grocery Item
9	Cup	Fruit, Grapes, raw

Creamy Lemon Coleslaw

Quantity		Grocery Item
0.125	Cup	Vegetable, Onions
2	Packet	True Lemon packet
6	Tablespoon	Miracle Whip Light
6	Each	Sugar Substitute Packet, Equal
0.5	teaspoon	Salt, Kosher
1	Each	Vegetable, Cabbage Head

Oven Fries

Quantity		Grocery Item
3	Each	Egg White
3	each	Vegetable, Potato
1	Teaspoon	Spice, Mrs. Dash

Chicken with Sherry Soy Sauce GDM Meal

Chicken with Sherry Soy Sauce

Quantity		Grocery Item
0.25	tsp	Salt
3	Teaspoon	Sweet, Sugar, granulated, white
2	Tablespoon	Soy Sauce, Low Sodium
0.25	teaspoon	Spice, Red Pepper
24	ounces	Chicken, Breast Boneless
0.25	Cup	Vegetable, Onions, Young Green, raw
3	Ounces	Wine, table, red - dry sherry
1	Teaspoon	Oil, Sesame Oil
0.25	tsp	Spice, Black Pepper
6	Teaspoon	Vinegar, Red Wine

Warm Bulgur Salad

Quantity		Grocery Item
0.15	Cup	Cheese, Feta
0.25	tsp	Spice, Black Pepper
1	ounces	Lemon Juice, Bottled
1	Cup	Vegetable, Tomato, Red, Cherry
3	Cup	Bulgar
0.75	Ounces	Vegetable, Spinach, raw, torn
2	Tablespoon	Oil, Vegetable or Olive

231

Baked Fish Filet GDM Meal

Easy Baked Fish Fillet

Quantity		Grocery Item
1.5	tablespoon	Butter, Light w/no added salt
0.5	Cup	Breadcrumbs, Plain, Grated, Dry
4	Tablespoon	Lime Juice
0.5	Teaspoon	Spice, Onion Powder
2	Tablespoon	Herb, Parsley, Raw, Chopped
24	oz	Fish, Cod, Pacific, Raw
1	tablespoon	Salad Dressing, Mayo, LT/Kraft
0.15	tsp	Spice, Black Pepper

Creamy Herbed Mashed Potatoes

Quantity		Grocery Item
4	fluid ounces	Milk, Nonfat/Skim
1	Tablespoons	Cream, Sour, Reduced Fat
3	tablespoon	Butter, Light w/no added salt
0.5	tsp	Salt
0.5	tsp	Spice, Black Pepper
4	Cup	Vegetable, Potato, Flesh only, diced, raw
4	Springs	Herb, Parsley, Raw, Fresh
3	Tablespoon	Herb, Chives, raw

Roasted Acorn Squash

Quantity		Grocery Item
32	Ounces	Vegetable, Squash, Acorn, peeled, raw
0.5	tsp	Salt
0.25	tsp	Spice, Black Pepper
2	Teaspoon	Oil, Olive

Black-Eyed Peas

Quantity		Grocery Item
1	Cup	Vegetable, Pepper, Green
2	Teaspoon	Herb, Garlic, Raw
6	Teaspoon	Oil, Olive
0.5	Teaspoon	Spice, Pepper, Cayenne
30	Ounces	Vegetable, Peas, Black Eyed, Canned

Brussel Sprouts and Bacon

Quantity		Grocery Item
2	Teaspoon	Herb, Garlic, Raw
1	teaspoon	Spice, Red Pepper
0.06	Cup	Nuts, Almond Sliced
1	Pounds	Vegetable, Brussels Sprouts, raw
4	Slices	Pork Bacon, Cured or Smoked, lower
1	tsp	Spice, Black Pepper
0.5	tsp	Salt

Broccoli Casserole

Quantity		Grocery Item
0.5	Cup	Cheese, Cheddar reduced fat
4	fluid ounces	Milk, Nonfat/Skim
6	Ounces	Soup, Cream of Celery, Fat Free
4	Cup	Vegetable, Broccoli Florets, Raw
0.125	tsp	Spice, Black Pepper

Garden Coleslaw With Almonds

Quantity		Grocery Item
1	ounces	Honey
6	Teaspoon	Oil, Olive
0.4	Tablespoon	Dijon Mustard
1	Cup	Vegetable, Carrots
0.25	tsp	Spice, Black Pepper
1	Each	Vegetable, Cabbage Head
9	Teaspoon	Vinegar, rice
2	ounces	Yogurt, Greek Non Fat
0.25	Cup	Nuts, Almond Sliced

Beef Ribs with Cilantro Relish GDM Meal

Beef Ribs with Cilantro Relish

Quantity		Grocery Item
0.75	Cup	Herb, Cilantro Raw
1	Each	Vegetable, Pepper, Jalapeno, raw
0.5	teaspoon	Fruit, Lemon Peel, Raw
0.5	teaspoon	Salt, Kosher
1	Cup	Vegetable, Onions
0.25	tsp	Spice, Cumin, Ground
0.5	ounces	Lemon Juice, Bottled
0.25	tsp	Spice, Black Pepper
3	Teaspoon	Oil, Olive
16	Ounce	Beef, Ribs lean

Greek Sandwich GDM Meal

Greek Sandwich On Sourdough

Quantity		Grocery Item
0.5	Cup	Vegetable, Cucumber, peeled, raw
0.25	tsp	Spice, Black Pepper
8	Each	Bread, Sourdough
0.5	Teaspoon	Sweet, Sugar, granulated, white
3	cup	Vegetable, Lettuce, arugula, raw
0.15	Cup	Cheese, Feta
0.25	Teaspoon	Herb, Garlic, Raw
8	Tablespoon	Vegetable, Onions, Red
1	Cup	Vegetable, Tomato Red Raw
1	ounces	Lemon Juice, Bottled
3	Teaspoon	Oil, Olive
2	Tablespoon	Vegetable, Olives, Kalamata
0.5	Teaspoon	Herb, Oregano, Ground

Cucumber and Tomato Salad

Quantity		Grocery Item
6	Teaspoon	Vinegar, Red Wine
0.25	tsp	Spice, Black Pepper
2	Cup	Vegetable, Tomato Red Raw
2	Cup	Vegetable, Cucumber, peeled, raw
3	Teaspoon	Oil, Olive
0.5	tsp	Salt

Oven Fries

Quantity		Grocery Item
3	each	Vegetable, Potato
1	Teaspoon	Spice, Mrs. Dash
3	Each	Egg White

Down Home Baked Beans

Quantity		Grocery Item
1	Cup	Vegetable, Kale, raw
1	Cup	Beans, Cannellini White, canned
0.25	Teaspoon	Spice, Dry Mustard
8	Tablespoon	Sauce, BBQ
1	tablespoon	Bacon Bits
0.33	Cup	Vegetable, Onions

Ratatouille

Quantity		Grocery Item
1	Cup	Vegetable, Pepper, Green
3	Teaspoon	Oil, Olive
8	ounces	Vegetable, Tomato, Red Canned, No Added
1.5	Cup	Vegetable, Zucchini, slices
1	Each	Vegetable, Eggplant
0.25	tsp	Spice, Black Pepper
0.5	tsp	Salt
2	Teaspoon	Herb, Garlic, Raw

Tomato Ranch Salad

Quantity		Grocery Item
12	Tablespoon	Salad dressing, ranch dressing, reduced fat
4.5	Cup	Vegetable, Lettuce, Iceberg, head, raw
2	Cup	Vegetable, Tomato Red Raw

Moroccan Pork GDM Meal

Moroccan Pork with Carmelized Radicchio

Quantity		Grocery Item
0.25	Teaspoon	Spice, Cinnamon, ground
1	Teaspoon	Sweet, Sugar, granulated, white
0.25	tsp	Spice, Black Pepper
16	ounces	Pork, Center Rib Chop
1	tsp	Spice, Cumin, Ground
1	teaspoon	Spice, Paprika
2	Teaspoon	Oil, Olive
2	Cup	Vegetable, Radicchio, raw
0.5	tsp	Salt
0.25	Teaspoon	Spice, Pepper, Cayenne
0.25	teaspoons	Spice, Mustard Powder

Rosemary Roasted Potatoes

Quantity		Grocery Item
2	teaspoon	Spice, Paprika
0.75	Teaspoon	Herb, Garlic, Raw
1	Tablespoon	Oil, Vegetable or Olive
5	each	Vegetable, Potato
3	teaspoon	Herb, Rosemary, Dried

Turkey and White Bean Chili
GDM Meal

Turkey and White Bean Chili

Quantity		Grocery Item
8	Tablespoon	Vegetable, Onions, chopped, raw
3	teaspoon	Spice, Chili Powder
1	cup	Soup, Chicken Broth Low Sodium
1	tsp	Spice, Cumin, Ground
2	Teaspoon	Herb, Garlic, Raw
12	Ounces	Vegetable, Tomatoes, canned, stewed
2	Cup	Beans, Cannellini White, canned
3	Teaspoon	Oil, Olive
1	Pound	Turkey, Ground Raw

Spring Salad with Craisins

Quantity		Grocery Item
12	Tablespoons	Salad Dressing, Dijon Vinaigrette,
4.5	Cups	Vegetables, Mixed salad greens, raw
0.5	Cups	Fruit, Cranberries, dried - Craisins

Steamed Carrots

Quantity		Grocery Item
3	Cup	Vegetable, Carrots
1	Teaspoon	Spice, Mrs. Dash

Warm Bulgur Salad

Quantity		Grocery Item
0.15	Cup	Cheese, Feta
0.25	tsp	Spice, Black Pepper
1	ounces	Lemon Juice, Bottled
2	Tablespoon	Oil, Vegetable or Olive
1	Cup	Vegetable, Tomato, Red, Cherry
0.75	Ounces	Vegetable, Spinach, raw, torn
3	Cup	Bulgar

Dessert Recipes

Banana Chocolate Chip Bread

Baked Apple

Caramel Brownie Sundae

Chocolate Mousse Pie

Chunky Monkey Ice Cream

Pretzel and Strawberry Delight

Lemon Poppyseed Bundt Cake

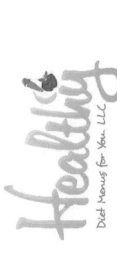

Meal Plan

www.healthydietmenusforyou.com

Diet: *GDM Desserts*

Meal: *Banana Choc Chip Bread Dessert*

Recipe	Ingredients	Instructions	Nutritionals			
Dessert Recipe Main		Desserts serve more than the normal number of people, so portion correctly.	Calories .	Sodium: .	Protein: .	Phos .
Serves: 0			Fat: .	Carbs: .	Chol: .	Pot: .
Serving Size: 0			Sat Fat: .	Fiber: .		
				Sugar: .		

Recipe	Ingredients		Instructions	Nutritionals			
Banana Chocolate Chip Bread	2	1 Fruit, Banana	Makes 16 servings. Prep time is 15 min. Preheat Oven to 350°. Lightly spray and 8 x 14" loaf pan with cooking spray. In a medium bowl, combine bananas, oil, buttermilk and egg whites; mix well. Set aside. In a large bowl, combine flour, oats, sugar, baking powder, baking soda and salt. Make a well in the center of the dry ingredients. Add banana mixture to the dry ingredients, all at once and mix well. Stir in 1/3 cup, less 1 tablespoon, chocolate chips to batter. Pour batter into loaf pan. Sprinkle 1 tablespoon chocolate chips on top of batter. Bake 50 to 60 min. or until toothpick inserted in center comes out clean.	Calories 133.2	Sodium: 231.1	Protein: 2.951	Phos 49.7
Serves: 16	6 Teaspoon	Oil, Olive		Fat: 3.165	Carbs: 24.4	Chol: 0.153	Pot: 129.9
Serving Size: 1 slice	2 ounces	Milk, Buttermilk Lowfat		Sat Fat: 0.963	Fiber: 1.334		
	4 Each	Egg White			Sugar: 11.1		
	24 Tablespoo	Flour, White bleached enriched					
	24 Teaspoon	Sweet, Sugar, granulated, white					
	0.5 Cup	Cereal, Rolled Oats Quick or Regular					
	0.5 tsp	Salt					
	2 Teaspoon	Baking Powder					
	0.5 Teaspoon	Baking Soda					
	0.333 Cup	Candy, Chocolate Chips, Mini, Semisweet					

Meal Plan

www.healthydietmenusforyou.com

Healthy
Diet Menus for You LLC

Diet: GDM Desserts

Meal: **Baked Apple Dessert**

Recipe	Ingredients	Instructions	Nutritionals				
Dessert Recipe Main		Desserts serve more than the normal number of people, so portion correctly.	Calories .	Sodium:	Protein:	Phos .	
Serves: 0			Fat:	Carbs:	Chol:	Pot:	
Serving Size: 0			Sat Fat:	Fiber:			
				Sugar:			

Recipe	Ingredients		Instructions	Nutritionals				
Baked Apple	4 Each	Fruit, Apple w/skin, raw	Preheat oven to 375°. Place cored Apples in a baking dish lightly coated with nonstick cooking spray. Apple can be left, whole, or sliced. Mix cinnamon and sugar substitute, then sprinkle with mixture evenly. Cover with aluminum foil. Bake for 45 to 50 min.	Calories 101.2	Sodium: 1.95	Protein: 0.525	Phos 20.9
Serves: 4	2 Teaspoon	Spice, Cinnamon, ground		Fat: 0.326	Carbs: 27.1	Chol: 0	Pot: 200.4
Serving Size: 1 Apple	4 Each	Sweeteners, sucralose, SPLENDA packets		Sat Fat: 0.055	Fiber: 5.058		
					Sugar: 19.7		

239

Meal Plan

www.healthydietmenusforyou.com

Healthy
Diet Menus for You, LLC

Meal: *Caramel Brownie Sundae GDM Dessert*

Recipe	Ingredients	Instructions	Nutritionals			
Dessert Recipe Main		Desserts serve more than the normal number of people, so portion correctly.	Calories .	Sodium: .	Protein: .	Phos .
Serves: 0			Fat:	Carbs:	Chol:	Pot:
Serving Size: 0			Sat Fat:	Fiber:		
				Sugar:		

Recipe	Ingredients		Instructions	Nutritionals			
Caramel Brownie Sundae	2 oz	Water	Preheat oven to 350°. Coat an 11 x 7" pan with cooking spray. In a large bowl, stir in Brownie mix, water, oil, applesauce, egg, and egg whites until well blended. Spread in pan and bake 30 to 40 min. or until toothpick inserted 2 inches from side of pan comes out almost clean. Cool. Cut brownies into 20 slices. Put one Brownie in bowl and top with 1/3 cup, ice cream and 2 teaspoons caramel sauce. Repeat for remaining servings. Makes 20 servings.	Calories 282.3	Sodium: 174.2	Protein: 4.767	Phos 66
Serves: 20	4 tablespoon	Oil, Canola		.	Fat: 8.994	Chol: 46.4	.
	1 Each	Egg, Whole		Fat:	Carbs: 25.1		Pot: 132
Serving Size: 1 Brownie Sunday	2 Each	Egg White		Sat Fat: 2.596	Fiber: 0.304		
	20 Ounces	Fudge Brownie Mix, dry			Sugar: 34.2		
	0.25 Cup	Fruit, Applesauce, canned, unsweetened					
	7 Cup	Ice Cream, Vanilla, Light					
	0.75 Cup	Topping, Caramel					

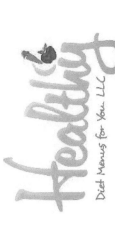

Meal Plan

www.healthydietmenusforyou.com

Diet: *GDM Desserts*

Meal: *Chocolate Mousse Pie Dessert*

Recipe	Ingredients	Instructions	Nutritionals			
Dessert Recipe Main		Desserts serve more than the normal number of people, so portion correctly.	Calories .	Sodium: .	Protein: .	Phos .
Serves: 0			Fat: .	Carbs: .	Chol: .	Pot: .
Serving Size: 0			Sat Fat: .	Fiber: .		
				Sugar: .		

Recipe		Ingredients	Instructions	Nutritionals			
Chocolate Mousse Pie	14 fluid ounce	Milk, Nonfat/Skim	Makes 8 Servings. Prep time is 5 min. In a medium bowl, whisk pudding mix and milk. Fold half of whipped topping into pudding mixture and mix gently until fully blended. Spread pudding mixture into pie crust and top with remaining whipped topping. Sprinkle top with chocolate chips. Cut into 8 pieces and serve.	Calories 270.7 .	Sodium: 408	Protein: 3.885	Phos 250. ?
Serves: 8	1 Each	Pie Crust, Cookie-type, Graham Cracker, Ready Crust		Fat: 13.9	Carbs: 33.3	Chol: 1.021	Pot: 248.4
Serving Size: 8	2.8 Ounces	Puddings, chocolate flavor, low calorie, instant		Sat Fat: 7.926	Fiber: 1.204		
	1 Cup	Candy, Chocolate Chips, Mini, Semisweet			Sugar: 14.8		
	8 Ounces	Whipped topping, nondairy, frozen - Cool Whip					

Meal Plan

www.healthydietmenusforyou.com

Healthy
Diet Menus for You, LLC

Meal: *Chunky Monkey Ice Cream Dessert*

Recipe	Ingredients	Instructions	Nutritionals				
			Calories	Sodium:	Protein:	Phos
Dessert Recipe Main		Desserts serve more than the normal number of people, so portion correctly.	Fat:	Carbs:	Chol:	Pot:
Serves: 0			Sat Fat:	Fiber:		
Serving Size: 0				Sugar:		

Recipe	Ingredients	Instructions	Nutritionals				
			Calories 152.1	Sodium: 6.339	Protein: 2.224	Phos 53
Chunky Monkey Ice Cream	6 1 Fruit, Banana	Puree the bananas, milk, and Nutella in a food processor or blender until smooth. Add the walnuts and chocolate chunks and pulse until mixed in. Serve immediately or freeze for later consumption. Yield: 4 cups (8 servings; 1/2 cup each).	Fat: 5.471	Carbs: 26.9	Chol: 0.153	Pot: 380.2
	2 fluid ounces Milk, Nonfat/Skim		Sat Fat: 2.366	Fiber: 3.071		
Serves: 8	0.25 Cup Chocolate Chips, semisweet			Sugar: 16.3		
Serving Size: 1/2 cup	0.25 cup Nuts, Walnut					
	2 Tablespoon Chocolate flavored hazelnut spread - Nutella					

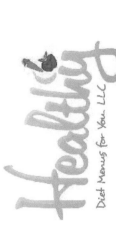

Healthy
Diet Menus for You, LLC

Meal Plan

www.healthydietmenusforyou.com

Diet: GDM Desserts

Meal: Pretzel and Strawberry Dessert

Recipe	Ingredients	Instructions	Nutritionals				
			Calories .	Sodium:	Protein:	Phos .	
Dessert Recipe Main		Desserts serve more than the normal number of people, so portion correctly.	Fat:	Carbs:	Chol:	Pot:	
Serves: 0			Sat Fat:	Fiber:			
Serving Size: 0				Sugar:			

Recipe	Ingredients	Instructions	Nutritionals				
Pretzel and Strawberry Delight	24 Teaspoon Sweet, Sugar, granulated, white	Makes 16 servings. 1/16 of a recipe. Prep time is 40 min. preheat oven to 400°. In a medium bowl, mix together pretzels, margarine and 1 tablespoon sugar. Pour mixture into a 9 x 13" glass baking dish and press to cover bottom of pan. Bake 8 to 10 min. Remove from oven and let cool. In a medium bowl, beat 1/2 cup sugar and cream cheese with electric mixer on high until creamy and smooth. Fold in whipped topping. Pour cream cheese mixture around edge of pretzel layer in baking dish and use a flat spatula to spread mixture evenly and gently towards the center. Refrigerate. In a large bowl, add 2 cups boiling water to gelatin mix and stir constantly for 2 min. or until dissolved. Stir in 1 cup cold water and refrigerate 30 min. Remove gelatin from refrigerator and stir in strawberries refrigerate another 30 min. Pour gelatin over cream cheese layer and refrigerate dessert 2 to 3 hours.	Calories 128.4 .	Sodium: 88.8	Protein: 2.811	Phos 44.2 .	Pot: 83.1
	8 Ounces Cheese Spread, Light Cream Cheese		Fat: 4.283	Carbs: 20.4	Chol: 7.938		
Serves: 16	3 Cup Fruit, Strawberries, halves/slices, raw		Sat Fat: 1.902	Fiber: 0.832			
Serving Size: 1/16 of the recipe	3 Ounces Sweet, Gelatin, dry mix strawberry flavor			Sugar: 12.5			
	2 Tablespoon Margarine, regular, stick, unsalted						
	2 Cup Pretzel, hard, unsalted - pretzels labeled "lowfat"						

247

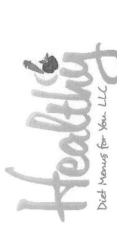

Meal Plan

www.healthydietmenusforyou.com

Diet: *GDM Desserts*

Meal: *Lemon Poppy Seed Cake GDM Dessert*

Recipe	Ingredients	Instructions	Nutritionals			
Dessert Recipe Main		Desserts serve more than the normal number of people, so portion correctly.	Calories .	Sodium: .	Protein: .	Phos .
Serves: 0			Fat: .	Carbs: .	Chol: .	Pot: .
Serving Size: 0			Sat Fat: .	Fiber: .		
				Sugar: .		

Recipe	Ingredients		Instructions	Nutritionals			
Lemon Poppy Seed Bundt Cake	1.5 Teaspoon	Baking Powder	Preheat oven to 325°. Coat a bunt pan with cooking spray. In a medium bowl, sift together flour, baking powder, and salt. Set aside. In a large bowl, beat sugar and margarine with an electric mixer at medium speed until well blended. Add eggs and egg white, one at a time. Beat well. Get the zest off of lemon until you have about a tablespoons worth. Add vanilla, lemon rind, and lemon juice; beat 30 seconds. Add part of flour mixture to sugar mixture and beat. Add part of sour cream to sugar mixture and beat. Continue alternating flour and sour cream to sugar mixture. Beat at low speed until well blended. Stir in Poppy seeds. Spoon batter into pan and bake for 35 min. or until toothpick inserted in center comes out clean. Let cool. In a small bowl, whisk together powdered sugar, lemon juice and water until glaze consistency is formed. Drizzle glaze over cooled cake. Make sure the cake is completely cool before you. Drizzle the glaze over it; otherwise, the glaze will melt into the cake. Cut into 16 servings.	Calories 216.3	Sodium: 98.6	Protein: 3.088	Phos 53.9
	0.25 tsp	Salt		Fat: 7.004	Carbs: 35.8	Chol: 26.8	Pot: 50.5
Serves: 16	4 Tablespoon	Margarine, regular, stick, unsalted		Sat Fat: 1.402	Fiber: 0.684		
	2 Each	Egg, Whole			Sugar: 22.9		
Serving Size: 1 slice	1 Each	Egg White					
	1 ounces	Lemon Juice, Bottled					
	2 Tablespoon	Spice, Poppy Seed					
	0.15 oz	Water					
	2 Cup	Flour, Wheat, White, All Purpose, unbleached, enriched					
	2 Cup	Sugar, granulated, white					
	1.5 Teaspoon	Extract, Vanilla					
	0 Cup	Cream, Sour, Fat Free					
	0.5 Cup	Sweet, Sugar, Powdered, White					
	3 Teaspoon	Lemon, Rind					

Meal Patterns For Gestational Diabetes

On the next few pages, you will find the meal patterns that allow you to create your own meals for gestational diabetes. Now that you know how many calories you need – in the range of 2,000 to 2,400 calories per day – you can choose your daily meals to build the right sets of foods to make a healthy and gestational diabetic friendly meal.

Start with either the 2,000 or 2,400-calorie meal plan that lists out the entire day's worth of meals. Then, you have your breakfast, lunch, and dinner counts as well as snacks. Now, take the exchanges on the list, and go to the meal you need to build. For example, you can go to the breakfast meal and see your plan at the top. You just have to look at the lists of food and choose the number of items it tells you and create your meals. Then you have the ability to create the 3 snack you need as well. Using these in conjunction with the variety of meals you just saw in the last 200+ pages makes you into the expert in no time at all.

Remember that everyone is different, and these patterns may not be just right for you. You might have to adjust them based on your meals, daily activity, and blood glucose levels. I wish you a happy, healthy pregnancy!

Here is a sample meal plan for a day for 2400 calories using the meal patterns:

Breakfast:

Breakfast Meal—No Juice or Fruit for Breakfast / Low Carbohydrates

2 Starches [1 starch svg = 15 g CHO, 3 g Pro, 1 g Fat, 80 calories]

2 ounces Medium Fat Meat [1 ounce medium fat meat = 7 g Pro, 5 g Fat, 75 calories]

1 Fat [1 fat svg = 5 g Fat, 45 calories]

Stick to 30 grams CHO at Breakfast

---

1 slice wheat bread + 1 cup skim milk (2 starches)

2 eggs (2 ounces meat)

1 ½-teaspoon peanut butter (1 fat)

AM Snack:

Morning Snack — No Juice or Fruit
[2hr after Breakfast]

1 Starches [1 starch svg = 15 g CHO, 3 g Pro, 1 g Fat, 80 calories]

1 ounces Lean Fat Meat [1 ounce lean fat meat = 7 g Pro, 3 g Fat, 55 calories]

1 Fat [1 fat svg = 5 g Fat, 45 calories]

| 3 Graham Cracker Squares |
| 1 Ounce Lean Deli Meat |
| 1 ½-teaspoon Peanut Butter |

Lunch:

Lunch Meal

3 Starches [1 starch svg = 15 g CHO, 3 g Pro, 1 g Fat, 80 calories]

3 ounces Medium Fat Meat [1 ounce medium fat meat = 7 g Pro, 5 g Fat, 75 calories]

1 Vegetable [1 vegetable svg = 5 g CHO, 2 g Pro, 25 calories]

1 Fruit [1 fruit svg = 15 g CHO, 60 calories]

1 Skim Milk [12 g CHO, 8 g Pro, 1 g Fat, 90—100 calories]

2 Fats [1 fat svg = 5 g Fat, 45 calories]

1 Hamburger Bun (2 starches) + 3 ounce burger patty (3 ounces meat)

¾ ounce Baked Potato Chips (small bag – 1 starch)

Small Side Salad (1 cup lettuce mixed with cucumbers and tomatoes) (1 vegetable)

½ Banana (1 Fruit)

1-cup skim milk (1 milk)

1-tablespoon sunflower seeds + 1 tablespoon regular salad dressing (2 fats)

Midday Snack:

Midday Snack — [2hr after Lunch]

1 Starches [1 starch svg = 15 g CHO, 3 g Pro, 1 g Fat, 80 calories]

1 Fruit [1 fruit svg = 15 g CHO, 60 calories]

1 Skim Milk [12 g CHO, 8 g Pro, 1 g Fat, 90—100 calories]

6 Saltine Crackers (1 Starch)

1 Orange (1 Fruit)

6 ounces Yogurt, Non Fat, Artificially Sweetened (1 Skim Milk)

Evening Meal:

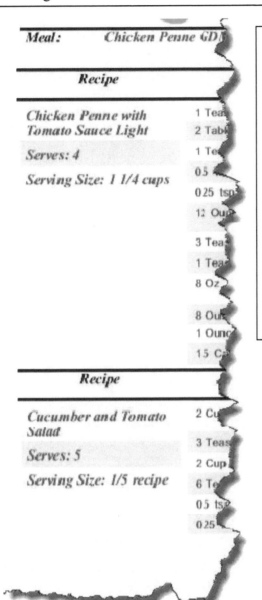

Meal:	Chicken Penne GD

Recipe	
Chicken Penne with Tomato Sauce Light	1 Tea
	2 Tab
Serves: 4	1 Te
Serving Size: 1 1/4 cups	0.5
	0.25 tsp
	12 Ou
	3 Tea
	1 Tea
	8 Oz
	8 Ou
	1 Ounc
	1.5 C

Recipe	
Cucumber and Tomato Salad	2 Cu
	3 Teas
Serves: 5	2 Cup
Serving Size: 1/5 recipe	6 Te
	0.5 tsp
	0.25

Dinner is using a meal from the meal listings:

Target for the evening meal is:

67 gm Carbohydrate, 46 gm Protein, 25 gm Fat and 680 calories according to the Daily Meal Plan Pattern for 2400 Calorie Gestational Diabetes on the upper right side of the page under the supper line.

This meal contains:

69.6 gm Carbohydrate, 24 gm Protein, 22 gm Fat and 610 calories for each serving of this meal. The only place it is a little short is the protein, but this meal happens to be a vegetarian meal so it does not have a high protein content. You should focus on meeting the carbohydrate counts first.

Evening Snack:

Evening Snack — [2hr before Bed]
1 Starches [1 starch svg = 15 g CHO, 3 g Pro, 1 g Fat, 80 calories]
1 ounce Medium Fat Meat [1 ounce medium fat meat = 7 g Pro, 5 g Fat, 75 calories]
1 Fat [1 fat svg = 5 g Fat, 45 calories]

½ English Muffin (1 starch)

1 egg (fried) (1 meat)

1 Tablespoon Tub Margarine Spreadable (1 fat)

(Make into a sandwich)

DAILY MEAL PLAN PATTERN
FOR 2000 CALORIE
GESTATIONAL DIABETES DIET

Meal	Grams - CHO	% Calories	Grams - Protein	% Calories	Grams - Fat	% Calories
Breakfast	30	34%	20	23%	17	43%
AM Snack	15	33%	10	22%	9	45%
Lunch	77	46%	33	20%	24	32%
Midday Snack	15	75%	3	15%	1	11%
Supper	67	39%	46	27%	25	33%
PM Snack	15	75%	3	15%	1	11%
Totals	219	43%	115	23%	77	34%

Breakfast Meal—No Juice or Fruit for Breakfast / Low Carbohydrates

2 Starches [1 starch svg = 15 g CHO, 3 g Pro, 1 g Fat, 80 calories]

2 ounces Medium Fat Meat [1 ounce medium fat meat = 7 g Pro, 5 g Fat, 75 calories]

1 Fat [1 fat svg = 5 g Fat, 45 calories]

Morning Snack — No Juice or Fruit [2hr after Breakfast]

1 Starches [1 starch svg = 15 g CHO, 3 g Pro, 1 g Fat, 80 calories]

1 ounces Lean Fat Meat [1 ounce lean fat meat = 7 g Pro, 3 g Fat, 55 calories]

1 Fat [1 fat svg = 5 g Fat, 45 calories]

Midday Snack — [2hr after Lunch]

1 Starches [1 starch svg = 15 g CHO, 3 g Pro, 1 g Fat, 80 calories]

CHO = Carbohydrate Pro = Protein Svg = Serving

Evening Snack — [2hr before Bed]

1 Starches [1 starch svg = 15 g CHO, 3 g Pro, 1 g Fat, 80 calories]

Lunch Meal

3 Starches [1 starch svg = 15 g CHO, 3 g Pro, 1 g Fat, 80 calories]

2 ounces Medium Fat Meat [1 ounce medium fat meat = 7 g Pro, 5 g Fat, 75 calories]

1 Vegetable [1 vegetable svg = 5 g CHO, 2 g Pro, 25 calories]

1 Fruit [1 fruit svg = 15 g CHO, 60 calories]

1 Skim Milk [12 g CHO, 8 g Pro, 1 g Fat, 90—100 calories]

2 Fats [1 fat svg = 5 g Fat, 45 calories]

Dinner/ Evening Meal

2 Starches [1 starch svg = 15 g CHO, 3 g Pro, 1 g Fat, 80 calories]

4 ounces Medium Fat Meat [1 ounce medium fat meat = 7 g Pro, 5 g Fat, 75 calories]

2 Vegetable [1 vegetable svg = 5 g CHO, 2 g Pro, 25 calories]

1 Fruit [1 fruit svg = 15 g CHO, 60 calories]

1 Skim Milk [12 g CHO, 8 g Pro, 1 g Fat, 90—100 calories]

2 Fats [1 fat svg = 5 g Fat, 45 calories]

DAILY MEAL PLAN PATTERN FOR 2400 CALORIE GESTATIONAL DIABETES DIET

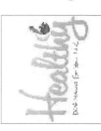

Meal	Grams - CHO	% Calories	Grams - Protein	% Calories	Grams - Fat	% Calories	Calories
Breakfast	30	34%	20	23%	17	43%	355
AM Snack	15	33%	10	22%	9	45%	180
Lunch	77	42%	40	22%	29	35%	740
Midday Snack	42	70%	11	18%	2	8%	240
Supper	67	39%	46	27%	25	33%	680
PM Snack	15	30%	10	20%	11	50%	200
Totals	246	41%	137	23%	93	35%	2395

Breakfast Meal – No Juice or Fruit for Breakfast / Low Carbohydrates

2 Starches [1 starch svg = 15 g CHO, 3 g Pro, 1 g Fat, 80 calories]

2 ounces Medium Fat Meat [1 ounce medium fat meat = 7 g Pro, 5 g Fat, 75 calories]

1 Fat [1 fat svg = 5 g Fat, 45 calories]

Morning Snack – No Juice or Fruit [2hr after Breakfast]

1 Starches [1 starch svg = 15 g CHO, 3 g Pro, 1 g Fat, 80 calories]

1 ounces Lean Fat Meat [1 ounce lean fat meat = 7 g Pro, 3 g Fat, 55 calories]

1 Fat [1 fat svg = 5 g Fat, 45 calories]

Lunch Meal

3 Starches [1 starch svg = 15 g CHO, 3 g Pro, 1 g Fat, 80 calories]

3 ounces Medium Fat Meat [1 ounce medium fat meat = 7 g Pro, 5 g Fat, 75 calories]

1 Vegetable [1 vegetable svg = 5 g CHO, 2 g Pro, 25 calories]

1 Fruit [1 fruit svg = 15 g CHO, 60 calories]

1 Skim Milk [12 g CHO, 8 g Pro, 1 g Fat, 90–100 calories]

2 Fats [1 fat svg = 5 g Fat, 45 calories]

Midday Snack – [2hr after Lunch]

1 Starches [1 starch svg = 15 g CHO, 3 g Pro, 1 g Fat, 80 calories]

1 Fruit [1 fruit svg = 15 g CHO, 60 calories]

1 Skim Milk [12 g CHO, 8 g Pro, 1 g Fat, 90–100 calories]

Dinner/ Evening Meal

2 Starches [1 starch svg = 15 g CHO, 3 g Pro, 1 g Fat, 80 calories]

4 ounces Medium Fat Meat [1 ounce medium fat meat = 7 g Pro, 5 g Fat, 75 calories]

2 Vegetable [1 vegetable svg = 5 g CHO, 2 g Pro, 25 calories]

1 Fruit [1 fruit svg = 15 g CHO, 60 calories]

1 Skim Milk [12 g CHO, 8 g Pro, 1 g Fat, 90–100 calories]

2 Fats [1 fat svg = 5 g Fat, 45 calories]

Evening Snack – [2hr before Bed]

1 Starches [1 starch svg = 15 g CHO, 3 g Pro, 1 g Fat, 80 calories]

1 ounce Medium Fat Meat [1 ounce medium fat meat = 7 g Pro, 5 g Fat, 75 calories]

1 Fat [1 fat svg = 5 g Fat, 45 calories]

CHO = Carbohydrate Pro = Protein Svg = Serving

BREAKFAST PLAN PATTERN GESTATIONAL DIABETES DIET

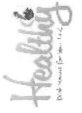

Breakfast Meal—No Juice or Fruit for Breakfast / Low Carbohydrates

2 Starches [1 starch svg = 15 g CHO, 3 g Pro, 1 g Fat, 80 calories]

2 ounces Medium Fat Meat [1 ounce medium fat meat = 7 g Pro, 5 g Fat, 75 calories]

1 Fat [1 fat svg = 5 g Fat, 45 calories]

CHO = Carbohydrate Pro = Protein

Svg = Serving

Stick to 30 grams CHO at Breakfast

Starch Options (Choose 2)

1/2 cup Cooked Oatmeal

1/2 cup Cooked Cream of Wheat

1/2 cup Bran Flakes

3/4 cup Cornflakes

3/4 cup Rice Crispies

1 cup Skim Milk

1/4 Large Bagel

1 slice , White or Wheat Bread

2 slices Reduced Calorie, White or
Wheat Bread

1 Toaster Waffle

1/2 English Muffin

6 ounces Yogurt Sweetened with
Splenda or NutraSweet

6 ounces Yogurt Nonfat or Plain

2 Tablespoons Light Pancake Syrup

1 Tablespoon Regular Pancake Syrup

1/2 Doughnut (3 3/4 in Diameter)

1 6 inch Flour Tortilla

Meat/Protein Options (Choose 1)

2 ounces Canadian Bacon

2 ounces Ham

1/2 cup Cottage Cheese, Lowfat

2 Eggs

2 ounces American Cheese

3 Egg Whites

2 Tablespoons Peanut Butter (in this
amount it is both Meat and Fat for meal)

Fat Options (Choose 1)

1 teaspoon Olive Oil

1 1/2 teaspoon Peanut Butter

1 tablespoon Tub Margarine, Spreadable

1 tablespoon Sunflower Seeds

1 slice Bacon

2 teaspoon Whipped Butter

1 tablespoon Cream Cheese

Free Foods

20 Cal or less per Svg

1/2 cup Sugar Free Gelatin

2 tablespoons Sugar-Free Syrup

2 teaspoons Low Calorie Jelly

1 tablespoon Fat-Free Cream Cheese

1 teaspoon Light Margarine Spreadable

1 tablespoon Ketchup

1/4 cup Salsa

Read Your Labels

On Packaged foods, always
double check the label for the
serving size.

Based on the information in
the overall pattern, you can
branch out and get other items
to eat at breakfast using food
labels.

LUNCH PLAN PATTERN GESTATIONAL DIABETES DIET

Read Your Labels

On Packaged foods, always double check the label for the serving size.

Based on the information in th overall pattern, you can branch out and get other items to eat at meals and snacks

Lunch Meal

3 Starches [1 starch svg = 15 g CHO, 3 g Pro, 1 g Fat, 80 calories]

3 ounces Medium Fat Meat [1 ounce medium fat meat = 7 g Pro, 5 g Fat, 75 calories]

1 Vegetable [1 vegetable svg = 5 g CHO, 2 g Pro, 25 calories]

1 Fruit [1 fruit svg = 15 g CHO, 60 calories]

1 Skim Milk [12 g CHO, 8 g Pro, 1 g Fat, 90—100 calories]

2 Fats [1 fat svg = 5 g Fat, 45 calories]

CHO = Carbohydrate

Pro = Protein

Svg = Serving

Starch Options (Choose 3)

1 Biscuit (2 1/2 in)

2 slices, Reduced Calorie, White or Wheat Bread

1 slice, White or Wheat Bread

1/2 Hamburger Bun, or Hot Dog Bun

1 Dinner Roll (1 ounce)

2 Medium Taco Shells

1 Six-Inch Flour Tortilla

1/3 cup Cooked Rice or Couscous

1/2 cup Cooked Macaroni or Pasta

6 Saltine crackers

3/4 ounce Baked Potato Chips

1/2 cup Canned or Frozen Corn, Peas Or Potatoes

1/3 cup Yams or Sweet Potatoes

1/3 cup Beans

6 Saltine Crackers

3 Graham Cracker Squares

Meat/Protein Options (Choose 1)

3 ounces Skinless Chicken or Turkey

3 ounces Lean Beef (90% lean)

3 ounces Lean Pork

3 ounces Fish

6 ounces shrimp

3/4 cup Tuna Canned in Water

3/4 Cup Cottage Cheese

3 Eggs

3 ounces, Lowfat Cheese

3 ounces Lean Deli Meat (90%+ Fat Free)

Vegetable Options (Choose 1)

A serving is 1/2 cup of cooked vegetables, 1/2 cup of vegetable juice, or 1 cup of raw vegetables.

Starchy vegetables like potatoes corn and peas are listed with starches and breads.

Beans (green, waxed, Italian, snap)

Beets

Broccoli

Carrots

Greens/Lettuce

Mushrooms

Okra

Onion

Pea Pods Or Snow Peas

Peppers

Sauerkraut

Spinach

Squash (Summer squash, zucchini)

Tomato Or Tomato Juice

Fruit Options (Choose 1)

1 Small Apple

1/2 Medium Banana

1 cup Berries

1 cup Cantaloupe or Honeydew Melon

15 Grapes

1/2 cup Fruit Juice

1 Orange

2 Tablespoons Raisins

1 Peach Or Pear (2 3/4")

3/4 cup Pineapple

Skim Milk (Choose 1)

8 ounces Skim or 1% Milk

6 ounces Yogurt, Non-fat Plain, Artificially Sweetened

8 Ounces Lowfat Buttermilk

Fat Options (Choose 1)

1 teaspoon Olive Oil

1 1/2 teaspoon Peanut Butter

1 tablespoon Tub Margarine, Spreadable

1 tablespoon Sunflower Seeds

2 teaspoon Whipped Butter

1 tablespoon Regular Salad Dressing

2 tablespoons, Reduced Calorie Salad Dressing

Free Foods
20 Cal or less per Svg

1/2 cup Sugar Free Gelatin

1 teaspoon Light Margarine Spreadable

1 tablespoon Ketchup

1/4 cup Salsa

1 cup Lettuce

1/2 cup Cucumber

1 teaspoon, Reduced Fat Mayonnaise

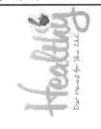

SNACK OPTIONS PATTERN GESTATIONAL DIABETES DIET

CHO = Carbohydrate

Pro = Protein

Svg = Serving

Snack Meal Patterns

<u>Review your meal pattern carefully</u>

The 2000 and 2400 Calorie Meal Patterns have <u>different</u> snacks

<u>Morning Snack – No Juice or</u> Fruit

[2hr after Breakfast]

1 Starches [1 starch svg = 15 g CHO, 3 g Pro, 1 g Fat, 80 calories]

1 ounces Lean Fat Meat [1 ounce lean fat meat = 7 g Pro, 3 g Fat, 55 calories]

1 Fat [1 fat svg = 5 g Fat, 45 calories]

<u>Midday Snack – [2hr after</u> Lunch]

1 Starches [1 starch svg = 15 g CHO, 3 g Pro, 1 g Fat, 80 calories]

Add for 2400 Calorie:

1 Fruit [1 fruit svg = 15 g CHO, 60 calories]

1 Skim Milk [12 g CHO, 8 g Pro, 1 g Fat, 90—100 calories]

<u>Evening Snack – [2hr before</u> Bed]

1 Starches [1 starch svg = 15 g CHO, 3 g Pro, 1 g Fat, 80 calories]

Add for 2400 Calorie:

1 ounce Medium Fat Meat [1 ounce medium fat meat = 7 g Pro, 5 g Fat, 75 calories]

1 Fat [1 fat svg = 5 g Fat, 45 calories]

<u>Starch Options</u>

1 Biscuit (2 1/2 in)

2 slices, Reduced Calorie, White or Wheat Bread

1 slice, White or Wheat Bread

1/2 Hamburger Bun, or Hot Dog Bun

1 Dinner Roll (1 ounce)

2 Medium Taco Shells

1 Six-Inch Flour Tortilla

1/3 cup Cooked Rice or Couscous

1/2 cup Cooked Macaroni or Pasta

6 Saltine crackers

3/4 ounce Baked Potato Chips

1/2 cup Canned or Frozen Corn, Peas Or Potatoes

1/3 cup Yams, Sweet Potatoes, or Beans

6 Saltine Crackers

3 Graham Cracker Squares

1/2 cup Bran Flakes

3/4 cup Cornflakes

3/4 cup Rice Crispies

1/2 English Muffin

<u>Meat/Protein Options</u>

1 ounce Skinless Chicken or Turkey

1 ounce Lean Beef (90% lean)

1 ounce Lean Pork

1 ounce Fish

2 ounces shrimp

1/4 cup Tuna Canned in Water

1/4 cup Cottage Cheese

1 Egg

1 ounce, Lowfat Cheese

1 ounce Lean Deli Meat (90%+ Fat Free)

<u>Skim Milk</u>

8 ounces Skim or 1% Milk

6 ounces Yogurt, Nonfat Plain, Artificially Sweetened

8 Ounces Lowfat Buttermilk

<u>Fruit Options</u>

1 Small Apple

1/2 Medium Banana

1 cup Berries

1 cup Cantaloupe or Honeydew Melon

15 Grapes

1/2 cup Fruit Juice

1 Orange

2 Tablespoons Raisins

1 Peach Or Pear (2 3/4")

3/4 cup Pineapple

<u>Fat Options</u>

1 teaspoon Olive Oil

1 1/2 teaspoon Peanut Butter

1 tablespoon Tub Margarine, Spreadable

1 tablespoon Sunflower Seeds

2 teaspoon Whipped Butter

1 tablespoon Regular Salad Dressing

2 tablespoons, Reduced Calorie Salad Salad

<u>Free Foods</u>

20 Cal or less per Svg

1/2 cup Sugar Free Gelatin

1 teaspoon Light Margarine Spreadable

1 tablespoon Ketchup

1/4 cup Salsa

1 cup Lettuce

1/2 cup Cucumber

1 teaspoon, Reduced Fat Mayonnaise

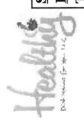

264

Entrée Index

Turkey Kielbasa Apple Pasta Bake, 105

Turkey Quesadilla w/ Cranberry Salsa, 192

Turkey w/ White Bean Chili, 228

Vegetarian

Baked Asparagus Omelet, 50

Baked Ziti and Veggies, 66

Banana Oat Pancakes, 33

Bow Ties w/ Tomatoes, Feta and Balsamic Dressing, 137

Cauliflower, Broccoli and Spinach Casserole, 108

Chipotle Bean Burrito, 182

Creamy Stove Top Macaroni and Cheese, 80

Fried Rice, 149

Greek Sandwich on Sourdough, 227

Meatless Skillet Lasagna, 36

Orzo Salad w/ Feta Vinaigrette, 164

Pasta w/ Tomato Basil Sauce, 123

Red Pepper Frittata, 92

Spinach Linguine, 195

Vegetable Bean Chili, 39

Made in United States
Troutdale, OR
04/03/2024

18918526R00151